Breast Cancer: A Guide to Clinical Practice

Breast Cancer: A Guide to Clinical Practice

Editor: Eliza Harrison

MURPHY & MOORE
www.murphy-moorepublishing.com

www.murphy-moorepublishing.com

MURPHY & MOORE

Cataloging-in-Publication Data

Breast cancer : a guide to clinical practice / edited by Eliza Harrison.
p. cm.
Includes bibliographical references and index.
ISBN 978-1-63987-084-4
1. Breast--Cancer. 2. Breast--Cancer--Diagnosis--Guidebooks. 3. Breast--Cancer--Treatment--Guidebooks. I. Harrison, Eliza.
RC280.B8 B74 2022
616.994 49--dc23

Murphy & Moore Publishing,
1 Rockefeller Plaza,
New York City, NY 10020, USA

ISBN 978-1-63987-084-4 (Hardback)

Contents

Preface

The cancer which occurs when breast cells begin to grow in an abnormal manner is known as breast cancer. Some of the major symptoms of breast cancer are a lump in the breast or in an armpit, inverted nipple, persistent pain in the breast or armpits, and discharge from the nipple. It generally begins in the inner lining of the milk ducts and then spreads to other body parts. The two major types of breast cancer are ductal carcinoma and lobular carcinoma. It can be diagnosed through biopsy and imaging tests. Determining the stage of the cancer is one of the most important aspects of diagnosis. This book unravels the recent studies on breast cancer. From theories to research to practical applications, case studies related to all contemporary topics of relevance to this field have been included in it. This book aims to equip students and experts with the advanced topics and upcoming concepts in this area.

The information contained in this book is the result of intensive hard work done by researchers in this field. All due efforts have been made to make this book serve as a complete guiding source for students and researchers. The topics in this book have been comprehensively explained to help readers understand the growing trends in the field.

I would like to thank the entire group of writers who made sincere efforts in this book and my family who supported me in my efforts of working on this book. I take this opportunity to thank all those who have been a guiding force throughout my life.

Editor

1

Felt Needs for Rehabilitation After Breast Cancer Treatment in Mexico

Viveka Hammelin, Luz María Tejada-Tayabas,
Dulce María Galarza-Tejada and
Joel Monárrez-Espino

Abstract

Breast cancer (BC) is the most frequent type of malignancy among women worldwide and the most common cause of mortality, particularly in low and middle-income countries. As detection and treatment have improved, a larger number of surviving women need adequate rehabilitation after treatment. However, awareness among affected patients remains low. Thus, the aim of this study was to explore the needs and expectations concerning rehabilitation among Mexican women after breast surgery. An ethnographic approach was used. Eight focus groups were conducted in the north-central state of San Luis Potosí, Mexico, in 2014, in which women under treatment and survivors participated. Results showed that women had insufficient and misleading information concerning the need for rehabilitation from health care authorities. Women seemed to focus more on survival than on quality of life after treatment even though impairments limiting their daily life activities caused frustration and feelings of uselessness. In conclusion, many women perceived the need for rehabilitation, but information was largely lacking. Public health services fail to provide rehabilitation services, which are now partially covered by private organizations. Treatment for breast cancer should be accompanied by rehabilitation. Awareness, availability and access to physiotherapy services need to be put in place.

Keywords: breast cancer, physiotherapy, Mexico, postsurgery care, rehabilitation

1. Introduction

Breast cancer (BC) is one of the most common malignancies in the world [1]. In Mexico, it is the most frequent cancer among women, with incidence and mortality rates of 25 and 14 cases per 100,000 person-years, respectively [2]. Between 2007 and 2014, the incidence of BC has been increasing steadily reaching 29 cases per 100,000 women [3] with a large proportion being diagnosed in stages III and IV, which are associated with a more complex treatment and a lower survival probability [4].

The central-northern state of San Luis Potosí (SLP), where this study was carried out, is one of the most affected areas by this tumor [5]. During 2013, BC was the main cause of hospital discharge among women aged 20 years or more and it accounted for 24.6% of all reported malignancies, becoming the first cause of hospital morbidity with 55% of all registered cases of women aged 40–59 years old [5].

Timely diagnosis remains a major concern, especially in poor and marginalized women, due to the limited availability and access to preventive health services [6, 7]. Therefore, when women are detected with BC, it is often at an advanced stage when surgery is the primary treatment modality [8].

Mastectomy [9], but also chemo and radiotherapy [10, 11], often results in decreased motion of the affected extremity and along with pain and edema impairs the mobility and reduces the strength of the upper limb [10] affecting the women's quality of life (QoL) [10, 12]. The occurrence of these conditions can vary depending on who is assessing them (e.g., physiotherapist or self-reported), the treatment modality (e.g., surgery with or without chemo/radiotherapy) and the time elapsed since the surgery [11, 13].

Some relatively common consequences derived from the operation are difficult to deal with, especially if physiotherapy is lacking. For instance, lymphedema arising from the resection of lymph nodes can develop in 15–25% of the women after 1–5 years of surgery [13]. In such cases, physiotherapy can decrease edema by using manual lymph drainage or by compressing garments. Pain, another complaint affecting up to 50% of women surviving cancer [14], can also be relieved through physical means. Thus, postsurgical care should involve physical rehabilitation to help women recover the motion of her upper limbs and to reduce the edema and pain associated [15].

However, many women from low- and middle-income countries, who undergo a mastectomy, do not receive physiotherapy [16, 17]. This could be due to various reasons, including the fact that women are not aware of the existence and relevance of physical therapy after surgery [17], or because availability and access to rehabilitation services is constrained [18, 19].

In Mexico, health care services offered for BC patients include those provided by social security institutions, those covered by the people's health insurance (PHI) run by the Ministry of Health and the costly private medical care [20]. One of the free public programs prioritized by the national health system is the "specific action program for BC," which covers both diagnosis and treatment, but pays little attention to rehabilitation care [21].

As detection and treatment have improved during the last decades, a larger number of women now survive who need adequate physiotherapy after treatment [22, 23]. However, awareness among affected patients still remains low, especially among poor women [13, 24].

So far, there is limited knowledge and understanding of the importance and use of physiotherapy after BC treatment in Mexican women [25]. Thus, this study aims at filling this gap by exploring the needs and expectations concerning rehabilitation after surgery. This information could be of value to better design and implement rehabilitation programs that can translate into a better QoL.

2. Methodology

The study presented here was part of a larger evaluation of the BC program in SLP, Mexico [26]. An ethnographic approach was used [27] with a purposive sample [28] of women diagnosed with BC who were either receiving or had received treatment at a public facility, though few family members were also included. Participants were contacted through the group RETO (i.e., total recovery in Spanish, but also means "challenge"), a nongovernmental organization (NGO) that provides social assistance to women with BC at SLP public Central Hospital. Eight focus groups (FGs) [29] comprising four to twelve participants were conducted (**Table 1**). FGs took place at the Faculty of Nursing and Nutrition of SLP Autonomous University between February and March 2014 by one of the coauthors trained and skilled in FG interviews (LMTT) until saturation was reached [30, 31]. Sessions lasted between 29 and 110 min and followed an interview guide that covered various themes dealing with experiences, limitations, strategies, needs and expectations concerning rehabilitation. FGs were audio-taped with the consent of participants. In some cases, family members also participated (this was differentiated in the transcriptions).

ID	Participants (relative)[1]	Duration in min	Age mean (min-max)
FG1	11 (2F)	82	51 (33–69)
FG2	4 (1F)	57	58 (49–76)
FG3	7	110	48 (27–74)
FG4	4 (2F)	51	57 (48–62)
FG5	4 (2M)	46	51 (45–57)
FG6	5 (1F)	36	53 (29–75)
FG7	12	29	44 (34–60)
FG8	5 (1F)	47	41 (36–50)

[1]Number and sex of family member(s) who participated in the group.

Table 1. Description of the focus groups.

Prior to the FGs, women filled in a questionnaire to obtain socio-demographic data. The disability of arm shoulder hand (DASH) questionnaire, a self-reported function validated and reliable instrument was used to determine the women's upper limb motion after surgery [32]. Thereafter, a clinical examination was carried out by one of the authors (VH), a professional physiotherapist, to examine the functional status of the shoulder and arm to identify the presence of limitations that hamper mobility among these women.

Women were examined in a sitting position where the active range of motion (ROM) of the shoulder was measured using a goniometer [33]. The arm volume was determined using the circumference of the arm to compute the volume of a cone [34]. Impaired ROM was defined as an inter-limb difference of more than 10° [35]. Observations made during the clinical examinations were recorded as field notes [36] and used in order to understand the context during the data analysis.

FG data was examined using content analysis, interpreting both manifest and latent content in order to understand both the context and subjectivity in the material [37]. Systematic codification and categorization were made using an inductive approach.

The full process included the following steps: (1) verbatim transcriptions of the FGs, (2) translation from Spanish into English, (3) systematic codification, (4) grouping into categories, (5) second codification of the segments to identify narrative consistency and variability and (6) final discussion among authors to reach consensus about the findings. The software ATLAS.ti 5.2 was used for the analytical process.

Ethical principles were followed concerning self-determination, anonymity and confidentiality. All participants signed an informed consent form using standard practices.

3. Findings

Women included in the study were between the ages of 26 and 76 years with a mean age of 50. Their overall socioeconomic status was low. Most were married, were housewives and had one or more children. About half of them went to secondary school and one in four completed college. Most women were affiliated to the PHI (the free public medical service for the lower-income segment of the population), but still reported having made personal payments for the health care received. The average time elapsed from the surgery to the survey date was nearly 3 years, ranging from 1 month to 23 years.

More than half of the women had impaired flexion and abduction and almost one-third of women had impaired lateral rotation of the shoulder. One in four had lymphedema and nearly all reported difficulties in performing tasks in daily life to a more or less severe extent.

The following sections present the findings using five relevant categories that arose from the data analyses: (1) functional limitations in daily life, (2) reasons for limitations and discomfort, (3) strategies to deal with impairments, (4) felt needs for information and (5) expectations of rehabilitation from the health care services.

3.1. Functional limitations in daily life

The limitations the women referred to after treatment included problems moving their arm and the lack of strength on the affected side, which hindered them from lifting and carrying heavy objects. This problem occurred in various degrees depending on the time elapsed since the breast surgery, being more severe the shorter the time elapsed. For instance, from 3 to 4 weeks after surgery, the limitation was complete resulting in difficulties even to perform basic personal hygiene actions, which made them rely on others. Yet, many household chores, such as doing the laundry or squeezing the mop, which are commonly performed by hand by these relatively poor women, were still constrained even after 6 months of treatment.

> *"For me it was very difficult. At first I couldn't do anything, like for half a year, I couldn't for example squeeze the mop [by hand]. I couldn't, it hurt in this hand and it hurt in the whole arm. It took me half a year until I had the strength to squeeze it, to be able to really squeeze it." (Woman FG 1)*

The impact of the limitation depended upon the specific context of every woman; while some received support from family members, others felt obliged to fulfill their household duties on their own in whatever way possible. For instance, a mother with young children was forced to move her arm to be able to care for her family.

> *"For me personally, I have my little girls, I need to move on, to continue doing things, that's why you do it, for the girls really, for the girls and the husband, you have to move on." (Woman FG 6)*

3.2. Reasons for limitations and discomfort

The women ascribed their limitations to both direct and indirect causes, which can be grouped into medical, emotional and idiosyncratic. While some described the limitations in medical terms, others referred them more simply as pain or weakness. Emotional reasons included the fear of moving the arm or unawareness of impairment. The role of culture and the perception of impairment in the Mexican context were also referred to by some women.

Sometimes the limitations were explained as a result of the extraction of lymph nodes and/or muscles and nerves being cut off. The bottom line was that these provided a logical explanation for the experienced sensations and difficulties. Women seemed to have obtained this information from their doctors, from members of the RETO group, or by reading educational materials.

> *"...because they take out the lymph nodes the circulation is insufficient, unlike it was before; they take out muscles, arteries and veins. For me it was a radical mastectomy, they took all the breast out, so it makes sense what I feel because some muscles and nerves die..." (Woman FG 4)*

The main discomforts mentioned by the women included pain, numbness, weakness, swelling of the arm and the feeling of having a heavy arm. Both women working at home and those with professional careers emphasized the impact that these problems had on their ability to perform daily tasks. Activities such as lifting heavy objects or working in the computer for various hours resulted in pain and exhaustion leading to feelings of incompetence.

> *"I felt incapable, I felt incapable of not being able to, like use a pen, an eraser..." (Woman FG 5)*

Some women reported being reluctant to move their arm out of fear that the wound would open, potentially damaging the neighboring anatomic structures and others were worried about the chance that the movement could increase the pain. Thus, the lack of information regarding the motion possibilities of their upper extremities resulted in fear, making some women overly cautious and over protective of their arms.

> *"...I was scared, mostly regarding the exercises. I thought that maybe they [the doctors] told me not to move the arm, as I might hurt myself and the wound could open... I was scared." (Woman FG 5)*

Another reason for the limitations faced was the acceptance of the impairment; a sense of normality concerning the discomfort, which they assumed would not require any therapeutic measure. Some women were not even aware of their inability to lift their arms until they were about to receive radiotherapy, as this was a requirement to get such treatment. Until then, some women had not even tried to improve their arms' mobility.

> *"I have gone every week [to the doctor] since February 10, but the doctor didn't tell me that I had to move my arm. I had the first radiation session yesterday, but I couldn't lift the arm; now I have to go next Tuesday to see if I can lift it for the radiation, otherwise I will have to wait week after week." (Woman FG 7)*

The local idiosyncrasy also seemed to play a role for preventing women from recognizing impartments as disabilities at least until they are completely unable to perform conventional tasks. Some discomfort and/or limitations were often seen as natural and justified as part of the normal healing process by both patients and doctors themselves.

> *"My arm has been fine; it hasn't hurt at all. I can lift it perfectly, like I don't feel anything. I only feel it when I'm carrying something. But if I forget and carry something heavy, then later I feel it; it's normal." (Woman FG 2)*

Fear of recurrence and feelings of loss of femininity due to the removal of the breast were heavy burdens to women. Consequently, many women expressed the need for psychological assistance and ascribed psychological rehabilitation more value than to physiotherapy.

> *"...we need information, but also psychological care; we need it a lot, really, because we women are very strong, but sometimes it knocks you down, really, it does." (Woman FG 2)*

3.3. Strategies to deal with impairments

Women used various strategies to decrease their impairment. While few used the available medical services, for the majority, this was not a feasible option due to financial constraints and geographic difficulties accessing rehabilitation services. For those unable to receive professional medical therapy, the alternative was to perform exercises at home and to adjust their daily tasks to their condition. Women also discussed about the relevance of keeping a good attitude toward recovery and the importance of being motivated to do so.

The use of medical services varied and ranged from the utilization of compression garments, manual lymphatic drainage and physiotherapy to the use of prosthetic devices and medications such as diuretics. Those using a prosthesis saw it more as an aesthetic device rather than as a functional implement; thus, women tended to use just the cloth without weight or nothing at all. Many women got in contact with the providers of these services through RETO or received help directly from this organization.

> *"...at RETO they gave me advice and a lot of help; they told me how to do many exercises. They sent me to lymphatic drainage because my arm had started to get swollen and heavy, but this drainage helped me a lot. They [RETO] also teach you how to do the massage." (Woman FG 3)*

In order to decrease the sense of impairment, many women made adjustments in their life. For instance, they would modify the way in which they use to perform a task or would just remove such activity from the agenda. Occasionally, women would receive help from their family or from close acquaintances, but this was rather exceptional. As a rule, women were responsible to take care of their children and other family members. Thus, to fulfill their chores they mentioned that they tried to plan their activities according to what could be done considering their limitations.

> *"... I have constant pain in my arm. This is because of the physical activities I do when I work at home with all my chores. I have to plan according to what my arm allows. If it goes well one day I sweep and I mop. But I always do the dishes and fix the food. I know that I have to do the daily tasks, but I plan for doing the laundry and to sweep because these are the things that cause most trouble; it's very heavy to mop." (Woman FG 2)*

Being able to manage household chores, work and to a smaller extent to perform recreational activities were often reasons for moving or exercising. Some women emphasized that their children and spouses provided motivation to continue fighting and to overcome their limitations.

> *"...I was 40 years old, so I still had a life, I had to fight for my kids, for my husband..." (Woman FG 4)*

Some women mentioned that feeling like a disabled person that has to cope with her reality worked as a motivator to become more active. For many, there was no alternative but to help themselves improve, as they have to support their families, which were already living on scarce means. Therefore, recovery became a necessity.

> *"...my doctor told me that I was going to have like a disability, well, he didn't say it like that and then I thought 'how will I make a living?'" (Woman FG 4)*

3.4. Felt needs for information

Women described functional limitations as a consequence of the lack of adequate information, exercise, or movement. Limited knowledge was often a source of insecurity. However, they also emphasized the value of the help received from RETO and highlighted the importance of the assistance of such NGOs for women during the course of treatment and thereafter.

After surgery many women left the hospital with bandages attaching their affected arm to the torso without knowing what they could or could not do. Some of them were actually told not to move their arm, even after the bandages had been taken off to avoid the opening of the wound, which resulted in fear and insecurity.

> *"... I liked to have the arm here [attached to the body]. I didn't move it and until today; I still cannot lift it very high, because I liked to walk with the arm here. The doctor said: 'leave it like that' [laughs]; I was scared to lift it." (Woman FG 1)*

Some women mentioned that few doctors and nurses gave them good and adequate information and advice. Yet, for the most part, it was lacking, contradictory, or failed to sufficiently clarify things for them and to provide full understanding of the issues involved. Consequently, the fear and insecurity persisted.

> *"I get scared of getting close to the stove because, who knows what could happen to me? I never got a clear explanation, not at any point after the operation. They never explained to me at any stage what kind of things I could do or not." (Woman FG 4)*

The most frequent support for rehabilitation was the instructions provided by RETO, which contained general information and guidelines for exercise and for the lymphatic drainage. These instructions were generally given in the form of a brochure that was handed out when leaving the hospital after the surgery. In fact, the support of RETO was often the only organization providing some kind of rehabilitation information for women.

> *"I went looking for information; I had to know what was going to come after [the surgery]. I took the little brochure and then at RETO they explained everything to you: how to do the exercises, how to start, how many days and all, everything. I got the information about that from them." (Woman FG 5)*

However, the presence of RETO at the hospital somehow also prevented the public health services to offer additional information and support concerning rehabilitation.

> *"...apart from the RETO group, I think that the doctors, well, here at the hospital it's like they think, or I don't know, that if the RETO group is helping us to survive then they are taking care of our needs." (Woman FG 1)*

3.5. Expectations of rehabilitation from the health care services

Women's views regarding the care that they believe BC patients should be given were also explored along with suggestions on how to do this. The presence of family members in the discussions shed additional light in topics such as the unequal access to care.

While the medical and surgical treatment for BC was covered by the popular health insurance, women mentioned financial and logistic obstacles to access adequate and comprehensive care that included rehabilitation. For instance, one spouse commented on the possible effect of not paying for services could have affected the coverage and quality of care of his wife.

> *"...well, I don't know, maybe it's because one doesn't pay, because it's given for free (...) and I guess it's that, because for the most part I don't contribute with anything economically that they leave you like that. You get your surgery and that's enough for you to be satisfied and then the rest is up to God to help you (...) because if one could pay, I guess they would say 'come on, let's go'."(Male relative, FG 5)*

Conversely, posttreatment care, including physical therapy, lymphatic drainage and the provision of assistive devices (e.g., prosthesis) are not covered by the PHI. Thus, since for most women were unable to pay out of their pocket for rehabilitation care, then they just had to rely on charitable assistance such as the one provided by RETO or simply receive no care whatsoever.

> *"...I didn't have the possibility [to get rehabilitation]; in fact, they didn't say anything to me about rehabilitating exercises, nothing, even though I wanted that. At that time, that year, my husband was out of work and God knows, you have to eat, so for one, paying rehabilitation, was impossible for one, we had to pay rent (...) it's impossible." (Woman FG 3)*

The financial problems were paired with the logistic access to rehabilitation services. This was particularly relevant for those women living in marginalized or rural areas where means of transportations became the main concern.

> *"...the truth is that I didn't, I didn't have rehabilitation of my arm. Yes, the oncologist sent me to rehabilitation, but it was very difficult for me because I lived two hours from Tampico [a major city where the service was available]. I needed to go every day and so this was one of the things that I couldn't do, thank you very much, but I couldn't do it." (Woman FG 2)*

Most women suggested additional public clinics and doctors that can spend more time with each patient. However, since women were not informed about the treatment procedures and the consequences thereof, they did not have a clear picture of what kind of care they could ask for. Some suggested seminars to inform and guide patients and their families about BC treatment and posttreatment care.

> *"We have to become people who demand and ask for better care, like 'you are going to take care of me because it's your job and I pay you for it and you have to do it'." (Woman FG 7)*

4. Discussion

This study aimed to explore the needs and expectations concerning rehabilitation among Mexican women after BC surgery. Due to insufficient and sometimes misleading information from the health care services, the actual need for posttreatment care is neither met nor acknowledged. However, the positive attitude found among women toward rehabilitation is an important resource for future interventions. How these women perceive their right to comprehensive health care seems to be affected by the structure of the health care services and the Mexican idiosyncrasy.

The study provides in-depth information about the rehabilitation needs and expectations of BC survivors from a middle-size central Mexican city. Various themes emerged that underlie factors associated with the lack of rehabilitation care for most women such as the absence of free- or low-cost public facilities that provide such services, as previously observed [18].

A relevant issue was the lack of knowledge concerning the various aspects of treatment and posttreatment care. There was a general unawareness of the impairments as such or a belief that the discomforts were part of the normal healing process. Contrary to previous findings showing that the needs and complications reported by patients tend to be greater than those reported by clinicians [38], the women in this study seemed to give less importance to the functional limitations than to what their actual clinical assessment revealed (nearly all women included in this study had significant functional motion restrictions as assessed by a physiotherapist; data not presented). Yet, most of those experiencing limitations after surgery did not even try to seek rehabilitation care in agreement with others studies reporting that just few women are aware of the importance of posttreatment rehabilitation, especially in poor settings [17, 39, 40].

The findings of this study are also added to the evidence that there is a dissatisfaction regarding the information and support given by physicians and health care personnel after BC surgery. Fear, insecurity and confusion are generated by absent or misleading information [16, 39] which makes women have an overtly protective attitude toward the movement of their affected arms. Advice to keep the arm still and to avoid heavy lifting led to the belief that strenuous activity can have a negative effect on movement and volume, when studies suggesting the opposite [41, 42]. The motion restrictions advised by the health care personnel seemed to derive from outdated information concerning the effects of arm movement after surgery [41] which points to the need to update physicians and health professionals on the current physiotherapy guidelines for BC patients.

Most women were not informed about the procedures or the consequences that the treatment entailed. In particular, they were neither told nor they themselves requested for rehabilitation care for the experienced discomfort. In accordance with previous studies [43, 44], many women tried to handle their bothers either by changing the usual way in which they carried out an activity, by modifying their work schedule, or by eliminating tasks considered too difficult to perform. The relatively lack of assistance from spouse, family members, or friends to carry out daily activities also needs to be considered, as it can affect the interaction of this women with their family and social environment [43].

Cancer brings negative consequences associated with both the disease and the medical and surgical treatment [45]. As women experience the cancer process, some of them develop a fatalist attitude with a loss of hope that results in less energy and motivation to continue fighting the disease [46, 47]. This can in turn prevent women from trying to improve their welfare while alive, which partially explains why they do not prioritize their rehabilitation. However, the disease can also result in a positive proactive attitude [48], as it was observed among many of the women interviewed here whereby they try to keep themselves alive in optimal conditions for their children and husbands. A positive mindset and the will to fight the disease with the hope to survive are also part of the survival strategies used by BC women [49]. Unfortunately, these women still lack the information and support needed to face their physical limitations and many end up prioritizing the needs of others at the expense of their physical rehabilitation.

While taking care of the close family can grow in relevance among BC women [50] becoming a key issue to face the disease, it seems that there can also have a negative effect when it comes to paying attention to their physical rehabilitation.

One must also consider the importance of providing social support to these women during this stage of the disease [51], including that of spouse, grown-up children and other family members, which is crucial to take appropriate decisions with respect to rehabilitation [52].

It is important that the public health services pay attention to the rehabilitation needs of BC women after surgery by designing and implementing follow-up programs that have been proven successful [53] involving family members that provide support [54] and optimizing the resources and offering benefits that translate into a better quality of life.

Since the survival rate for BC is increasing, so it is the importance of posttreatment care. As it is the case in many other low- and middle-income countries, there is no institutional public program available in Mexico that provides free coverage for rehabilitation services to BC women after surgery [55]. At present, the health system mainly focuses on survival, namely, on primary and adjuvant treatment [56, 57] whereby posttreatment care is left to NGOs such as the RETO group that provide information, exercise programs, lymphatic drainage and other activities to support women during the rehabilitation period. Yet, this study and others [16, 17, 39, 40] illustrate the need of rehabilitation and psychological therapy in addition to surgical treatment and radiotherapy for BC women.

During the discussions, economic and logistic issues were brought up as reasons limiting the access to comprehensive care. Those few women referred for rehabilitation found significant barriers to access those services either because of the high cost involved and/or due to distance and transportation difficulties. Differential accessibility to health services has been acknowledged in Mexico by health authorities who have even called for strong patients' advocacy groups to improve cancer care [58]. Unfortunately, the notion that survival is the main and almost only goal of treatment seems to prevail among both, patients and health personnel and so far little attention is being paid to the provision of better care after BC surgery [57].

The structure and recent evolution of the Mexican health system has had an impact on how the right to health care is looked upon by the population. The PHI, implemented in 2003 with the aim of providing comprehensive health care to those uninsured, entitled nearly 50 million Mexicans to a regulated and structured health care service. Thus, it is important to considered that many of the women interviewed here would have received an even more limited health care service prior to the inclusion of BC treatment in the insurance policies of 2007 [8, 55, 56]. However, the inclusion of posttreatment rehabilitation is yet to be part of such insurance to achieve a more humane comprehensive care for these women.

It is worth noting that while the public health services in SLP have insufficient human resources and infrastructure to rehabilitate BC women after surgery, the health authorities fail to even provide women with relevant information concerning the benefits of motility and physical exercise after surgery and during chemo and radiotherapy; instead, women have to rely upon the support and guidance of a NGO for that purpose [18]. Governmental authorities must be aware of this and as a result take a more active role rehabilitating these women. The same logic applies to the psycho-emotional support, which is commonly overlooked, as both BC women and health professionals are mostly focused on survival, but far less on the women's quality of life.

Altogether the findings of this study stress the pain and difficulties of BC women have to go through, which affect their quality of life significantly, including their social interaction with those dearest and nearest to them. However, the positive attitude of most women in their will to improve their functionality after surgery should be seen as an opportunity to design and implement effective rehabilitation programs with high adherence to its guidelines.

5. Conclusion

Many women perceived the need for rehabilitation, but information is still largely lacking. At present, public health services fail to provide rehabilitation services, which are now partially covered by private organizations. Treatment for BC should be accompanied by adequate rehabilitation. Therefore, awareness, availability and access to physiotherapy services need to be put in place.

Abbreviation list

BC	Breast cancer
DASH	Disability of arm shoulder hand
FG	Focus groups
NGO	Nongovernmental organization
PHI	People's health insurance
RETO	Recuperación total (total recovery)
ROM	Range of motion
SLP	San Luis Potosí

Author details

Viveka Hammelin, Luz María Tejada-Tayabas, Dulce María Galarza-Tejada and Joel Monárrez-Espino*

*Address all correspondence to: joel.monarrez-espino@ki.se

Department of Public Health Sciences, Karolinska Institutet, Stockholm, Sweden

References

[1] Torre L, Bray F, Siegel R, Ferlay J, Lortet-Tieulent J, Jemal A. Global cancer statistics, 2012. CA: A Cancer Journal for clinicians 2015, 65(2):87–108. Available from: http://onlinelibrary.wiley.com/doi/10.3322/caac.21262/epdf

[2] Soto-Perez-de-Celis E, Chavarri-Guerra Y. National and regional breast cancer incidence and mortality trends in Mexico 2001–2011: Analysis of a population-based database. *Cancer Epidemiol*, 2016. 41: 24–33. DOI: http://dx.doi.org/10.1016/j.canep.2016.01.007

[3] Ministry of Health. Statistical information. Statistics on Breast Cancer and Uterine Cervical Cancer [internet]. Available from: http://www.gob.mx/salud/acciones-y-programas/informacion-estadistica

[4] Caplan L. Delay in breast cancer: Implications for stage at diagnosis and survival. *Front PublicHealth*, 2014. 2: 87.

[5] National Institute of Statistics and Geography (INEGI). Statistics on the international day against breast cancer, 2013. Available from: http://www.inegi.org.mx/saladeprensa/aproposito/2016/mama2016_0.pdf

[6] Cruz-Castillo AB, Hernández-Valero MA, Hovick S, Campuzano-González ME, Karam-Calderón MA. Bustamante-Monte P. A study on the knowledge, perception and use of breast cancer screening methods and quality of care among women from central Mexico. *J Cancer Educ*, 2015. 30(3): 453–459.

[7] Lee CI, Bogart A, Germino J, et al. Availability of advanced breast imaging at screening facilities serving vulnerable populations. *J Med Screen*, 2016. 23: 24–30.

[8] Chavarri-Guerra, Y, Villarreal-Garza C, Liedke P, et al. Breast cancer in Mexico: A growing challenge to health and the health system. *Lancet Oncol*, 2012. 13(8): 335–343.

[9] Inger-Lise N, Alv AD, Løkkevik E, Mengshoel AM, fossá SD. Arm and shoulder morbidity in breast cancer patients after breast-conserving therapy versus mastectomy, Acta Oncologica, 2008. 47(5): 835–842. Available from: http://dx.doi.org/10.1080/02841860801961257

[10] Campbell KL, Pusic KL, Zucker D, et al. A prospective model of care for breast cancer rehabilitation: Function. *Cancer*, 2012. 118: 2300–2311. Available from: http://onlinelibrary.wiley.com/doi/10.1002/cncr.27464/pdf

[11] Lee TS, Kilbreath S, Refshauge K, et al. Prognosis of the upper limb following surgery and radiation for breast cancer. *Breast Cancer Res Treat*, 2008. 110: 19–37.

[12] Rietman JS, Dijkstra PU, Hoekstra HJ, et al. Late morbidity after treatment of breast cancer in relation to daily activities and quality of life: a systematic review. *Eur J Surg Oncol*, 2003. 29(3): 229–238.

[13] Ewertz M, & Jensen AB. Late effects of breast cancer treatment and potentials for rehabilitation. *Acta Oncol*, 2011. 50(2): 187–193.

[14] Kurita GP, & Sjogren P. Pain management in cancer survivorship. *Acta Oncol*, 2015. 54(5): 629–634.

[15] Van Dijck S, Nelissen P, Verbelen H. et al. The effects of physical self-management on quality of life in breast cancer patients: A systematic review. *The Breast*, 2016. 28: 20–28.

[16] Binkley JM, Harris SR, Levangie P, et al. Patient perspectives on breast cancer treatment side effects and the prospective surveillance model for physical rehabilitation for women with breast cancer. *Cancer*, 2012. 118(Suppl 8): 2207–2216. Available from: http://onlinelibrary.wiley.com/doi/10.1002/cncr.27469/pdf

[17] Ganz PA, Yip Ch, Gralow J, et al. Supportive care after curative treatment for breast cancer (survivorship care): Resource allocations in low- and middle-income countries. A Breast Health Global Initiative 2013 consensus statement. *The Breast*, 2013. 22: 606–615.

[18] Tejada-Tayabas, L.M., Amell, L., Monárrez-Espino, J. Medical therapeutic itineraries of women with breast cancer diagnosis affiliated to the people's health insurance in San Luis Potosí, central Mexico. *Cad Saúde Pública*, 2015. 31(1): 60–70. Available from:http://www.scielo.br/pdf/csp/v31n1/0102-311X-csp-31-01-00060.pdf

[19] Borman P, Yaman A, Yasrebi S, et al. The importance of awareness and education in patients with breast cancer-related lymphedem. *J Canc Educ*, 2016. Apr 6 [Epub ahead of print]. Available from: http://link.springer.com/article/10.1007/s13187-016-1026-1/fulltext.html

[20] Pauwels, EE. Charlier C, De Bourdeaudhuij I, Lechner L, Van Hoof E. Care needs after primary breast cancer treatment. Survivors' associated sociodemographic and medical characteristics. *Psychooncology*, 2013, 22(1): 125–132.

[21] Gómez-Dantes, O., Sesma, S., Becerril, V.M., Knaul, F.M., Arreola, H., Frenk, J. Sistema de salud de México. *Salud Publica Mex*, 2011. 53(Suppl 2): 220–232. Available from: http://www.scielosp.org/pdf/spm/v53s2/17.pdf

[22] Ministry of Health. Specific Action Program for the Prevention and Control of Breast Cancer 2013–2018. 1st ed. 2014. Mexico City. National Health System. Available from:

http://cnegsr.salud.gob.mx/contenidos/descargas/cama/PrevencionyControldelCancerdelaMujer_2013_2018.pdf

[23] Anaya-Ruiz M, Vallejo-Ruiz V, Flores-Mendoza L, Perez-Santos M. Female breast cancer incidence and mortality in Mexico, 2000–2010. *Asian Pac J Cancer Prev*, 2014. 15(3): 1477–1479. Available from: http://ocean.kisti.re.kr/downfile/volume/apocp/POCPA9/2014/v15n3/POCPA9_2014_v15n3_1477.pdf

[24] Schmitz KH, Stout NL, PT andrews A, et al. Prospective evaluation of physical rehabilitation needs in breast cancer survivors. *Cancer*, 2012. 118(Suppl 58): 2187–2190. Available from: http://onlinelibrary.wiley.com/doi/10.1002/cncr.27471/pdf

[25] Systematization of the Navigation´s Experience (support) of Breast Cancer Patients. 2012, Heredia, National University of Costa Rica. Available from: http://www.kerwa.ucr.ac.cr/handle/10669/1408

[26] Tejada-Tayabas LM, Castillo T, Monarrez-Espino J. Qualitative evaluation, a interpretive and critical approach to improving programs and health services. *Int J Qualitative Stud Health Well-Being*, 2014, 9: 24417. http://dx.doi.org/10.3402/qhw.v9.24417

[27] Cook KE. Using critical ethnography to explore issues in health promotion. *Qual Health Res*, 2005. 15: 129–138.

[28] Suri H. Purposeful sampling in qualitative research synthesis. *Qual Res J*, 2011. 11(2): 63–75. Available from: http://www.emeraldinsight.com/doi/pdfplus/10.3316/QRJ1102063

[29] Morgan DL, Krueger RA. Planning focus groups. Focus group Kit 2. United States of America: SAGE publications India Pvt. Ltd, 1998.

[30] Guest G, Bunce A, & Johnson L. How many interviews are enough? An experiment with data saturation and variability. *Field methods*, 2006. 18: 59–82.

[31] Kerr C, Nixon A, & Wild D. Assessing and demonstrating data saturation in qualitative inquiry supporting patient-reported outcomes research. *Expert Rev Pharmacoecon Outcomes Res*, 2010. 10(3): 269–281.

[32] Gummesson C, Ward MM, Atroshi I. The shortened disabilities of the arm, shoulder and hand questionnaire (QuickDASH): validity and reliability based on responses within the full-length DASH. *BMC Musculoskelet Disord*, 2006. 7: 44. Available from: http://bmcmusculoskeletdisord.biomedcentral.com/articles/10.1186/1471-2474-7-44

[33] Muir SW, Corea CL, Beaupre L. Evaluating change in clinical status: Reliability and measures of agreement for the assessment of glenohumeral range of motion. *N Am J Sports Phys Ther*, 2010. 5(3): 98–110.

[34] Brorson H, & Hoijer P. Standardised measurements used to order compression garments can be used to calculate arm volumes to evaluate lymphoedema treatment. *J Plast Surg Hand Surg*, 2012. 46(6): 410–415.

[35] Thomas-Maclean RL, Thomas H, Winkle K, et al. Arm morbidity and disability after breast cancer: New directions for care. *Oncol Nurs Forum*, 2008. 35(1): 65–71.

[36] Emerson, R.M., Fretz, R.I. & Shaw, L.L. Writing ethnographic fieldnotes. Chicago: University of Chicago Press, 1995.

[37] Graneheim UH, & Lundman B. Qualitative content analysis in nursing research: concepts, procedures and measures to achieve trustworthiness. *Nurse Educ Today*, 2004. 24(2): 105–112.

[38] Cheville AL, Beck LA, Petersen TL, Marks RS. The detection and treatment of cancer-related functional problems in an outpatient setting. *Support Care Cancer*, 2009. 17(1): 61–67.

[39] Ridner S, Rhoten B, Radina E, et al. Breast cancer survivors' perspectives of critical lymphedema self-care support needs. Supportive Care in Cancer, 2016, 24(6): 2743–2750. Available from: http://link.springer.com/article/10.1007/s00520-016-3089-2

[40] Keast DH, Despatis M, Allen JO, Brassard A. Chronic edema/lymphoedema: Under-recognised and under-treoated. *Int Wound*, 2015. 12(3): 328–333.

[41] Lee TS. Kilbreath S, Sullivan G. et al. Factors that affect intention to avoid strenuous arm activity after breast cancer surgery. *Oncology nursing forum*, 2009. 36(4): 2454–2462.

[42] McNeely ML, Binkley M, Pusic AL, et al. A prospective model of care for breast cancer rehabilitation: Postoperative and postreconstructive issues. *Cancer*, 2012. 118: 2226–2236. Available from: http://onlinelibrary.wiley.com/doi/10.1002/cncr.27468/pdf

[43] Thomas–MacLean R, et al. "This is a kind of betrayal": A qualitative study of disability after breast cancer. *Curr Oncol*, 2009. 16(3): 26–32.

[44] Tiedtke, C. Dierckx B, Rijkc A et al. Breast cancer treatment and work disability: Patient perspectives. *Breast*, 2011. 20(6): 534–538.

[45] Khan F, Amatya B, Pallant JF, Rajapaksa I. Factors associated with long-term functional outcomes and psychological sequelae in women after breast cancer. *The Breast*, 2012. 21(3): 314–320.

[46] Curtis R, Groarke A, McSharry J, Kerin M. Experience of breast cancer: burden, benefit, or both? *Cancer Nurs*, 2014. 37(3): E21-E30.

[47] Nakatani Y, Iwamitsu Y, Kuranami M, Okazaki S, Yamamoto K, Watanabe M, Miyaoka H. Predictors of psychological distress in breast cancer patients after surgery. *Kitasato Med J*, 2013. 43: 49–58.

[48] Scheffold K, Mehnert A, Muller V, Koch U, Harter M, Vehling S. Sources of meaning in cancer patients—influences on global meaning, anxiety and depression in a longitudinal study. *Eur J Cancer Care*, 2014. 23(4): 472–480.

[49] Rotegard AK, Fagermoen MS, Ruland CM. Cancer patients' experiences of their personal strengths through illness and recovery. *Cancer Nurs*, 2012, 35(1): E8–E17.

[50] Salander P, Lilliehorn S, Hamberg K, Kero A. The impact of breast cancer on living an everyday life 4.5-5 years post-diagnosis — A qualitative prospective study of 39 women. *Acta Oncol*, 2011. 50(3): 399–407.

[51] Drageset S, Lindstrom TC, Giske T, Underlid K. "The support I need": Women's experiences of social support after having received breast Cancer diagnosis and awaiting surgery. *Cancer Nurs*, 2012. 35(6): E39-E47.

[52] Jensen CG, Elsass P, Neustrup L, et al. What to listen for in the consultation. Breast cancer patients' own focus on talking about acceptance-based psychological coping predicts decreased psychological distress and depression. *Patient Educ Couns*, 2014. 97(2): 165–172.

[53] Stanley S, Arriola KJ, Smith S, Hurlbert M, Ricci C, Escoffery C. Reducing barriers to breast cancer care through a patient navigation programs. *J Public Health Manag Pract*, 2013. 19(5): 461–467.

[54] Marshall CA, Badger TA, Curran MA, Koerner SS, Larkey LK, Weihs KL, et al. Un abrazo para la familia: Providing low-income Hispanics with education and skills in coping with breast cancer and caregiving. *Psychooncology*, 2013. 22(2): 470–474.

[55] Kaul FM. et al. The quest for universal health coverage: achieving social protection for all in Mexico. *The Lancet*, 2012. 380(9849): 1259–1279

[56] Gonzalez-Robledo MC, Wong R, Arreola H, Knaul F. Costs of breast cancer care in Mexico: analysis of two insurance coverage scenarios. *Ecancermedicalscience*, 2015. 9: 587.

[57] Yip CH. Cazap E anderson B, et al. Breast cancer management in middle-resource countries (MRCs): Consensus statement from the breast health global initiative. *The Breast*, 2011. 20(2): 12–19.

[58] Chertorivski S. Planning cancer control — A Mexican perspective. *The lancet oncol*, 2013. 14(5): 386–387.

2

Machine Learning Methods for Breast Cancer Diagnostic

Shahnorbanun Sahran, Ashwaq Qasem,
Khairuddin Omar, Dheeb Albashih, Afzan Adam,
Siti Norul Huda Sheikh Abdullah, Azizi Abdullah,
Rizuana Iqbal Hussain, Fuad Ismail, Norlia Abdullah,
Suria Hayati Md Pauzi and Nurdashima Abd Shukor

Abstract

This chapter discusses radio-pathological correlation with recent imaging advances such as machine learning (ML) with the use of technical methods such as mammography and histopathology. Although criteria for diagnostic categories for radiology and pathology are well established, manual detection and grading, respectively, are tedious and subjective processes and thus suffer from inter-observer and intra-observer variations. Two most popular techniques that use ML, computer aided detection (CADe) and computer aided diagnosis (CADx), are presented. CADe is a rejection model based on SVM algorithm which is used to reduce the False Positive (FP) of the output of the Chan-Vese segmentation algorithm that was initialized by the marker controller watershed (MCWS) algorithm. CADx method applies the ensemble framework, consisting of four-base SVM (RBF) classifiers, where each base classifier is a specialist and is trained to use the selected features of a particular tissue component. In general, both proposed methods offer alternative decision-making ability and are able to assist the medical expert in giving second opinion on more precise nodule detection. Hence, it reduces FP rate that causes over segmentation and improves the performance for detection and diagnosis of the breast cancer and is able to create a platform that integrates diagnostic reporting system.

Keywords: computer-aided detection, computer-aided diagnosis, support vector machine, false positive, grading

1. Introduction

Breast cancer is one of the most dangerous and common reproductive cancers that affect mostly women. The oldest documented cases of breast cancer were in Egypt in 3000 BC [1]. Breast tumor is an abnormal growth of tissues in the breast, and it may be felt as a lump or nipple discharge or change of skin texture around the nipple region. Cancers are abnormal cells that divide uncontrollably and are able to invade other tissues. Cancer cells have the ability to spread to other parts of the body through the blood and lymphatic systems [1]. It is the leading cause of death among middle aged and older women [1]. According to cancer statistics, breast cancer is the second most common and the leading cause of cancer deaths among women, second only to lung cancer [1]. Around 1 in 36 (3%) women dies due to breast cancer [2]. It has become a major health issue in the past 50 years, and its incidence has increased in recent years [1]; in Malaysia, breast cancer is the most frequent type of cancer among women. It has an incidence rate of about 26% (more than 4400 women) among cancer affecting women. Around 40% of the women who suffered from breast cancer in Malaysia have died (IARC). Hence, determining the right decision from a right diagnosis is crucial.

In today's world with the advent of personalized medicine, it increases the workload and complexity of the doctors in cancer diagnosis. Radiologic and pathology are the key players in making decision for cancer diagnosis. Based on the radiology diagnosis, the results will be submitted to pathology for further diagnosis. Pathology and radiology form the core of cancer diagnosis, yet based on our observation at our studied hospital and under current process of diagnostic medicine, the communication among them remained on papers. That paper contains their respective report of the case on the same patient. This scenario is in parallel with what James et al. [3] had highlighted in their paper. The working flows of both specialties remain ad hoc and occur in separate "silos," with no direct linkage between their case accessioning and/or reporting systems, even when both departments belong to the same host institution. Since both radiologists' and pathologists' data are essential to make correct diagnoses and appropriate patient management and treatment decisions, the isolation of radiology and pathology work flows can be detrimental to the quality and outcomes of patient care. These detrimental effects underscore the need for pathology and radiology work flow integration and for systems that facilitate the synthesis of all data produced by both specialties. With the enormous technological advances currently occurring in both fields, the opportunity has emerged to develop an integrated diagnostic reporting system that supports both specialties and, therefore, improves the overall quality of patient care. In this chapter, we are focusing on breast cancer diagnostic for data collected from UKMMC. Hence, breast radio-pathological correlation is essential. The covered topics would include radio-pathological correlation with recent imaging advances such as machine learning with use of technical methods such as mammography and histopathology.

As a standard, the current diagnostic screening consists of a mammography to identify suspicious regions of the breast, followed by a biopsy of potentially cancerous areas. A breast biopsy is a diagnostic procedure that can determine if the suspicious area is malignant or benign [4–6]. Although criteria for diagnostic categories of radiologic and pathology are well established, manually detection and grading respectively is a tedious and subjective process and thus suffers from inter-observer and intra-observer variations. Early detection via mammography increases breast cancer treatment options and the survival rate. However, mammography is not perfect. Detection of suspicious abnormalities is a repetitive and fatiguing task. For every thousand cases analyzed by a radiologist, only three to four are cancerous, and thus an abnormality may be overlooked. As a result, radiologists fail to detect 10–30% of cancers. Approximately two thirds of these false-negative results are due to missed lesions that are evident retrospectively. Due to the considerable amount of overlap in the appearance of malignant and benign abnormalities, mammography has a positive predictive value (PPV) of less than 35%, where the PPV is defined as the percentage of lesions subjected to biopsy that were found to be cancer. Thus, a high proportion of biopsies are performed on benign lesions. Avoiding benign biopsies would spare women anxiety, discomfort, and expense [7]. As mentioned earlier, with the advent of personalized medicine, the process becomes more complex. Not only that, the emerging of 4th Industrial Revolution (4IR) technology allowed huge amount of data to be captured, and this contributes to the complexity of the radiology and pathology workload. To address these challenges, many researchers are leveraging artificial intelligence to improve medical diagnostics. Machine learning is a sub discipline in the field of artificial intelligence (AI) that explores the study and design of algorithms that can learn from data [8].

2. Machine learning

ML comprises a broad class of statistical analysis algorithms that iteratively improve in response to training data to build models for autonomous predictions. In other words, computer program performance improves automatically with experience [9]. ML algorithm's aim is to develop a mathematical model that fits the data. It comprises of two types of learning which are supervised and unsupervised. Supervised learning algorithm required the data to be labeled for training purposes. For example, in training a set of medical images to identify a specific breast tumor type, the label would be tumor pathologic results or genomic information. These labels, also known as ground truth, can be as specific or general as needed to answer the question. The ML algorithm is exposed to enough of these labeled data to allow them to move into a model designed to answer the question of interest. Because of the large number of well-labeled images required to train models, curating these data sets is often laborious and expensive [10]. Unsupervised ML clusters the data that have similar characteristics, and the unlabeled data are exposed to the algorithm with the goal of generating labels that will meaningfully organize the data. This is typically done by identifying useful clusters of data based on one or more dimensions. Compared with supervised techniques, unsupervised learning sometimes requires much larger training data sets. Unsupervised learning is useful in identifying meaningful clustering labels that can then be used in supervised training to develop a useful ML algorithm. This blend of supervised and unsupervised learning is known as semi-supervised.

ML algorithms are to analyze any data set to extract data-driven model, prediction rule, or decision rule from the data set. Generally, in order to ensure the ML behave intelligently without human intervention, the system learns or extracts knowledge such as rules or patterns from a collection of input data or past experience. So the steps involved can be described as firstly, the system must acquire features from data. Elaboration of features is well explained in our previous work [11, 12]. Feature selection is very important as it contains information that can be used to train the system to identify specific patterns. The pixels are rich with qualitative abstractions or values of the input. Second step is analyzing all these features for detecting and classifying possible pattern or abnormality. Finally, the step is involving a ML algorithm to determine a best suitable model to represent the behavior or the pattern of the data [13].

Various machine learning algorithms are now used to develop high-performance medical image processing systems such as computer-aided detection (CADe) system that detects clinically significant objects from medical images and computer-aided diagnosis (CADx) system that quantifies malignancy of manually or automatically detected clinical objects [14]. Therefore, CADe for mass in mammogram detects the suspicious region in the mammogram then tries to reduce the false positive and finally classifies this region to a mass or nonmass. In CADx for mass in a mammogram, most researchers use a region of interest (ROI) that contains the mass as an input to the CADx. Then, CADx tries to classify it into benign or malignant and gives the appropriate recommendation to do biopsy or follow-up screening [15]. Recent studies have shown that CAD systems, when used as an aid, have improved radiologists' accuracy of detection of breast cancer and also pathology decision [1, 7, 16]. It is worthwhile to distinguish ML from traditional computer-aided detection (CAD) algorithms. Traditional CAD algorithms are mathematical models that identify the presence or absence of image features known to be associated with a disease state. One of the examples is a microcalcification on a mammogram. Traditional CAD allows the developer to identify a feature explicitly and attempts to determine the presence or absence of that feature within a set of images. In contrast, ML techniques focus on a particular labeled outcome (ductal adenocarcinoma), and in the process of training, clusters of nodes evolve into algorithms for identifying features. The power and promise of the ML approach over traditional CAD is that useful features can exist

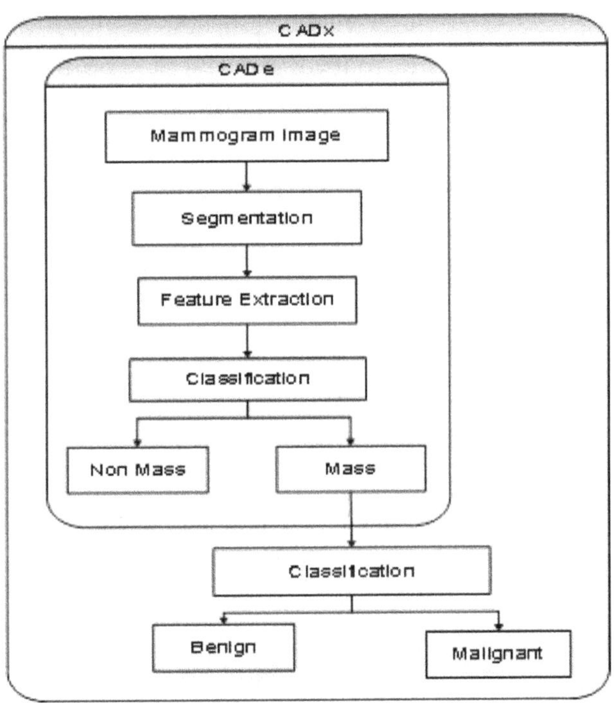

Figure 1. CADe vs. CADx. Source: Sampat et al. [7].

that are not currently known or are beyond the limit of human detection [10]. **Figure 1** shows the difference between CADe and CADx.

In **Figure 1**, ML algorithm is implemented at the segmentation, feature extraction, and classification steps. One of the most popular and powerful ML algorithm for all the steps is support vector machine (SVM). SVMs are useful for taking a large number of features and discriminating inputs into one of two classes. SVMs, once trained, show the line or border that provides the greatest margin of separation. This concept can be extrapolated to a larger number of features (or dimensions), whereby the line of separation becomes an irregular plane known as a hyperplane. Because of the large number of features that can be combined mathematically, SVMs have been found useful for image processing. This chapter is focusing on SVMs for both CADe for radiology and CADx for pathology diagnostics.

3. Computer-aided detection

Digital medical image recognition (DMIR) might give a promising solution. DMIR is considered as an essential aspect of artificial intelligence. DMIR techniques aim to extract specific information from medical images to assist doctors in diagnosing certain diseases and follow their progress. Many image processing techniques have been utilized in DMIR, such as segmentation, object detection, and classification. DMIR is concerned with numerous imaging modalities in the field of diagnosis including computed tomography (CT), digital mammography, magnetic resonance imaging (MRI), and microscopic histopathological images [16, 17]. Depending on the type of breast tissue, breast mass appears different in a mammogram. While it appears as solid block in dense breast, it appears as a roundish pie in a fatty breast. The mass may be alone or with microcalcifications [1]. In some cases, healthy breasts are also diagnosed as suspicious of cancer by the radiologist, and unfortunately, unnecessary biopsy is performed on them. Knowing that there are many possibilities of masses in breast cancer, detecting these features and localizing them are important. In general, localizing the mass is important in computer-aided detection, where it searches for the location in the mammogram images and segments it. Refs. [1, 18] examine the most important approaches used for mass segmentation in mammogram. In general, localizing the mass is important in computer-aided detection where it searches for the location in the mammogram images and do segmentation. Cheng et al. [18] examine the most important approaches used for mass segmentation in mammogram. Image segmentation using thresholding is the simplest way to isolate the object from its background when the image has a distinct gray level distribution. Segmentation separates the regions by assuming that the region that have gray levels below a specific value, called the threshold, as a background and the region with gray levels higher than the threshold as the object or vice versa. Identifying the threshold value is the key point in this algorithm. By selecting a representable threshold, object extraction will be more accurate. Mostly, image histogram is used to identify the threshold value. Mass localization method is discussed in this chapter. This section is based on our previous work on SVM rejection model for breast cancer. This method is a rejection model based on SVM algorithm used to reduce the FP of the output of the Chan-Vese segmentation algorithm that was initialized by the MCWS algorithm.

Abnormal findings on screening mammograms lead to recall for further assessment, which includes additional imaging procedures and if considered necessary fine needle aspiration cytology, core needle biopsy, or surgical biopsy. Women recalled for further assessment without having a breast cancer diagnosed are considered to have had a FP screening result. FP results are a concern of mammographic screening as they might cause distress, anxiety, and other psychological problems to the women [19, 20]. It also implies additional hospital visits and diagnostic tests, as well as additional costs [21, 22]. The rates of FP screening results depend on the screening performance and organization, such as the screening interval, single versus double reading, participation patterns, sensitivity of the radiologists performance, equipment, and characteristics related to the screening population [22–26]. From image segmentation perspective, the FP is an over-segment result where the noncancerous pixel is segmented as a cancer pixel. The FP rate is considered a challenge in localizing masses in mammogram images. Hence, in this section, a rejection model is proposed by using SVM.

The goal of the rejection model which is based on SVM is the reduction of FP rate in segmenting mammogram through the Chan-Vese method, which is initialized by the MCWS algorithm. The MCWS algorithm is utilized for segmentation of a mammogram image. The segmentation is subsequently refined through the Chan-Vese method, followed by the development of the proposed SVM rejection model with different window size as well as its application in eliminating incorrect segmented nodules MCWS algorithm. SVM rejection model consists of three important stages: (i) initial segmentation, (ii) segmentation using Chan-Vese, and (iii) refined segmentation using SVM rejection model. First, the source image is cropped to remove any unnecessary parts in an image. Based on the high dimensionality in digital mammogram images, the image is then resized to speed up the subsequent processes. Second, completing the pre-processing stage, the SVM rejection model is built to reduce the FP rate. Presegmentation and postsegmentation enhancement for Chan-Vese level set algorithm is then proposed to localize masse in the mammogram. The key to achieve a good segmentation result using Chan-Vese is the initial contour. Instead of getting the initial contour from the expert, here, MCWS algorithm is used to obtain the initial contour, as well as to eliminate the noise. This makes the proposed method fully automated and reduces the time of interference. Lastly, localization of mass in mammogram, Chan-Vese active contour-based algorithm was used. Chan-Vese can find and maximize the convergence ranges, as well as treat the topological change. This ensures that Chan-Vese performs well in image segmentation. Support vector machine is a learning machine algorithm expounded by Cortes and Vapnik [15] at the AT&T Bell Laboratories that strives to address the issues pertaining to a two-group classification. The underlying working principle of this algorithm is to search for the optimal hyperplane that sets positive classes (+1) apart from negative classes (−1). In this context, the two classes are the nodules and the nonnodules of breast images, of which the provided training data were used for the SVM to build a model in predicting the target values of the two test data attributes. In this work, the radial basis function (RBF) kernel is employed in complementary with the SVM. The two best parameters, C and γ, are prerequisites for the generation of an accurate breast nodule and nonnodule classification by the RBF kernel. The SVM rejection model has three phases: extracting teacher image, training, and testing as shown in **Figure 2**. The grid has been used as a straightforward search on the training data to find the best parameters, and the reason for using the grid search instead of other

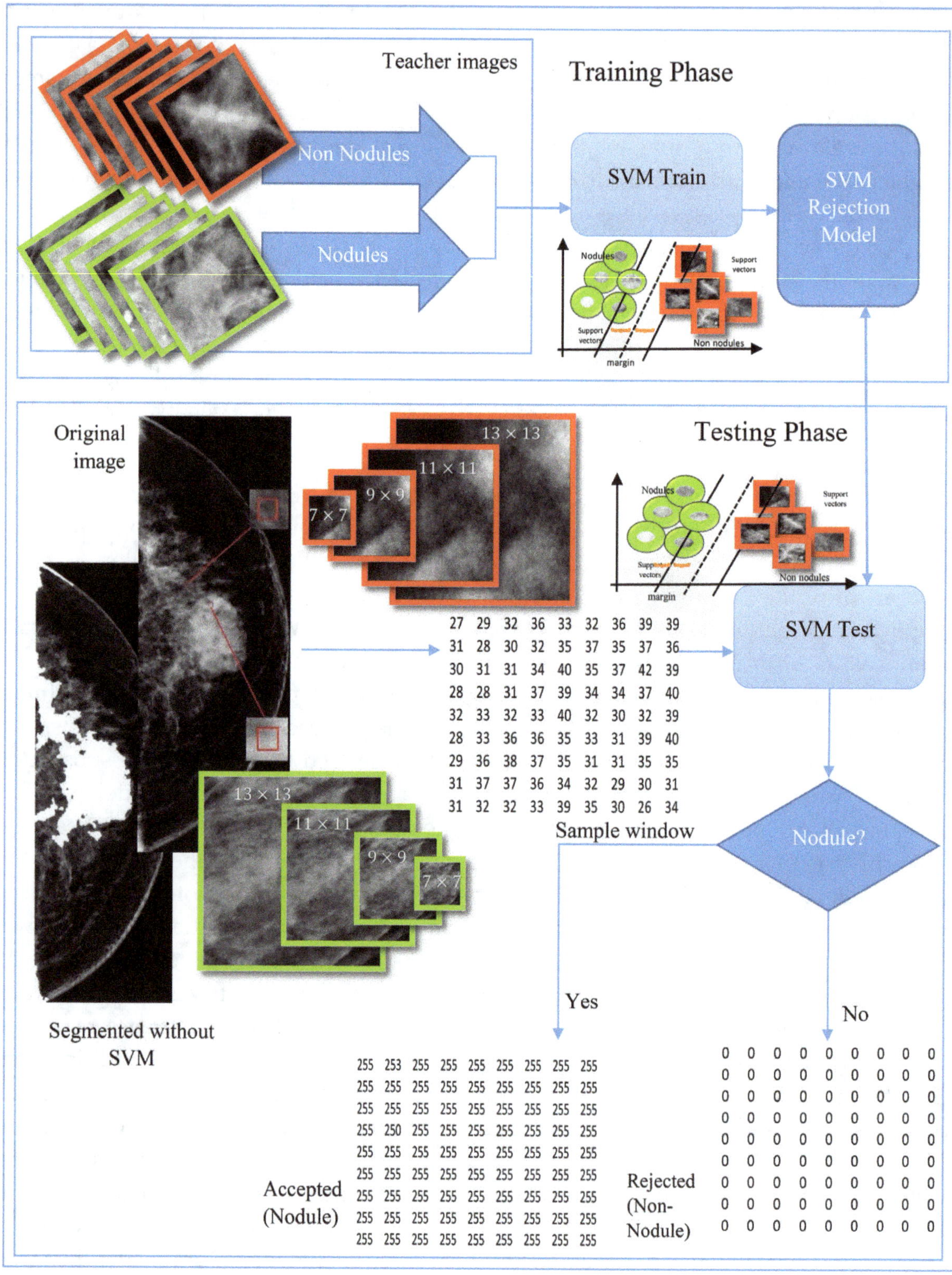

Figure 2. The process of SVM rejection model.

search algorithms is because of its short computation time. Additionally, the grid search can be easily parallelized because it is independent. The search spaces used in this research are $\{2^{-5}, 2^{10}\}$. It is important to note that this study used the strategy of dividing the data set into two parts, of which one is considered unknown. The prediction accuracy obtained from the unknown set will reflect on the classification performance of the independent data set. This procedure is known as cross validation. Its goal is to divide the training set into v subsets of equal size. One subset will be tested using the classifier trained on the remaining subsets. Subsequently, each instance of the training set will be predicted once. This is to ensure that the cross-validation accuracy is the percentage of data that have been correctly classified. The training data (teacher images) for the rejection model were manually extracted from the mammogram images by analyzing the false positives (FP) and true positives (TP) of the Chan-Vese segmentation result. After the teacher images were extracted, they were resized using the same factor for the original image. Next, depending on the window size that considered the number of inputs to SVM rejection model, the teacher image was resized. Based on the experiment, either a window size of (7 × 7), (9 × 9), (11 × 11), or (13 × 13) was taken into consideration. After that, the image was transferred to a vector and then written into the training data file. This file contained two variables, x and y. The first variable x is a matrix containing rows of window pixel values for the teacher images. Each row represented one image. The length of the rows depended on the window size. The number of rows in this variable depended on the number of teacher images. The other variable y is a vector containing the class for each image. The class may be "1" for nodule images or "0" for nonnodule images. Before proceeding with the SVM rejection training, training data were used to obtain the best values for parameters C, γ. As previously mentioned, the grid search was used as a straightforward search on the training data to obtain these values. Cross validation was also applied to spill the training data 10-fold into training and testing. Depending on the best accuracy value returned by SVM, the best C and best γ values were chosen. The SVM rejection model was built using the selected C and γ values and the training data set.

Based on model in **Figure 2**, each row in the training data (x_i) represents an observation, and each column represents features. Class labels (y_i) represent the class label for the corresponding row in the training data.

3.1. Results and evaluation

About 170 mammogram images from 109 patients were collected from the UKM Medical Centre (UKMMC). **Table 1** and **Figure 3** show training and testing data that have been used in the experiment. The teacher images extracted from the training data based on the segmentation result contained 35 nodule images and 35 nonnodule images extracted from the training data set. The SVM rejection model was run 10 times with a standard deviation of 0.0001, and the results showed the effectiveness of using the rejection model compared with the ground

	Training data		Testing data	
	Nodule	Nonnodule	Nodule	Nonnodule
Number of images	11	17	46	96
Total number of images	28		142	

Table 1. Data set for training and testing.

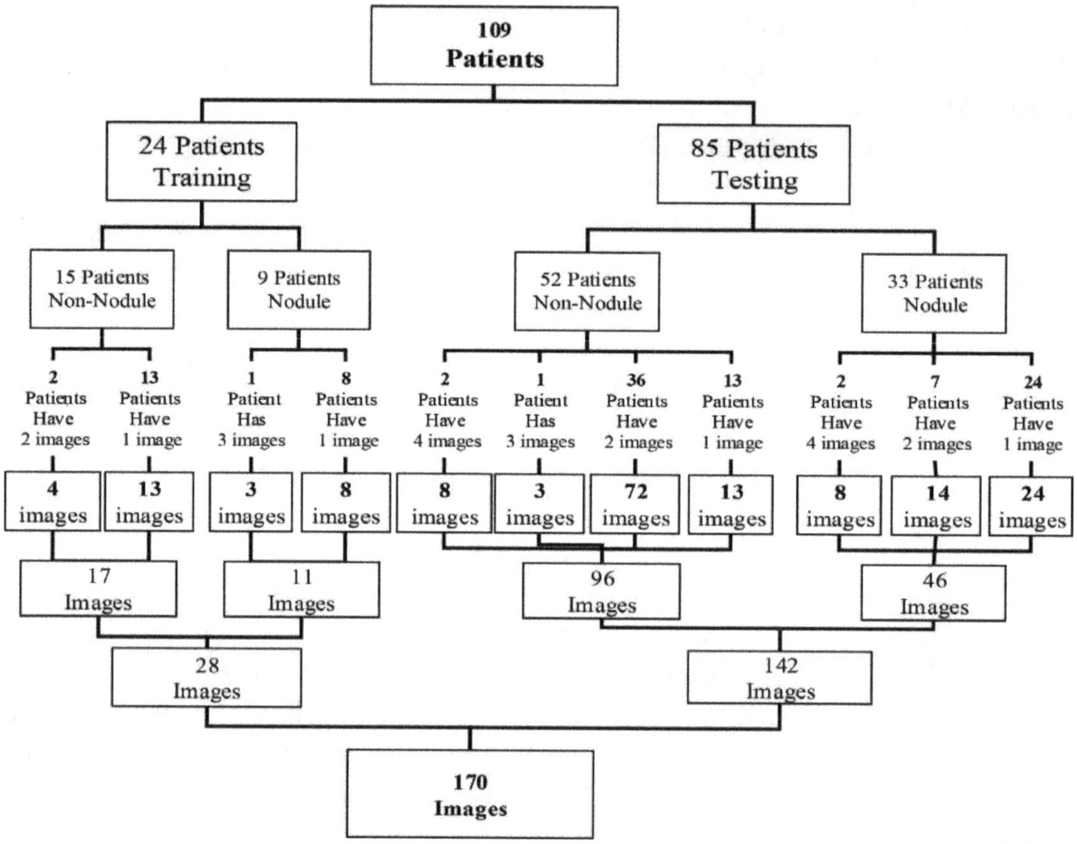

Figure 3. Hierarchy of UKMMC data set.

truth. As mentioned earlier, the grid search was used as a straightforward search on the training data to determine the best parameters C, γ. **Table 2** shows values of C, γ using various window sizes (7 × 7), (9 × 9), (11 × 11), and (13 × 13).

Accuracy denotes the proportion of the correct result and it can be calculated as shown in the following Eqs. (1)–(7), where TP is true positives, TN is true negatives, FP is false positives (type 1 error), and FN is false negatives (type 2 error). In mass localization, the concept of the confusion matrix that is in **Table 2** represents the correctly segmented nodule and nonnodule with the miss segment. TP and TN are the correctly localized nodule and nonnodule, respectively, while FP is the incorrectly segmented nonnodule as a nodule and FN is incorrectly segmented nodule as a nonnodule.

	Result (predicted)	
	Nodule pixel	**Nonnodule pixel**
Ground truth (actual)		
Nodule pixel	TP	FN
Nonnodule pixel	FP	TN

Table 2. Confusion matrix.

Specificity is also known as TN rate, and it represents the ability of the method to identify the nonnodule and avoiding false positives.

Sensitivity, which is also known as TP rate or recall, represents the ability to identify the nodule and avoid false negatives.

The FP rate shows the nonnodule pixel, which is segmented as nodule. It is an over segmented pixel. The FN rate shows the nodule pixel, which is segmented as nonnodule. It is the miss segmented.

$$Accuracy = \frac{TP+TN}{TP+FP+TN+FN} \quad (1)$$

$$Specificity\ (SP) = \frac{TN}{TN+FP} \quad (2)$$

$$Sensitivity\,(SE) = \frac{TP}{TP+FN} \quad (3)$$

$$FP\ rate = \frac{FP}{FP+TN} \quad (4)$$

$$FN\ rate = \frac{FN}{FN+TN} \quad (5)$$

$$Negative\ Rate\ Matric\ (NRM) = \frac{FP\ rate + FN\ rate}{2} \quad (6)$$

The NRM shows the mismatch between the predicted results and the actual ground truth. Our method was evaluated by comparing the segmented images to the ground truth. To show the effectiveness of the method, a comparison was done before and after the rejection model, as shown in **Figure 4**. This process was performed first by comparing each pixel in the resulting image with the corresponding pixel in the ground truth image. Then, objective evaluation was used to evaluate the method by calculating the confusion matrix as in **Table 2**, based on the prediction result and the actual ground truth. **Table 3** and **Figure 4** show the quantitative analysis of the results and sample of the result. The effectiveness of our method can be proven by comparing the result before and after using the rejection model. **Table 3** shows the FP rate of the rejection model is inversely proportionate to the window size. On the other hand, the specificity rate of the rejection model is linearly proportional to window size.

This section discussed on reducing the FP rate based on SVM machine learning. The SVM rejection model was built to reduce the FP rate after segmentation. Our method has three steps in the segmentation phase: first, MCWS was used to obtain the initial contour by segmenting the mammogram image. Then, the output of MCWS was used as an initial contour to the Chan-Vese algorithm. Finally, the rejection model based on SVM was used in order to reduce the FP rate. The SVM rejection model has three steps in the following order: extracting teacher images, training the rejection model, and testing the model. The FP rate reduction by means of SVM machine learning been put forth, wherein the FP rate, upon segmentation, had been reduced by the developed SVM rejection model. The segmentation of the mass in mammogram

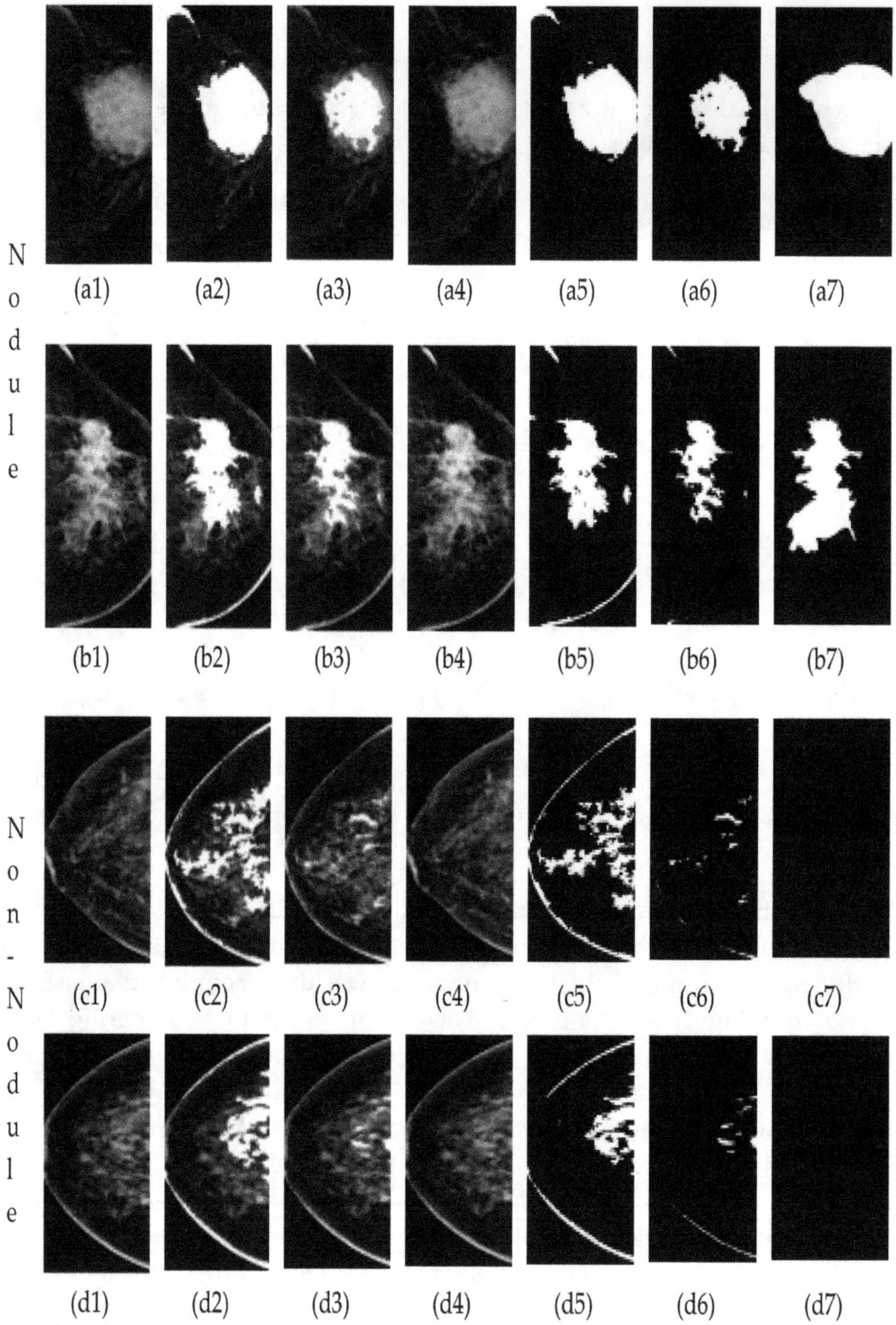

Figure 4. Result before and after using SVM model. (a1, b1, c1, and d1) original nonnodule and nodule images. (a2, b2, c2, and d2) segmentation result without using SVM rejection model, (a3, b3, c3, and d3) segmentation result after reducing the FP rate using SVM rejection model, (a4, b4, c4, and d4) ground truth images,. (a5, b5, c5, and d5) binary segmentation result without using SVM rejection model (a6, b6, c6, and d6) binary segmentation result after reducing the FP rate using SVM rejection model (a7, b7, c7, and d7) ground truth images.

images as well as the extraction of the initial contour was performed through MCWS, of which the proposed method comprises. The Chan-Vese algorithm is employed as the initial contour to enhance the result of the segmentation. The three steps of the SVM rejection model are in

	FP rate	SP	AC	NRM	OVERLAP
Without the rejection model	0.196	0.803	0.803	0.099	0.800
With the rejection Model (7 × 7 × 7 × 7)	0.058	0.941	0.938	0.031	0.933
With the rejection model (9 × 9 × 9 × 9)	0.051	0.948	0.944	0.028	0.940
With the rejection model (11 × 11 × 11 × 11)	0.044	0.955	0.950	0.025	0.946
With the rejection model (13 × 13 × 13 × 13)	0.040	0.959	0.954	0.023	0.950

Table 3. Quantitative analysis.

the following sequence: extracting teacher images, training the rejection model, and testing the model. Credence can be given to the MCWS algorithm in surmounting the challenges associated with the Chan-Vase algorithm. The Chan-Vese algorithm can be made more autonomous and converge faster by using a good initialization generated by MCWS.

Nevertheless, the reliance mammogram segmentation on the divergence and convergence of the intensity value of the image pixels is the constraint factor for this algorithm. The tendency has been toward segmenting the outlier component as part of the contour component, resulting in an incremental FP rate of the selected contour pixels. Accordingly, to overcome this issue, the SVM rejection model is geared toward reducing the FP rate. T-test was performed to determine the mean difference of two samples, that is, the accuracy before and after using rejection model with the best window size, which is (13 × 13). The T-test was applied to determine if there was a difference before and after applying the rejection model. The hypothesized mean difference of T-test was set to value 0, also named as null hypothesis. That means, assuming that there was no difference in the result whether using the rejection model. The alpha was set to value 0.05. The concept of T-test states that if the P value is less than the assumed alpha, the null hypothesis is not correct and there is a difference between the mean of the two samples. T-test result shows that the proposed method is considered statistically significant with ($P = 0.00001 < 0.05$). Furthermore, the proposed rejection models also showed less standard deviation (0.0001) and yields to stability in its performance. In general, this proposed method offers alternative decision-making ability and is able to assist the medical expert in giving second opinion on more precise nodule detection. Hence, it reduces FP rate that causes over segmentation.

4. Computer aided diagnosis for pathology

This section focuses on the histopathological grading step in the breast diagnosis, the procedure used to grade a certain tissue by examining the tissue slide biopsy, which must undergo a preparation step prior to the grading.

4.1. Tissue preparation

Breast tissue biopsy is a piece of tumorous tissue taken from the breast to investigate the occurrence of cancer. After the biopsy is extracted, it is enclosed in a fixative to prevent it from decaying. Then, the tissue is sectioned into fragile slices (e.g., 2–15 μm) using a microtome machine, which creates very thin slices. The slices are then arranged on the glass slide before being stained. The tissue is stained using certain pigments to reveal the tissue components (e.g., lumen, nuclei, cytoplasm, and stroma). This helps the pathologist to view the individual tissue component more clearly. This procedure is called cells marker. The pathologists use different methods of staining depending on the diagnostic process at hand. Among the common staining types, Hematoxylin and Eosin combination H&E is the most popular for diagnosis and grading. After staining the tissue slide, the pathologist evaluates the tissue slide using the microscope as in UKMMC or through a digital scanner used to produce digital pathology images. In UKMMC, a specific type of microscope (Olympus BX50 microscope) is used for the diagnosis [16]. This microscope has a camera to capture images of the region of interest. The next subsection will explain the image acquisition steps involved in the creation of the prostate and breast cancer data sets required for this study. Subsequent subsections will present a brief overview of the devices required for the image acquisition and image acquisition flow.

4.2. Image acquisition devices

In this study, prostate histological images were captured from tissue slides. All the images were viewed using an Olympus BX50 microscope (Olympus Corporation, Japan), and images were captured using a DP72 digital camera (Olympus Corporation) and cellSens Life Science imaging software, version 1.6 (Olympus Corporation) [16]. The sensitivity of the illumination source and camera's intensity were kept constant. The microscopes were adjusted manually to form clear magnified images, and the cameras were controlled through desktop computers to capture color digital images. Before image acquisition, the pathologists in UKMMC had selected the ROIs under the microscope. However, this requires substantial time and effort from pathologists, and more importantly, a subjective choice of the ROIs could introduce biases into the database and harm the generalizability of the developed computer CAD system.

4.3. Image acquisition work flow

Prior to acquiring the images, the microscope components, such as the light condenser, diffusing screen, and objective lens, were properly cleaned to remove any dust in the light path, which might badly affect the clarity of the acquired image. The focal plane was adjusted manually for clear images and was readjusted before every new image was taken. A light condenser was used to increase the light intensity for high-resolution image acquisition. To acquire an image from an ROI, the pathologist in UKMMC first reviewed the tissue section at a low magnification (e.g., 1× or 4×) to locate the ROI at the center of the image's field of view [16]. Usually, fine tuning is needed at higher magnification (40× magnification) to ensure a region with a typical Gleason pattern in the ROI is selected. The focal plane was then adjusted to produce a sharp image, and the light intensity was tuned so that the largest pixel value was slightly lower than the upper limit of the pixel's dynamic range. When all those adjustments were satisfactory, a still image was captured and saved onto the desktop computer as a color RGB digital image with a (tiff) extension. This process was repeated for all images that were captured for breast pathologists.

4.4. Self-collected data set from UKMMC

This data set contains self-collected breast tissue region images stained using the H&E procedure and captured from tissue slides of needle biopsies taken from 32 breast carcinoma cases. These tissue region images were digitized at 40× magnification, yielding high resolution images (4140 × 3096 pixels) in (tiff) format. The diagnosis assigned to each region image is based on the Bloom–Richardson grading system [16]. Each image was annotated as low grade (Grade 1) or high grade (Grade 3) by three expert pathologists from the HUKM center [16]. The total number of collected images is 100. These can be classified into 56 low-grade cases and 54 high-grade cases. **Figure 5** shows some sample images taken from this data set.

4.5. Ensemble learning of tissue components for histopathology image grading

This section explains the ensemble framework that we used for the classification of breast cancer and Gleason grading using the tissue components of the H&E histopathological region images. This project has been carried out from our previous work [16]. The framework is based on the ensemble learning approach from machine learning and medical tissue components (lumen, nuclei, cytoplasm, and stroma), both of which are of semantic meanings to pathologists. The framework extracts a set of textural features for each tissue component, which creates four independent sub data sets, and the diversity demonstrated by these data sets is then used to create an ensemble framework that is able to classify and grade breast cancer. Our framework consists of five phases: segmentation of four tissue components, feature extraction, feature selection, base classifiers of the framework, and ensemble fusion phase, as per **Figure 5**.

The typical CAD for breast cancer grading extracts features directly from histopathological images. Then, a single classifier is used to train these features to classify unknown patterns (e.g., image). Unlike this typical CAD, our project uses the concept ensemble learning (**Figures 5** and **6**).

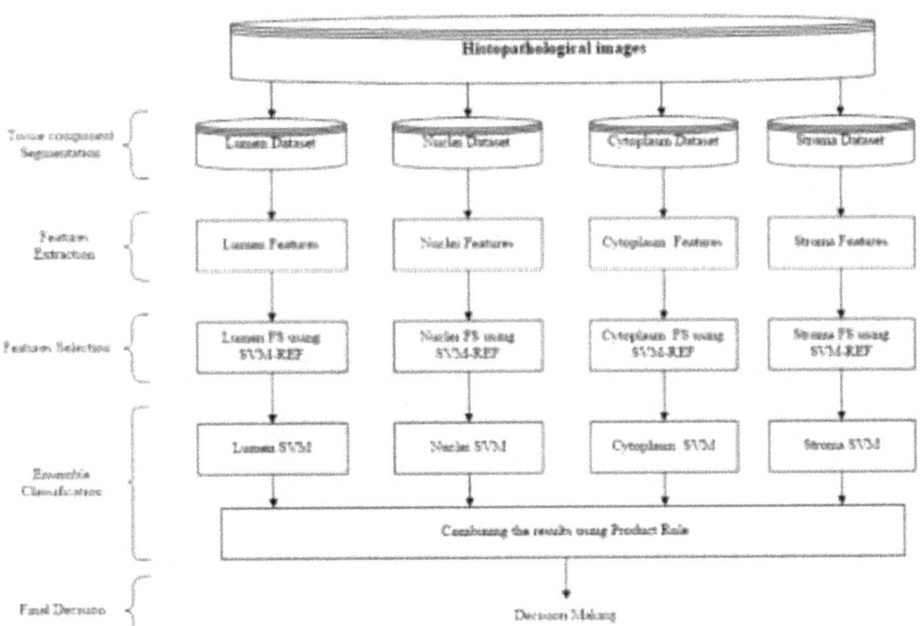

Figure 5. Ensemble framework for breast tissue image diagnosis and grading.

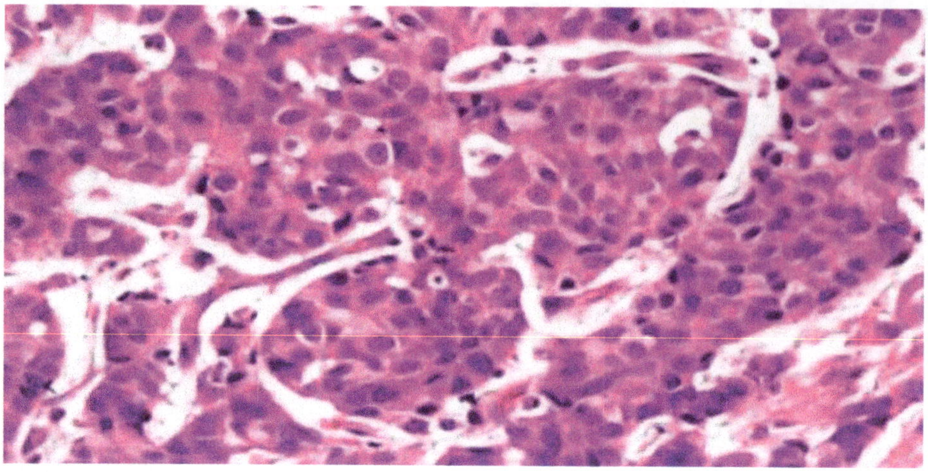

(a)

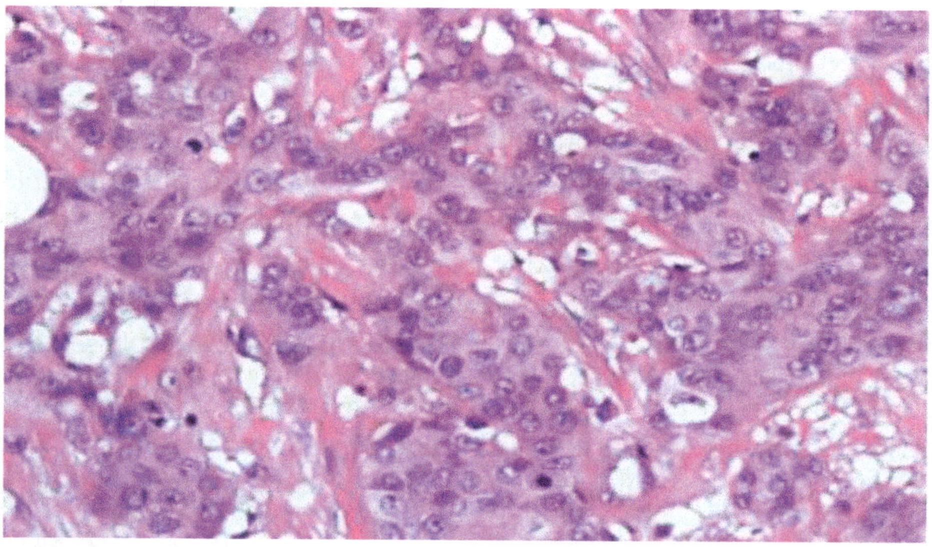

(b)

Figure 6. Two types of tissue classes of interest for the breast grading problem: (a) Grade 1 (low grade) tissue and (b) Grade 3 (high grade) tissue.

Due to the diversity of the tissue components, four different training data sets are created for the corresponding tissue components (lumen, nuclei, cytoplasm, and stroma). Thus, the diversity of the tissue components in ensemble learning is utilized to improve prostate diagnosis and grading. In this project, the ensemble framework, consisting of four-base SVM (RBF) classifiers, where each base classifier is a specialist, is trained to use the selected features of a particular tissue component. The decision function of SVM (RBF) with the top selected features (Ω) in the training model is defined as per (Eq. (7)):

$$(x\Omega) = \mathrm{sgn}\{(\mathrm{w} \,.\, x\Omega)\} = \mathrm{sgn}\{\propto i \; yi \; k(x\Omega, i, x\Omega) + b \; ni = 1\}, \tag{7}$$

where $x\Omega$ is the test sample with only Ω corresponding features, $x\Omega$, ii is that of sample i in the training set ($i = 1, 2, \ldots, n$) with only Ω features, $y_i \in$ {1 *bening*, 0 *malignant* (low *Grade or high Grade*)} is the class label of the training sample $x\Omega$, i, and k is the kernel function that is used to calculate the inner product between the Φ $x\Omega$, i and $\Phi(x\Omega)$ in the transformed space using nonlinear mapping Φ. The product rule Eq. (8) is utilized to produce the final decision for the proposed ensemble framework to combine the prediction outputs of all four base classifiers. The product rule is preferred in the ensemble when the single classifiers posterior probabilities are correctly estimated [16]. The final prediction (x) for the test image (x) based on product rule is computed using (Eq. (8))

$$class(x) = \max_{j=1}^{c=2} \prod \prod_{t=1}^{t=4} p_j^t(x) \quad (8)$$

4.6. Results and evaluation

In the ensemble framework, the stages of feature selection and classification are executed 50 times for each classification task. In each run, the data set of each base classifier (i.e., tissue component) is randomly divided into 50% training and 50% testing) after normalizing, as per [16]. It should be pointed out that in each run of the ensemble framework, similar numbers of selected features are used with all base classifiers. The base classifiers utilize the SVM with Radial-Basis-Function (RBF) kernel, while the SVM-RFE utilizes the linear SVM. To deploy RBF, one needs to set an appropriate value of the cost penalty, c, and gamma, γ. The grid search tool is one of the most common methods to identify suitable values for c and γ [1, 16]. The SVM implementation is utilized by the LibSVM toolbox [1, 16], while the C and γ in the SVM are estimated using a grid search with different internal threefold cross-validations on the training data set only from $\{2^{-20}, 2^{20}\}$. In this data set, the low vs. high grades classification task is dealt with, which is the most well-known task in state-of-the-art breast cancer analyses [1]. The results reported by this data set are shown in **Table 4**. As shown in **Table 4**, the proposed ensemble framework can effectively classify the low vs. high grades breast images. The AUC of low vs. high grade reached an average of 90.7%, which was greater than both the naïve and typical CAD. Moreover, when comparing the structure-method, the proposed method was far more superior. In using the proposed ensemble CAD, classification performance in the context of AUC can be substantially improved by 15% for the structure-based method. The results in **Figure 5** show that the ensemble framework was significantly quite accurate (90.8%) compared to the accuracy of each individual tissue components in the low vs. high grades in breast histopathology images. This framework has also been

Classification task Breast UKM	Measure	Proposed ensemble framework	Naïve approach	Typical CAD [22]	Significant of ensemble with	
					Naive	Typical CAD [22]
Low vs. high grade	AUC	90.7 ± 5.0	89.9 ± 4.8	89.8 ± 3.9	—	—
	Accuracy	90.8 ± 5.0	89.9 ± 4.8	89.8 ± 3.9	—	—
	Sensitivity	87.11 ± 8.4	87.1 ± 8.8	88.5 ± 7.7	—	—
	Specificity	94.3 ± 5.3	92.7 ± 6.3	91.1 ± 6.9	—	—

Table 4. The performance of the proposed ensemble framework on breast histopathology images data set.

validated using prostate and colon data set. Results proved that the ensemble framework can be utilized with other types of histopathology images if the main tissue components are visible in the image [7].

5. Discussion and conclusion

This chapter discusses how machine learning, particularly SVM can improve the performance for detection and diagnosing of breast cancer. SVM for now is one of the most powerful machine learning techniques that is able to model the human understanding of classifying data. It can find the relationship between data and segregates them accordingly. Using pixel values in mammogram images, SVM helps to improve the mass detection and segmentation of Chan-Vese algorithms by classifying correctly the false positive pixels. As a result, a sharper mass was detected with better estimation of its shapes and sizes. Hence, radiologist can give better diagnosis and biopsy location. Then, images of cell structure or tissue textures from the biopsy sample were examine by the pathologist. These pathology slides were analyzed under the pathologist sharp eyes to locate and identify any abnormal pattern of tissue texture or architecture. The process is tiring and subjective to the pathologist experience in interpreting the tissue condition. Thus, inter-observer and intra-observer variations exist. However, the proposed SVM algorithm can identify the different tissue component and model the pattern of relationship between these components spatially and statistically. The model is then used to grade any new pathology slides into its modified Bloom-Richardson grading, according to what the SVMs have learned from previous examples. Using the technique, it helps the radiologist and pathologist reducing their work load by automating the automation for decision making, especially for common and mundane cases. Radiologist and pathologist would have more time to spend on special or rare cases. The learning curve for young apprentice can

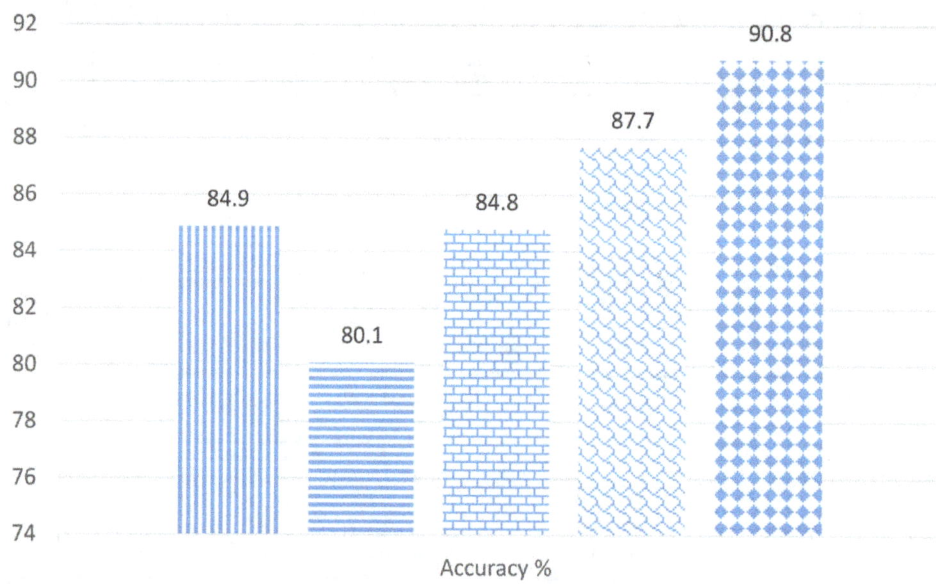

Figure 7. Single vs. ensemble classification results for low vs. high grade.

be steeper. The automate grading of breast cancer helps to reduce the variation of inter- and intra-observation by the pathologist. In our work, it should be noted that we are not using the identical patient data of mammogram and pathology due to some limitation. However, in the future it is possible to take the identical patient. Via the automatic decision making we are able to create a platform that integrate diagnostic reporting system that supports both specialties and, therefore, improves the overall quality of patient care (**Figure 7**).

However, combining these tissue components' features resulted in dense feature vectors, which suffers from overfitting. The use of the ensemble learning framework that allows prediction using several training subsets could help mitigate this problem. These different subsets are clearly shown in the proposed ensemble framework. The results indicate that proposed ensemble framework significantly outperformed the typical CAD, naïve approach, and structure-based method.

Acknowledgements

The authors thank the Faculty of Information Science and Technology, Universiti Kebangsaan Malaysia, for providing the facilities and financial support under "ETP-2013-053 diagnostic services nexus for breast cancer." Gratitude is also due to Human Life Advancement Foundation (HLAF) for its financial support. Ethics approval was obtained entitled "FF-338-2012 Breast Cancer Diagnostic Imaging System Using Mammogram and Ultrasound" from UKM Medical Center, Malaysia, for collecting and studying breast cancer patient records.

Author details

Shahnorbanun Sahran[1*], Ashwaq Qasem[1], Khairuddin Omar[1], Dheeb Albashih[2], Afzan Adam[1], Siti Norul Huda Sheikh Abdullah[1], Azizi Abdullah[1], Rizuana Iqbal Hussain[3], Fuad Ismail[4], Norlia Abdullah[5], Suria Hayati Md Pauzi[6] and Nurdashima Abd Shukor[6]

*Address all correspondence to: shahnorbanun@ukm.edu.my

1 Center for Artificial Intelligence Technology, Faculty of Information Science and Technology, Universiti Kebangsaan Malaysia, Bangi, Malaysia

2 Computer Science Department, Prince Abdullah Bin Ghazi Faculty of Information Technology, Al-Balqa Applied University, Jordan

3 Department of Radiology, Universiti Kebangsaan Malaysia Medical Center, Malaysia

4 Department of Oncology, Universiti Kebangsaan Malaysia Medical Center, Malaysia

5 Department of Surgeon, Universiti Kebangsaan Malaysia Medical center, Malaysia

6 Department of Pathology, Universiti Kebangsaan Malaysia Medical Center, Malaysia

References

[1] Ashwaq Q, Siti Norul Huda SA, Shahnorbanun S, Rizuana IH, Fuad I. An accurate rejection model for false positive reduction of mass localisation in mammogram. Pertanika Journal of Science and Technology. 2017;**25**(S):49-62

[2] The American Cancer Society. How Common Is Breast Cancer? 2017. Available from: https://www.cancer.org/cancer/breast-cancer/about/how-common-is-breast-cancer.html [Accessed: 22-01-2018]

[3] James S, Denise RA, Dena E, Silvana L, Ossama T, Dean WW. Integrating pathology and radiology disciplines: An emerging opportunity? BMC Medicine. 2012;**10**:100

[4] Ebert J, Xu Y, Smith G, Shen Y, Jiang J, Buchholz T, Hunt K, Black D, Giordano GW, Yang W, Shen C, Elting L, Smith B. Surgeon influence on use of needle biopsy in patient with breast cancer: A national medicare study. Journal of Clinical Oncology. 2014; **32**(21):2206-2216

[5] Adepoju L, Qu W, Kazan V, Nazzal M, Williams M, Sferra J. The evaluation of national time trends, quality of care and factors affecting the use of minimally invasive breast biopsy and open biopsy for diagnosis breast lesions. American Journal of Surgery. 2014;**208**(3):382-390

[6] Wan T, Cao J, Chen J, Qin Z. Automated grading of breast cancer histopathology using cascaded ensemble with combination of multi-level image features. Journal of Neurocomputing. 2017;**229**(C):34-44

[7] Sampat MP, Markey MK, Bovik AC. Computer-aided detection and diagnosis in mammography. Handbook of Image and Video Processing. 2005;**2**(1):1195-1217

[8] Anju J. Machine learning techniques for medical diagnosis: A review. In: 2nd International Conference on Science, Technology and Management. New Delhi; 27 September 2015

[9] Jordan MI, Mitchell TM. Machine learning: Trends, perspectives, and prospects. Science. 2015;**349**:255-260

[10] Marc K, Luciano MP, Ross WF, Geis JR. Implementing machine learning in radiology practice and research. American Journal of Roentgenology. 2017;**208**(4):754-760

[11] Afzan A,Khairuddin O. Computerized breast cancer diagnosis with Genetic Algorithm and Neural Network. In: Proceedings of the 3rd International Conference on Artificial Intelligence and Engineering Technology (ICAIET), Universiti Malaysia Sabah; 22-24 November 2006. pp. 533-538

[12] Shahnorbanun S, Albashish D, Azizi A, Nordashima AS, Suria HMP. Absolute cosine-based SVM-RFE feature selection method for prostate histopathological grading. Artificial Intelligence in Medicine. 2018;**87**:78-90

[13] Azizi A. Supervised Learning Algorithms for Visual Object Categorization. Netherlands: Universiteit Utrecht; 2010. ISBN: 978-90-393-5440-7

[14] Nemoto M, Masutani Y, Nomura Y, Hanaoka S, Miki S, Yoshikawa T, Hayashi N, Ootomo K. Machine learning for computer-aided diagnosis. Igaku Butsuri. 2016;**36**(1):29-34

[15] Cortes C, Vapnik V. Support-vector networks. Machine Learning. 1995;**20**(3):273-297

[16] Dheeb AA. Thesis of Embedded feature selection methods based on support vector machine for histopathology grading. Malaysia: Universiti Kebangsaan; 2017

[17] Pham DL, Xu C, Prince J. Current methods in medical image segmentation. Annual Review of Biomedical Engineering. 2000;**2**(1):315-337

[18] Cheng H, Shi X, Min R, Hu L, Cai X, Du H. Approaches for automated detection and classification of masses in mammograms. Pattern Recognition. 2006;**39**(4):646-668

[19] Brett J, Bankhead C, Henderson B, Watson E, Austoker J. The psychological impact of mammographic screening. A systematic review. Psychooncology. 2005;**14**:917-938

[20] Bond M, Pavey T, Welch K, Cooper C, Garside R, Dean S, et al. Systematic review of the psychological consequences of false-positive screening mammograms. Health Tech_nology Assessment (Winchester). 2013;**17**:1-170, v-vi

[21] Lerman C, Trock B, Rimer BK, Boyce A, Jepson C, Engstrom PF. Psychological and behavioral implications of abnormal mammograms. Annals of Internal Medicine. 1991; **114**:657-661

[22] Román M, Castells X, Hofvind S, von Euler-Chelpin M. Risk of breast cancer after false-positive results in mammographic screening. Cancer Medicine. 2016;**5**(6):1298-1306

[23] Roman R, Sala M, Salas D, Ascunce N, Zubizarreta R, Castells X. Effect of protocol-related variables and women's characteristics on the cumulative false-positive risk in breast cancer screening. Annals of Oncology. 2012;**23**:104-111

[24] Elmore JG, Miglioretti DL, Reisch LM, et al. Screening mammograms by community radiologists: Variability in false-positive rates. Journal of the National Cancer Institute. 2002;**94**:1373-1380

[25] Sala M, Salas D, Belvis F, et al. Reduction in false-positive results after introduction of digital mammography: Analysis from four population-based breast cancer screening programs in Spain. Radiology. 2011;**258**:388-395

[26] Utzon-Frank N, Vejborg I, von Euler-Chelpin M, Lynge E. Balancing sensitivity and specificity: Sixteen years of experience from the mammography screening programme in Copenhagen, Denmark. Cancer Epidemiology. 2011;**35**:393-398

3

Triple-Negative Breast Cancer: Expression of Hypoxia-Inducible Factor 1α in Triple-Negative Breast Cancer with Metastasis to Lymph Nodes

Anna Maria Badowska-Kozakiewicz and
Michał Piotr Budzik

Abstract

A great number of scientific studies have shown that the development of different TNBC forms is closely associated with the induction of various signaling pathways and that TNBC cells show greater sensitivity to different drugs. Recent studies showed hypoxia-inducible factor-1α (HIF-1α) was strongly correlated to clinicopathological features in many types of cancers. This molecule seems to play a significant role in the development of different tumors and breast cancer among them. The aim of this study was to evaluate the relationship between immunohistochemical expression of novel prognostic marker—HIF-1α—and clinicopathological features for patients with triple-negative breast cancer. Among 162 breast cancer patients, we identified 111 (68.5%) subjects with triple-negative breast cancer. In our study, TNBC was most commonly assessed as G2 and G3 (52.2%; 45.1%), pT1 and pT2 (34.2%; 62.1%), and pN1 and pN2 (45%; 41.4%). TNBC more often presented HIF-1α expression (43.2%) than non-TNBC (35.2%). TNBC subgroup demonstrated significant correlation between HIF-1α expression and tumor size (pT1–pT4) ($p = 0.021$), which may suggest that HIF-1 alpha expression in this group of patients may be an additional and significant marker in the evaluation of the advance of the disease, affecting therapeutic decisions.

Keywords: triple-negative breast cancer, hypoxia, immunohistochemistry

1. Introduction

Breast cancer is the most common cancer in women [1], and it comprises heterogeneous tumors with different biological features, clinical course, prognosis, and response to treatment [2].

With modern techniques, we can distinguish many molecular forms of breast cancer [3], which is important because the molecular classification of breast cancer enables effective, individualized treatment [4]. Based on cDNA microarray and immunohistochemical analysis, five basic molecular subtypes of breast cancer have been distinguished:

- luminal subtype A (ER+ and/or PR+, HER2–, CK5/6–)
- luminal subtype B (ER+ and/or PR+, HER2+, CK5/6–)
- basal-like subtype (ER–, PR–, HER2–, CK5/6+)
- subtype with overexpression of the *HER2* gene (ER–, PR–, HER2+, CK5/6–)
- subtype with expression of genes typical for cells of the normal mammary gland (normal breast-like)
- subtype with a decreased expression of genes coding proteins responsible for intercellular junctions and adhesion of epithelial cells (claudin and cadherin E) [5, 6]

On routine histology, breast cancer is defined based on immunohistochemical detection of three receptor proteins: estrogen receptor (ER), progesterone receptor (PR), and HER2 receptor with additional gene status analysis of the *HER2* gene (*in situ* hybridization). This immunohistochemical profiling shows that 25% of breast cancers consist of type A luminal cells; 32%, of type B/HER2– cells; 18.5%, of luminal B/HER+ cells; and 7%, of cells that express solely the HER2 protein [7]. Cancers of the luminal subtype A and B express genes characteristic for glandular cells, which form the inner layer of normal ducts and lobules of the breast. Moreover, the luminal subtypes of breast cancer express cytokeratins typical for glandular cells, such as cytokeratins 8, 18, and 19, as well as α 6 integrins and Bcl-2, Ep-CAM, and MUC1 proteins. The luminal subtype A is characterized by a high expression of genes for estrogen receptors and progesterone receptors and genes regulating the function of these receptors, i.e., *FOX1*, *GATA3*, *LIV*-1, and *XBP1*. The luminal subtype A breast cancer typically occurs in young patients; in contrast to the luminal subtype B, the luminal subtype A breast cancer has a good prognosis [8–10]. In recent years, among all the molecular subtypes of breast cancer, the triple-negative breast cancer (TNBC) has been studied most extensively.

2. Characterization of the triple-negative breast cancer

The TNBC is a subtype of breast cancer that lacks steroid receptors, i.e., estrogen and progesterone receptors, and does not overexpress the *HER2* gene. Eighty percent of patients with the TNBC have the basal type of breast cancer, according to the molecular classification [1, 3, 8]. About 15–20% of all patients with breast cancer have the TNBC, which is more common in patients younger than 50 years. The risk factors for the TNBC are as follows:

- young age at menarche
- obesity in the menopausal age
- family history of breast cancer

The TNBC has an aggressive course, grows fast, and metastasizes early, usually to the brain and lungs, and less commonly to the bones and liver. Compared with other breast cancers, the TNBC is poorly differentiated (G3) in the Bloom-Richardson classification [5, 6, 9]. In 2010, studies among 15,240 women with breast cancer, including 2500 with the TNBC, showed that patients with the TNBC had a worse prognosis than other patients [5, 6, 8–10].

The TNBC is also characterized by early recurrence, usually within 1–3 years after diagnosis [8]. Most patients with TNBCs have a poor prognosis because adjuvant therapy rarely leads to remission, and the presence of metastases is associated with a high resistance to chemotherapy and short survival [9]. Not all patients with TNBC, however, have a poor prognosis [6, 7, 9]. Numerous studies showed that the TNBC is related to the dysfunction of the *BRCA* genes and their protein products [9, 10]. According to Atchley et al. [10], TNBCs occur in 57% of patients with breast cancer and *BRCA1* mutations. Moreover, more than a half of TNBCs overexpress the MGFR receptor (c-Met growth factor receptor), which is associated with the signaling pathway initiating the epithelial-mesenchymal transformation [8, 9]. The TNBC is often associated with *P53* mutations, PTEN loss, activation of the PI3K/AKT signaling pathway, and loss of heterozygosity of the loci4p14, 4p15.3 m 5q11.1, 5q14, and 18q22–23 [11].

Although TNBC was initially detected in basal-like carcinoma, these two types of breast cancer are different from each other [12]. The basal-like carcinoma is diagnosed based on the immunohistochemical status of steroid receptors (ER, PR) and the HER2 receptor [4, 7, 9].

Molecularly, the TNBC comprises a heterogeneous group of tumors. Lehmann et al. [13] distinguished six types of the TNBC:

- basal-like 1 and basal-like 2 (BL1 and BL2)
- immunomodulatory (IM)
- mesenchymal (M)
- mesenchymal stem-like (MSL)
- luminal androgen receptor (LAR)
- unstable

Of all these TNBC subtypes, only the LAR TNBC does not express basal cytokeratins, such as CK5, CK6A, CK6B, CK14, CK16, CK17, CK23, and CK81, and it does not express proteins such as EGFR, p53, smooth muscle actin, P-cadherin, and c-Kit receptor [10, 11]. In contrast, the LAR TNBC expresses CK7, CK8, CK18, CK19, and the androgen receptor [12]. Moreover, the LAR TNBC expresses genes whose protein products regulate hormonal pathways and the gene for the androgen receptor and its co-activators [12, 13].

The BL1 TNBC expresses genes whose protein products are associated with cell cycle regulation, cell proliferation, repair process, and DNA replication [12].

The BL2 TNBC expresses genes whose protein products are involved in the signal transduction in the cell, through growth factors such as EGF, NGF, MET, Wnt/β-catenin, and IGF1R [12].

The IM TNBC is characterized by the expression of genes whose protein products are involved in immune reactions, such as signal transduction in Th1 and Th2 cells, natural killer cells, and dendritic cells [10, 12].

The M TNBC is characterized by the expression of genes whose protein products regulate cell mobility, interaction of cells with the extracellular matrix, and cell differentiation and growth [12].

The MSL TNBC expresses genes whose protein products are involved in angiogenesis and the signaling pathways of the ABC transporters [12, 13].

Most subtypes of the TNBC have the molecular profile typical for the basilar subtype of breast cancer, which lacks expression of ER, PR, and HER2 [8, 9, 12]. This molecular profile is observed mainly in subtypes BL1 (85%) and BL2 (31%), and subtypes IM (58%) and M (47%) [8, 12].

Usually, the LAR TNBC is a luminal A or B breast cancer (82%) [12–14]. Based on immunohistochemical studies, 50–80% of TNBCs are basal-like cancers, and conversely, 77–80% of basal-like breast cancers are TNBCs [9, 10, 12]. Molecular analyses indicate that TNBCs and the basal subtype of breast cancer are different cancers [13–15].

All the above-mentioned subtypes of the TNBC incur different prognoses; the longest recurrence-free survival is found in patients with the MSL TNBC, and the shortest recurrence-free survival, in patients with the LAR TNBC [15].

Histologically, the majority of TNBCs are luminal cancers (invasive carcinoma of no special type—IDC—NST) [15]. The TNBC occurs more commonly in patients with specific histological types of breast cancer, including the medullary breast cancer, metaplastic breast cancer, apocrine breast cancer, salivary gland-like breast cancer, secretory breast carcinoma, breast cancer derived from lipid-laded cells, and lobular breast carcinoma [16]. In patients with TNBCs, it is the histological type of the tumor that determines its biological properties; thus, patients with TNBCs do not always have rapid disease progression and poor prognosis [17, 18].

To identify a homogenous group of patients, Eiermann et al. [19] suggested that the tumors that become triple-negative after neoadjuvant treatment, and were not triple-negative before this treatment, should not be classified as TNBC. However, if the disease recurs as triple-negative metastases, the tumor should be considered as triple-negative although the primary tumor was not triple-negative [19]. According to these investigators, also rare histological subtypes of the TNBC, such as apocrine, glandular, or low-differentiated cancers, should be excluded from the group of triple-negative cancers [18, 20].

3. Treatment of patients with TNBC

Patients with the TNBC do not benefit from hormonal treatment or treatment with anti-HER2 antibodies (trastuzumab) because their tumors do not express the ER, PR, and HER2 receptors. Therefore, surgery, radiation therapy, and chemotherapy, used alone or in various combinations, are currently the only reliable therapeutic options for patients with TNBCs. However, recent research on TNBC has identified many receptors that could be used as future therapeutic targets. Until this is achieved, chemotherapy remains the mainstay of systemic treatment for patients with stage I to stage III TNBC. Currently, none of the standard chemotherapy regimens is considered superior for patients with TNBCs, and treatment of these patients is based on the same principles as that in patients with other subtypes of breast cancer. Most guidelines recommend a regimen based on the combination of an anthracycline with a taxane.

The therapeutic strategies for the management of TNBC are targeting the DNA repair complex (platinum compounds and taxanes), P53 (taxanes), and cell proliferation (anthracycline-containing regimens) [21]. Despite the aggressive clinical course, the TNBC's response to chemotherapy is good. However, despite achieving high rates of pathological complete response (pCR) with conventional chemotherapy, the TNBC phenotype is associated with higher recurrence rates than the ER+ and HER2+ breast cancers. This is known as the triple-negative paradox [22].

Since the first application of taxanes, used in adjuvant therapy for over 20 years, relatively few new treatments have appeared in recent years for patients with the TNBC. New therapeutic methods are still lacking despite numerous ongoing clinical trials. Many retrospective studies have demonstrated that tumor infiltrating lymphocytes (TILs) are of prognostic importance in patients with early-stage TNBC. Increased TIL numbers within the neoplastic milieu correlate with a better response to the standard treatment regimen with anthracyclines in neoadjuvant therapy [23].

However, it has still not been shown whether the presence of TILs identifies tumors that are more susceptible to treatment, or whether the presence of lymphocytes itself increases the effectiveness of treatment [23]. There are numerous reports on the benefits of using platinum derivatives in chemotherapy, in particular in cancers with the *BRCA1* mutation, which is much more frequent in TNBCs (about 30%) than in other cancers. Nearly 80% of tumors that develop in carriers of the *BRCA1* mutation are triple-negative. The *BRCA* mutation status is increasingly therapeutically relevant beyond consideration of prophylactic mastectomy/oophorectomy and surveillance. A recent randomized phase III trial demonstrated that in unselected patients with the metastatic TNBC, carboplatin and docetaxel were equal in efficacy as first-line treatments [24].

However, in the *BRCA* mutation-associated TNBC, carboplatin yielded a superior response rate and progression-free survival compared with docetaxel. The improvement in pCR attained with the addition of carboplatin to anthracycline/taxane chemotherapy comes at the cost of increased toxicity. Because of the molecular variability of TNBCs, the platinum derivatives improve prognosis only in some patients. Therefore, it is very important to identify those patients with TNBC who will have the greatest benefit [25]. The current highest pCR rates, about 40–45%, are achieved by taxane/anthracycline sequential chemotherapy regimens and inclusion of platinum drugs with the taxane component. Inclusion or substitution of other chemotherapy drugs (capecitabine, gemcitabine, vinorelbine, or ixabepilone) resulted in little or no improvement in pCR rates [26, 27]. To date, all clinical trials showed that the neoadjuvant chemotherapy was the preferred option for patients with TNBC who required systemic therapy. Neoadjuvant chemotherapy studies have consistently reported higher response rates in TNBC than in non-TNBC, and pCR has been shown to predict improved long-term outcomes for patients with TNBC. The specific adjuvant regimens that may be effective for TNBC are still being determined. Many large randomized trials have established the benefit of adjuvant anthracyclines and taxanes in breast cancer [28].

The evidence consistently shows that 10–20% of patients with TNBC who would not experience pCR following treatment with a current third-generation taxane and anthracycline will achieve pCR when a platinum drug is added to the regimen. However, because of the substantial added toxicity and predicted modest overall survival benefit across patient subgroups, carboplatin and cisplatin have not been routinely incorporated into neoadjuvant treatment [29].

The principles of local treatment in breast cancer, i.e., surgery and radiotherapy, are the same for the TNBC and all other types of breast cancer. Over the last several years, the percentage of patients operated on for breast cancer has increased; this trend has also been observed in patients with TNBC.

In patients with the TNBC, radiation therapy is given as in other types of breast cancer, i.e., after mastectomy or breast-conserving surgery. However, this approach to radiation therapy remains controversial because more and more patients have TNBCs, which has a fast local growth. The general rule that breast-conserving surgery followed by radiation therapy in early stage cancers ($T_{1\text{-}2}$ N_0) is the equivalent of mastectomy, in this case, has many limitations. Also the general consensus that post-mastectomy radiation therapy is not indicated for patients with node-negative tumors less than 5 cm in diameter should not be oversimplified in patients with triple-negative tumors [28].

4. Targeted therapy in TNBC

Although chemotherapy can be effective in patients with TNBCs, molecular studies could still improve treatment outcomes by giving new treatment targets. The molecular heterogeneity of TNBCs means that patients with TNBCs need personalized treatment because currently 60–70% of patients with TNBC do not respond fully to chemotherapy. Genomic analyses of the TNBC revealed large-scale transcriptional, mutational, and copy number heterogeneity, without any frequently recurrent mutations, other than *TP53*. Consistent with this molecular heterogeneity, most targeted agents, so far, have a very low activity in unselected TNBC, but important "basket" trials are ongoing. Therefore, there are promising opportunities for studying targeted therapy in appropriately selected patients with residual disease after neoadjuvant chemotherapy. Several ongoing phase I/II studies are investigating phosphatidylinositol-3-kinase (PI3K) inhibitors in advanced TNBC, and early-phase studies are also assessing Janus kinase 2 and cyclin-dependent kinase inhibitors in hormone-negative breast cancer [29].

At least some important discoveries made in recent years seem to be worth emphasizing in this textbook. The molecular pathways and receptors mentioned below might become new treatment targets for patients with the TNBC.

4.1. Anti-angiogenic factors

Blockage of angiogenesis has been one of the ways to treat patients with breast cancer. In patients with the TNBC, bevacizumab, among the drugs that interfere with angiogenesis, has been studied most extensively. In 2008, the Food and Drug Administration (FDA) approved bevacizumab in combination with a taxane (paclitaxel) as first-line therapy for metastatic HER2-negative breast cancer, including the TNBC [30]. A meta-analysis of phase III studies with bevacizumab showed an improvement in progression-free survival but not in overall survival in these patients. However, the addition of bevacizumab considerably increased treatment toxicity [31].

Based on these data, in 2011, the FDA withdrew bevacizumab as the treatment for metastatic breast cancer.

4.2. Immune checkpoint inhibitors

Because we know more and more about the interaction of inflammatory cells with cancer cells, in future, immunotherapy might be introduced for the treatment of breast cancer. Cancer cells use many mechanisms to avoid immune responses. For instance, in the TNBC, cancer cells express the PD-1 antigen and its ligands on cell surface. These proteins induce T lymphocyte tolerance. Preclinical studies showed that blocking the activity of the PD-1/PD-L1 might be used as treatment for TNBC. Both anti PD-1 antibodies (pembrolizumab and nivolumab) and an anti-PD-L1 antibody (atezolizumab) showed promise in preclinical studies [32].

4.3. PARPi

Poly-ADP-ribose polymerases (PARPs) are enzymes that are essential for cell survival. Cell damage activates PARPs, which, in turn, induces cell repair systems that maintain genome stability and regulation of transcription. Preclinical studies showed that PARPs are inhibited in cancer cells with pre-existing DNA repair defects, e.g. with the *BRCA1* mutations. The FDA has recently approved monotherapy with olaparib, a PARPi, as a first-in-class drug to treat germline *BRCA* mutation-associated advanced refractory breast cancer. Several ongoing studies are assessing the activity of PARPi alone or in combination with chemotherapy for germline BRCA-associated metastatic and early-stage breast cancers. Because a substantial proportion of TNBCs are thought to harbor DNA repair defects, it might be possible to extend the observation of PARPi sensitivity of germline BRCA-associated tumors to *BRCA* wild-type TNBCs that harbor a BRCAness phenotype. Accordingly, PARPi are being explored in the general population of patients with the TNBC [33].

4.4. PI3K/AKT/mTOR pathway inhibitors

The high frequency (about 50%) of PI3K pathway alterations in the TNBC makes this pathway a promising target for therapeutics, and inhibitors of PI3K, AKT, and/or mTOR are in clinical development. PI3K blockade promotes HR deficiency by downregulating BRCA1/2 and thus sensitizing BRCA-proficient tumors to PARP inhibition [34].

4.5. Histone deacetylase inhibitors

These drugs modulate gene expression through epigenetic regulation and can induce cell cycle arrest, differentiation, and apoptosis. Panobinostat is a potent pan-histone deacetylase inhibitor with preclinical activity in the TNBC. Several histone deacetylase inhibitors are currently being tested as treatment for metastatic TNBC in combination with chemotherapy or with immune checkpoint inhibitors [35].

4.6. Androgen-targeted therapy

TNBCs expressing the androgen receptor (AR-positive) account for about 10% of all TNBCs and are characterized by a more benign course [13]. These tumors express the AR, which can be detected by immunohistochemistry or the analysis of AR gene expression. AR-positive TNBCs have several common features with ER-positive breast tumors, including the expression of several estrogen-dependent genes and the frequent presence of PIK3CA mutations. Anti-androgens have been studied as potential drugs for these cancers. Few TNBCs express AR, and patients with AR-positive tumors were qualified for clinical trials with anti-androgens. Many molecules have been studied, but data on bicalutamide and enzalutamide are most extensive. Unfortunately, few patients responded to the treatment with these agents. Nonetheless, 20–35% of patients achieved disease stabilization [36]. It remains unclear whether these findings reflect the relatively mild nature of AR-positive TNBCs or whether they reflect the actual, but limited, activity of anti-androgens.

4.7. Other agents

New treatment targets for patients with cancer are being studied. These include, among others, reparixin (inhibitor of interleukin-8 activation of CXCR1/CXCR2 chemokine receptors), CXCR1/2 (stem cell pathway), cyclin-dependent kinases, c-Met pathway, aurora kinase inhibitor, death receptors, and CSF1 inhibitor (*colony stimulating factor 1*).

After over 20 years with relatively few new treatments for the TNBC, recent years have seen a growing interest in the TNBC among researchers. This is because more and more people with breast cancer have the TNBC, which is aggressive and tends to metastasize. Currently, studies are assessing different chemotherapy regimens and are testing the usefulness of new targeted therapies. In the early stages of the TNBC, standard neoadjuvant chemotherapy might save patients' lives; patients who receive standard neoadjuvant therapy can later receive adjuvant chemotherapy or be included in clinical trials if there is extensive residual cancer after neoadjuvant therapy. Growing evidence supports the benefit of adding cisplatin to the chemotherapy with taxanes/anthracyclines in patients with *BRCA* mutations [37].

Because many new targeted therapies for the TNBC are assessed in ongoing trials, we hope that the treatment of TNBC will soon be improved.

5. Hypoxia in TNBC

A great number of scientific studies have shown that the development of different TNBC forms is closely associated with the induction of various signaling pathways and that TNBC cells show greater sensitivity to different drugs. Recent studies showed hypoxia-inducible factor-1α (HIF-1α) was strongly correlated to clinicopathological features in many types of cancers. This molecule seems to play a significant role in the development of different tumors and breast cancer among them.

HIF-1α is responsible mainly for cellular adaptation to hypoxic conditions; therefore, genes triggered by this factor are responsible mainly for the improvement in oxygen supply (by increasing angiogenesis, broadening the lumen of existing vessels, increased erythropoiesis or increased iron consumption), adaptation of cells to anaerobic metabolism conditions as well as for other changes facilitating cell survival in insufficient oxygen availability and modifying the main metabolic pattern. Stimulation of angiogenesis promotes the increased risk of distant metastases. Better accessibility of blood vessels increases the chance of tumor cells finding their way into the bloodstream and being transported to niches allowing settlement and formation of a metastatic lesion [38].

Hypoxia-inducible factor 1 is a master transcriptional regulator of genes regulating oxygen homeostasis. The HIF-1 protein is composed of two HIF-1α and HIF-1β/aryl hydrocarbon receptor nuclear translocator subunits. The prognostic relevance of HIF-1α protein overexpression has been shown in breast cancer. The impact of HIF-1α alternative splice variant expression on breast cancer prognosis in terms of metastasis risk is not well known.

Therefore, Dales et al. [39] investigated the prognostic value of different HIF-1α transcript expression levels in breast cancer and found a significant relationship between either clinicopathological characteristics or patient metastasis-free survival. They proved mRNA expression of a $HIF\text{-}1\alpha^{TAG}$splice variant reflects a stage of breast cancer progression and is associated with a worse prognosis [39].

Due to the fact that TNBC frequently shows morphologic evidence of hypoxia (central fibrosis and necrosis) [40, 41] an augmented expression of HIF-1α in tumors with a triple-negative phenotype should be anticipated. In fact, this had been elegantly demonstrated through the preferential expression of HIF-1α in peri-necrotic tumor cells in TNBC and BRCA1 mutated breast cancers [42].

In contrast, Tan et al. [43] and Choi et al. [44] demonstrated in TNBC an increase of carbonic anhydrase IX, a downstream product of the hypoxic pathway, rather than an increase in HIF-1α per se. The authors did not dispute the likely contribution of hypoxia to the tumors' aggressive phenotype.

HIF-1α overexpression is an indicator of poor prognosis and significant survival time reduction in patients suffering from breast cancer [45]. HIF-1 upregulates transcription of angiogenic genes like erythropoietin (EPO) and vascular endothelial growth factor (VEGF), which induce sprouting of new vessels and in result they increase the risk of metastasis because they boost surface of contact between tumor cells and vasculature. HIF-1 induces transcription of cytoprotective proteins in malignant cells in hypoxic conditions. HIF-1α predicts poor prognosis breast cancer [46, 47].

The relationship between inflammation and tumor progression is widely accepted. This phenomenon is also well known in breast cancer, and is mediated by numerous interleukins.

Besides playing a central role in the induction of inflammatory processes, interleukin 1β (IL-1β) was also identified as a factor important for progression of the tumor and stimulation of angiogenesis as well as being responsible for the increase in the invasiveness of cancer lesions. Recently, there has been considerable interest in understanding the non-hypoxic upregulation of the hypoxia-inducible factor HIF-1α by IL-1 in neoplastic cells since aberrant expression of HIF-1α correlates with tumor progression. Naldini et al. [48] studied the effect of IL-1β on cell migration and HIF-1α accumulation in the human invasive breast cancer cell line MDA-MB-231.

It was found that hypoxia-independent induction of HIF-1α by IL-1β was associated with an increase in cell migration and a simultaneous increase in the activity of phosphorylated p38 MAPK and CXCR1 expression. Inhibition of HIF-1α by siRNA led to a significant reduction in CXCR1 expression and cell migration, confirming the role of HIF-1α in hypoxia-independent, IL-1β-induced migration of the MDA-MB-231 line cells. The results of the studies present a new role of IL-1 in breast cancer. The therapeutic approach focused on inhibition of IL-1β activity appears to be a new target for the research aimed at the development of novel methods to treat invasive breast cancer [48].

6. Aim

The first aim of our study was to evaluate the expression of ER, PR and HER2 in order to extract a group of TNBC and non-TNBC. The second aim of this study was to evaluate the relationship between immunohistochemical expression of novel prognostic marker—HIF-1α—and clinicopathological features for patients with triple-negative breast cancer.

7. Materials and methods

Studies were conducted in a group of 162 patients with breast carcinoma with lymph node metastasis (111 triple-negative breast cancer and 51 non-triple-negative breast cancer) in the Department of Pathology, Military Medical Institute in Warsaw. Material for the study came from biopsies, excisional biopsies and modified radical mastectomies. Tumor samples were fixed in 10% buffered formalin phosphate. After 24-h fixation, material was dehydrated using alcohol in gradually increasing concentrations and embedded in paraffin. Paraffin blocks were cut into serial sections 4 μm in thickness. They were then stained using standard methods. The tumors were classified and graded according to the WHO and the Nottingham modification of the Scarff-Bloom-Richardson systems. In the sections stained with routine H&E method, the following determinations were carried out: type of neoplasm (WHO classification), tumor grade including tubule formation, and intensity of division as well as the degree of neoplastic cell differentiation and mitotic index as a mean number of mitotic figures in neoplastic cells counted in 10 fields of vision at a 400× magnification (surface field 0.17 mm^2).

Paraffin sections on the slides covered with 2% saline solution in acetone at temperature of 42°C were used for immunohistochemical examination.

Routine tests were performed in order to determine immunohistochemical expression of basic profile of diagnostic markers, such as estrogen receptor (ER), progesterone receptor (PR) and HER2. Monoclonal antibodies against receptors for estrogen (Monoclonal Mouse Anti-Human Estrogen Receptor alpha, 1:50 dilution, Clone: 1D5, Code: IR654, DAKO) and progesterone (Monoclonal Mouse Anti-Human Progesteron Receptor, 1:400 dilution, Clone: PR636, Code: IR068, DAKO) were used in order to determine the expression of steroid receptors. Evaluation of the immunohistochemical markers was performed by two pathologists as follows: ER and PR were categorized as negative—(0%), low positive—(1–10%); nuclear staining in >10% of tumor cells was considered positive for ER and PR.

The study was conducted as follows: sections were incubated at 60°C overnight and subsequently dewaxed. The next step involved revealing the epitope by heating the slides in a buffer for 40 min. Subsequently, preparations were left at room temperature for 20 min. Preparations were rinsed in buffer and endogenous peroxidase was blocked by washing in 3% H_2O_2 for 10 min. In the next step, preparations were incubated with an appropriate antibody for 30 min. After incubation, preparations were rinsed in buffer for 10 min, and then incubated with the reagent (Visualization Reagent) for 30 min. After incubation with the reagent, preparations were washed in TBS (Tris-Buffered Saline, Code: S1968) with pH 7.6 for 10 min, and then incubated with 3,3′-diaminobenidine (DAB) (Substrate—Chromogen Solution) for 10 min to visualize the color of the reaction. At the end of the procedure, preparations were stained with hematoxylin.

HER2 expression was determined using HerceptTest™ DAKO test (Code: K5204). It enabled detection of HER2 expression using a polyclonal antibody against this protein (Rb A—Hu HER2—Rabbit Anti-Human HER2 Protein). Antigen retrieval for HER2 using HerceptTest was performed by immersing and incubating the slides in 10-mmol/L citrate buffer in a calibrated water bath (95–99°C) for 40 min (±1 min). After decanting the epitope-retrieving solution, sections were rinsed in the wash buffer and later, soaked in the buffer for 5–20 min before staining. The slides were loaded onto the autostainer using the HercepTest program, as described in the manufacturer's insert. In the autostainer, the slides were rinsed, placed in 200 μL of peroxidase-blocking reagent for 5 min, rinsed, placed in 200 μL of primary anti-HER2 protein (or negative control reagent) for 30 min, rinsed twice and immersed in 200 μL of substrate chromogen solution – DAB for 10 min. The slides were counterstained with hematoxylin and finally coverslipped. HER2 results were determined based on the maximum area of staining intensity according to the instruction in the package insert and the ASCO/CAP guidelines as follows: strong, circumferential membranous, staining in >30% of invasive carcinoma cell was scored 3+, moderate, circumferential, membranous staining in ≥10% of invasive tumor cells or 3+ staining in ≤30% of cells was designated as 2+ staining, weak and incomplete membranous staining in invasive tumor cells was scored 1+ and no staining was scored 0. Tumors with 0 and 1+ staining were considered negative.

A total of 162 cases of breast cancer with metastasis to lymph nodes were assessed for expression of HIF-1α (Monoclonal Mouse Anti-Human HIF-1α 1:50 dilution, Clone:28b, Santa Cruz Biotechnology®, Inc.). A visualization system ImmunoCruz™ Mouse ABC Staining System (Santa Cruz Biotechnology®, Inc.) was subsequently applied; tumor-cell immunoreactivity was scored according to both the extent of nuclear staining—relative number of HIF-1α

positive cells, and the intensity of the reaction: [–] not detected; [+] <1% positive cells; [+] 1–10% weakly to moderately stained cells; [++] 1–10% intensively stained cells or 10–50% weakly stained cells; [+++] 10–50% positive cells with moderate to marked staining; [++++] >50% positive cells [49]. Positive controls were HIF-1α immunoreactive breast cancer tissues. Negative controls were prepared with omission of primary antibodies.

8. Statistical analysis

All statistical analyses were performed with SPSS software v12.0. The Chi-square (χ^2) was used to assess the relationship between HIF-1α and degree of histological malignancy and clinical staging. The Fisher exact test was used when the expected cell counts were less than 5. The results were considered as statistically significant if the p value was less than 0.05 ($p < 0.05$).

9. Results

Histopathological examination was performed in tumors obtained from 162 patients suffering from breast cancer. Among 162 breast cancer patients we identified 111 (68.5%) subjects with triple-negative breast cancer (TNBC was identified as ER-negative, PR-negative, and HER2-negative) and 51 (31.5%) subjects with non-triple-negative breast cancer. Mean age of patients with TNBC was 47.8 and of patients with non-TNBC 60.4 years.

Histopathological subtyping of the 111 triple-negative breast cancers identified 89.1% invasive ductal carcinomas of no special type (IDC-NST) (**Figure 1**) and 10.9% other special types of cancers: invasive lobular carcinomas, mixed ductal and lobular types, metaplastic carcinomas (**Table 1**).

All cases of triple-negative breast cancer were grouped according to histological grading: 3 (2.7%) cases were grade 1 (G1), 58 (52.2%) cases were identified as grade 2 (G2) and 50 (45.1%)

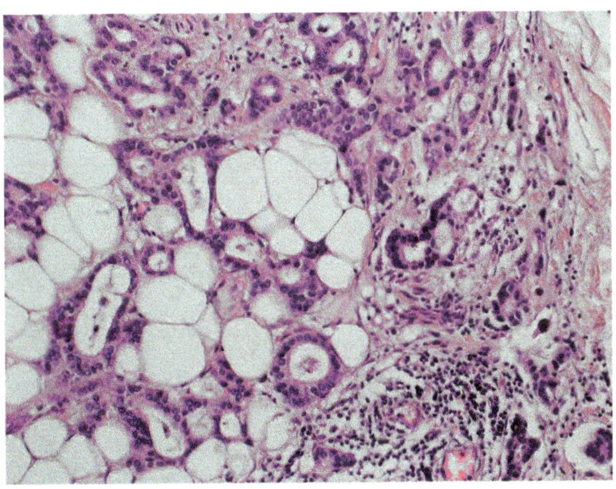

Figure 1. Triple negative breast cancer (TNBC) H&E.

Immunohistochemistry	Frequency n = 162	Prognostic parameters					
		Tumor necrosis			Histological type of invasive breast cancer		
		positive	negative	p-value	IDC-NST	other types	p-value
TNBC	111 (100%)	40 (36.0)	71 (64.0)	0.036*	99 (89.1)	12 (10.9)	0.858
non-TNBC	51 (100%)	10 (19.6)	41 (80.4)		45 (88.2)	6 (11.8)	

Table 1. Relationship between immunohistochemical profile (TNBC/non-TNBC) and prognostic parameters invasive breast cancer with metastasis to lymph bodes (*statistically significant results $p < 0.05$).

cases—grade 3 (G3). Given the histological grade of malignancy, G2 and G3 tumors comprised the largest group of triple-negative breast cancers.

In our study TNBC were most commonly assessed as G2 and G3 (52.2%; 45.1%), pT1 and pT2 (34.2%; 62.1%), and pN1, pN2 (45%; 41.4%). Respectively non-TNBC were most commonly assessed as G2 and G3 (47%; 47%), pT1 and pT2 (39.2%; 47%) and pN1 (52.9%). In our study a statistically significant association was found only between TNBC and non-TNBC tumor size (pT) ($p = 0.0011$). Furthermore in TNBC more commonly than in non-TNBC the presence of necrosis in the tumor mass was observed (36%; 19.6%) and statistically significant correlation between TNBC and non-TNBC in the presence of necrosis was demonstrated ($p = 0.036$) (**Table 1**).

In all examined breast cancers we also assessed the expression of HIF-1α but not statistically significant relationship between TNBC and non-TNBC was revealed. TNBC more often presented HIF-1α expression (43.2%) than non-TNBC (35.2%). In both groups we investigated correlation between the HIF-1α expression and features such as: tumor size (pT), histological grade (G1–G3) and the presence of lymph node metastasis (pN1–pN3). While TNBC subgroup demonstrated significant correlation between HIF-1α expression and tumor size (pT1–pT4) ($p = 0.021$). Detailed data and relationships between different parameters are presented in **Tables 2** and **3**.

Immunohistochemistry – basal panel for diagnosis of breast cancer	Frequency n = 162	HIF-1α expression		
		Negative (<10%)	Positive (>10%)	p-value
TNBC (ER-/PR-/HER2-)	111 (100%)	63 (56.8)	48 (43.2)	0.339
non-TNBC (ER+/PR+/HER2+)	51 (100%)	33 (64.8)	18 (35.2)	

Table 2. Relationship between basic immunohistochemical profile (ER, PR, HER2) and expression HIF-1α in invasive breast cancer with metastasis to lymph nodes (*statistically significant result $p < 0.05$).

Clinicopathological features of TNBC		HIF-1 α expression		
		Negative (<10%)	Positive (>10%)	p-value
Histological grade	G1	0	3	0.134
	G2	35	23	
	G3	28	22	
Tumor stage	pT1	16	22	0.021*
	pT2	46	23	
	pT3	1	2	
	pT4	0	1	
Nodal stage	pN1	30	20	0.821
	pN2	25	21	
	pN3	8	7	

Table 3. Clinicopathological features of TNBC and their relationship to expression of novel breast cancer marker - HIF-1α (*statistically significant result $p < 0.05$).

10. Discussion

A group of patients without the expression of any of the receptors qualifying for hormone therapy or targeted therapy against HER2 constitutes an important clinical problem in breast cancer treatment. Therefore, it seems important to undertake studies aimed at determining histopathological and immunohistochemical characteristics of this invasive group of triple-negative breast cancer (TNBC). Triple-negative breast cancer is most commonly found in patients less than 50 years of age [49, 50]. Our study also found that TNBC is most common among women before 50 years of age (mean age 47.8).

In our study, histopathological subtyping of 111 patients with identified TNBC yielded the following results: 89.1% of IDC-NST and 10.9% of other special types of cancers. Infiltrating ductal carcinoma of no special type (IDC-NST) was the predominant histopathological type. Similar results were obtained by other researchers, e.g., Nofech-Mozes et al. [51], Williams et al. [52], Atik et al. [53], Rao et al. [54], Osman et al. [55], Sood et al. [56] and Tawfik et al. [57] (92%, 91%, 27%, 88%, 85.7%, 80.56% and 81.9%), who found that IDC-NST is the dominant histological type in a group of triple-negative breast cancers. Given the histological grade of malignancy, the largest group of triple-negative breast cancers encompassed tumors given G2 and G3 grade. Statistical analysis showed no significant correlation between histological grade (G1–G3) and triple-negative tumor morphology ($p > 0.05$). The following authors obtained similar results: Atik et al. [53] assessing 75% of cancers in TNBC group as G3, Carey et al. [58], who found that in the TNBC group most cases are G3 cancers (26%). In a study on 16 cases of TNBC, Dabbs et al. [59] found that all tested tumors showed high degree of histological malignancy. Choi et al. [60] obtained similar results, stating that in a group of triple-negative cancers 63.1% were G3 tumors. Research by Zhou et al. [61] also showed that triple-negative G2 (51.6%) and G3 (45.2%) cancers were most numerous. Osman et al. [55] confirmed in their study that G3 carcinomas (61.9%) comprised the largest group of triple-negative tumors, while Sood et al. [56] pointed to G2 (47.22%) and G3 (38.89%) as most common tumors.

There are conflicting reports on the prevalence of lymph node metastases at the time of diagnosis among patients with TNBC. In our study we found that women without metastases to regional lymph nodes (pN0) comprised the largest group of all investigated patients with invasive triple-negative breast cancer (56.7%); no statistically significant relationship between lymph node status and histological type of TNBC-IC ($p > 0.05$) was noted. Lymph node status among patients with TNBC was reported as follows: 19.81%—N1, 19.81%—N2, 3.6%—N3. The study also showed no association between tumor size and presence of lymph node metastasis in patients with TNBC, which stood in contradiction to the findings of Thike et al. [62] who had demonstrated a relationship between tumor size and presence of nodal metastases. In studies by Rao et al. [54] lymph node metastases were found in 37 of 50 patients with TNBC (74% of cases), and TNBC was associated with higher rates of node-positive cases, which was in agreement with the findings of Carey Rakha et al. [58] and Rakha et al. [63].

In our study 30.9% of all tumors showed central necrosis. In TNBC more commonly than in non-TNBC the presence of necrosis was observed (36%; 19.6%). Yehia et al. [64] in their study divided breast cancers into three subgroups (TNBC, HER2+ and ER+/PR+). 15.3% of all tumors showed central fibrosis and tumor necrosis, which differed significantly among the three groups ($p = 0.019$). TNBC had the highest values among all groups even after adjusting the results for age. Respectively necrosis was observed in 25.8% TNBC, 9.4% HER2+ and 10.9% ER+/PR+ of cancers [64]. 62 TNBC, 64 HER2+, and 64 hormone-receptors positive breast cancers were evaluated also for HIF-1α expression. HIF-1α was expressed in 35.5% TNBC, 45.3% HER2+ and 25.0% ER+/PR+ ($p = 0.055$). In our study HIF-1α expression was observed in 43.2% TNBC and 35.3% non-TNBC.

Due to the fact that TNBC subtype frequently show morphologic evidence of hypoxia (central fibrosis and necrosis) [40, 41] an augmented expression of HIF-1α in tumors with a triple-negative phenotype was anticipated. In fact, this had been elegantly demonstrated through the preferential expression of HIF-1α in peri-necrotic tumor cells in TNBC and BRCA1 mutated breast cancers [42].

HIF-1α overexpression is an indicator of poor prognosis and significant survival time reduction in patients suffering from breast cancer [45]. HIF-1 upregulates transcription of angiogenic genes like EPO and vascular endothelial growth factor (VEGF), which induce sprouting of new vessels and in result they increase the risk of metastasis because they boost surface of contact between tumor cells and vasculature. HIF-1 induces transcription of cytoprotective proteins in malignant cells in hypoxic conditions. HIF-1α predicts poor prognosis breast cancer [46, 47].

11. Conclusions

Demonstration of statistically significant relationship between HIF-1 α expression and tumor size (pT) in patients diagnosed with triple-negative breast cancer with lymph node metastases, may suggest that HIF-1 α expression in this group of patients may be an additional and significant marker in the evaluation of advance of the disease, affecting therapeutic decisions.

Conflict of interests

The authors declare that there is no conflict of interests regarding the publication of this paper.

Author details

Anna Maria Badowska-Kozakiewicz* and Michał Piotr Budzik

*Address all correspondence to: abadowska@wum.edu.pl

Department of Biophysics and Human Physiology, Medical University of Warsaw, Warsaw, Poland

References

[1] Adkins FC, Gonzalez-Angulo AM, Lei X, et al. Triple-negative breast cancer is not a contraindication for breast conservation. Annals of Surgical Oncology. 2011;**18**:3164-3173

[2] Brenton JD, Carey LA, Ahmed AA, et al. Molecular classification and molecular forecasting of breast cancer: Ready for clinical application? Journal of Clinical Oncology. 2005;**23**:7350-7360

[3] Ogawa Y, Moriya T, Kato Y, et al. Immunohistochemical assessment for estrogen receptor and progesterone receptor status in breast cancer: Analysis for a cut-off point as the predictor for endocrine therapy. Breast Cancer. 2004;**11**:267-275

[4] Goldhirsch A, Wood WC, Coatest AS, et al. Strategies for subtypes dealing with the diversity of breast cancer highlights of the St.Gallen International Expert Consensus on the Primary Therapy of Early Breast Cancer 2011. Annals of Oncology. 2011;**22**:1736-1747

[5] Perou CM, Sørlie T, Eisen MB, et al. Molecular portraits of human breast tumours. Nature. 2000;**406**:746-752

[6] Prat A, Adamo B, Cheang MC, et al. Molecular characterization of basal-like and non-basal-like triple-negative breast cancer. The Oncologist. 2013;**18**:123-133

[7] Howland NK, Driver TD, Sedrak MP, et al. Lymph node involvement in immunohistochemistry-based molecular classification of breast cancer. The Journal of Surgical Research. 2013;**185**:697-703

[8] Montagna E, Maisonneuve P, Rotmensz N, et al. Heterogeneity of triple-negative breast cancer: Histologic subtyping to inform the outcome. Clinical Breast Cancer. 2013;**13**:31-39

[9] Somali I, Ustaoglu BY, Tarhan MO, et al. Clinicopathologic and demographic evaluation of triple-negative breast cancer patients among a Turkish patient population: A single center experience. Asian Pacific Journal of Cancer Prevention. 2013;**14**:6013-6017

[10] Atchley D, Albarracin C, Lopez A, et al. Clinical and pathologic characteristics of patients with BRCA-positive and BRCA-negative breast cancer. Journal of Clinical Oncology. 2008;**26**:4282-4288

[11] Bertucci F, Finetti P, Birnbaum D. Basal breast cancer: A complex and deadly molecular subtype. Current Molecular Medicine. 2012;**12**:96-110

[12] Rastelli F, Biancanelli S, Falzetta A, et al. Triple-negative breast cancer: Current state of the art. Tumori. 2010;**96**:875-888

[13] Lehmann BD, Bauer JA, Chen X, et al. Identification of human triple-negative breast cancer subtypes and preclinical models for selection of targeted therapies. The Journal of Clinical Investigation. 2011;**121**:2750-2767

[14] den Hollander P, Savage MI, Brown PH. Targeted therapy for breast cancer prevention. Frontiers in Oncology. 2013;**3**:250

[15] Lakhani SR, Ellis IO, Schnitt SJ, et al. editors. WHO Classification of Tumours of the Breast, Lyon. IARC; 2012

[16] Criscitiello C, Azim HA Jr, Schouten PC, et al. Understanding the biology of triple-negative breast cancer. Annals of Oncology. 2012;**23**(Suppl 6):vi13-vi18

[17] Rosen PP, Hoda SA. Breast Pathology. Diagnosis by Needle Core Biopsy.3rd ed. Philadelphia: Wolters Kluwer, Lippincott Wiliams & Wilkins; 2010

[18] Ridolfi RL, Rosen PP, Port A, et al. Medullary carcinoma of the breast: A clinicopathologic study with 10 year follow-up. Cancer. 1977;**40**:1365-1385

[19] Eiermann W, Bergh J, Cardoso F, et al. Triple negative breast cancer: Proposals for a pragmatis definition and implications for patient management and trial design. Breast. 2012;**21**:20-26

[20] Arpino G, Clark GM, Mohsin S, et al. Adenoid cystic carcinoma of the breast: Molecular markers, treatment, and clinical outcome. Cancer. 2002;**94**:2119-2127

[21] Sharma P. Biology and management of patients with triple-negative breast cancer. The Oncologist. 2016;**21**:1050-1062

[22] Carey LA, Dees EC, Sawyer L, et al. The triple negative paradox: Primary tumor chemosensitivity of breast cancer subtypes. Clinical Cancer Research. 2007;**13**:2329-2334

[23] Dieci MV, Criscitiello C, Goubar A, et al. Prognostic value of tumor-infiltrating lympho-

cytes on residual disease after primary chemotherapy for triple-negative breast cancer: A retrospective multicenter study. Annals of Oncology. 2015;**26**:1518

[24] Tutt A, Ellis P, Kilburn L, et al. The TNT trial: A randomized phase III trial of carboplatin (C) compared with docetaxel (D) for patients with metastatic or recurrent locally advanced triple negative or BRCA1/2 breast cancer (CRUK/07/012). Cancer Research. 2015;**75**:S3-S01

[25] Byrski T, Huzarski T, Dent R, et al. Pathologic complete response to neoadjuvantcisplatin in BRCA1-positive breast cancer patients. Breast Cancer Research and Treatment. 2014;**147**:401-405

[26] Medioni J, Huchon C, Le Frere-Belda MA, et al. Neoadjuvant dose-dense gemcitabine plus docetaxel and vinorelbine plus epirubicin for operable breast cancer: Improved prognosis in triple-negative tumors. Drugs in R&D. 2011;**11**:147-157

[27] Wahba HA, El-Hadaad HA. Current approaches in treatment of triple-negative breast cancer. Cancer Biology & Medicine. 2015;**12**:106-116

[28] Székely B, Silber AL, Pusztai L. New therapeutic strategies for triple-negative breast cancer. Oncology (Williston Park, N.Y.). 2017;**31**:130-137

[29] Gradishar WJ, Anderson BO, Balassanian R, et al. Invasive breast cancer version 1.2016, NCCN clinical practice guidelines in oncology. Journal of the National Comprehensive Cancer Network. 2016;**14**:324-354

[30] Miller K, Wang M, Gralow J, et al. Paclitaxel plus bevacizumab versus paclitaxel alone for metastatic breast cancer. The New England Journal of Medicine. 2007;**357**:2666-2676

[31] Rossari JR, Metzger-Filho O, Paesmans M, et al. Bevacizumab and breast cancer: A meta-analysis of first-line phase III studies and a critical reappraisal of available evidence. Journal of Oncology. 2012;**2012**:417673

[32] Soliman H, Khalil F, Antonia S. PD-L1 expression is increased in a subset of basal type breast cancer cells. PLoS One. 2014;**9**:e88557

[33] Meehan RS, Chen AP. New treatment option for ovarian cancer: PARP inhibitors. Gynecologic Oncology Research and Practice. 2016;**3**:3

[34] Juvekar A, Burga LN, Hu H, et al. Combining a PI3K inhibitor with a PARP inhibitor provides an effective therapy for BRCA1-related breast cancer. Cancer Discovery. 2012;**2**:1048-1063

[35] Garmpis N, Christos D, Garmpi A, et al. Histone deacetylases as new therapeutic targets in triple-negative breast cancer: Progress and promises. Cancer Genomics and Proteomics. 2017;**14**:299-313

[36] Traina TA, Miller K, Yardley DA, et al. Results from a phase 2 study of enzalutamide (ENZA), an androgen receptor (AR) inhibitor, in advanced AR+ triple-negative breast cancer (TNBC). Journal of Clinical Oncology. 2015;**33**(suppl):abstr 1003

[37] Masoud V, Pagès G. Targeted therapies in breast cancer: New challenges to fight against resistance. World Journal of Clinical Oncology. 2017;**8**:120-134

[38] Xin L, Yibin K. Hypoxia and hypoxia-inducible factors: Master regulators of metastasis. Clinical Cancer Research. 2010;**16**:5928-5935

[39] Dales JP, Beaufils N, Silvy M, et al. Hypoxia inducible factor 1α gene (HIF-1α) splice variants: Potential prognostic biomarkers in breast cancer. BMC Medicine. 2010;**8**:44

[40] Livasy CA, Karaca G, Nanda R, et al. Phenotypic evaluation of the basal-like subtype of invasive breast carcinoma. Modern Pathology. 2006;**19**:264-271

[41] Fulford LG, Easton DF, Reis-Filho JS, et al. Specific morphological features predictive for the basal phenotype in grade 3 invasive ductal carcinoma of breast. Histopathology. 2006;**49**:22-34

[42] Yan M, Rayoo M, Takano EA, et al. BRCA1 tumors correlate with a HIF-1alpha phenotype and have a poor prognosis through modulation of hydroxylase enzyme profile expression. British Journal of Cancer. 2009;**101**:1168-1174

[43] Tan EY, Yan M, Campo L, et al. The key hypoxia regulated gene CAIX is upregulated in basal-like breast tumors and is associated with resistance to chemotherapy. British Journal of Cancer. 2009;**100**:405-411

[44] Choi J, Jung WH, Koo JS. Metabolism-related proteins are differentially expressed according to the molecular subtype of invasive breast cancer defined by surrogate immunohistochemistry. Pathobiology. 2013;**80**:41-52

[45] Schindl M, Schoppmann SF, Samonigg H, et al. Overexpression of hypoxia-inducible factor 1alpha is associated with an unfavorable prognosis in lymph node-positive breast cancer. Clinical Cancer Research. 2002;**8**:1831-1837

[46] Dales JP, Garcia S, Meunier-Carpentier S, et al. Overexpression of hypoxia-inducible factor HIF-1alpha predicts early relapse in breast cancer: Retrospective study in a series of 745 patients. International Journal of Cancer. 2005;**116**:734-739

[47] Kronblad A, Jirstrom K, Ryden L, et al. Hypoxia inducible factor-1alpha is a prognostic marker in premenopausal patients with intermediate to highly differentiated breast cancer but not a predictive marker for tamoxifen response. International Journal of Cancer. 2006;**118**:2609-2616

[48] Naldini A, Filippi I, Miglietta D, et al. Interleukin-1b regulates the migratory potential of MDAMB231 breast cancer cells through the hypoxia-inducible factor-1α. European Journal of Cancer. 2010;**46**:3400-3408

[49] Seow A, Koh WP, Chia KS, et al. Trends in cancer incidence in Singapore 1968-2002. Singapore Cancer Registry Report. 2004:6

[50] Thike AA, Cheok PY, Jara-Lazaro AR, et al. Triple-negative breast cancer: Clinicopathological characteristics and relationship with basal-like breast cancer. Modern Pathology. 2010;**23**:123-133

[51] Nofech-Mozes S, Trudeau M, Kahn HK, et al. Patterns of recurrence in the basal and non-basal subtypes of triple—Negative breast cancers. Breast Cancer Research and Treatment. 2009;**118**:131-137

[52] Williams DJ, Cohen J, To TV, et al. Triple negative breast carcinoma in women from Vietnam and United States: Characterization of differential markers expression by tissue microarray. Human Pathology. 2009;**40**:1176-1181

[53] Atik E, Guray M, Ozgur T, et al. Characterization of immunohistochemical markers in triple negative breast carcinomas. JBUON. 2013;**18**:886-890

[54] Rao C, Shetty J, Krishan Prasad HL. Immunohistochemical profile and morphology in triple-negative breast cancers. Journal of Clinical and Diagnostic Research. 2013; **7**:1361-1365

[55] Osman NM, Chalabi N, Raboh NMA. Triple negative breast cancer: MRI features in comparison to other breast cancer subtypes with correlation to prognostic pathologic factors. Egyptian Journal of Radiology and Nuclear Medicine. 2014;**45**:1309-1316

[56] Sood N, Nigam JS. Correlation of CK5 and EGFR with clinicopathological profile of triple negative breast cancer. Pathology Research International. 2014; 6 p. Article ID: 141864. http://dx.doi.org/10.1155/2014/141864

[57] Tawfik O, Davis K, Kimler BF, et al. Clinicopathological characteristics of triple negative invasive mammary carcinomas in African-American versus Caucasian women. Annals of Clinical and Laboratory Science. 2010;**40**:315-323

[58] Carey LA, Perou CM, Livasy CA, et al. Race, breast cancer subtypes, and survival in the Carolina breast cancer study. Journal of the American Medical Association. 2006;**295**:2492-2502

[59] Dabbs DJ, Chivukula M, Carter G, et al. Basal phenotype of ductal carcinoma in situ: Recognition and immunohistologic profile. Modern Pathology. 2006;**19**:1506-1511

[60] Choi J, Jubg WH, Koo JS. Clinicopathologic features of molecular subtypes of triple negative breast cancer based on immunohistochemical markers. Histology and Histopathology. 2012;**27**:1481-1493

[61] Zhou L, Li K, Luo Y, et al. Novel prognostic markers for patients with triple – Negative breast cancer. Human Pathology. 2013;**44**:2180-2187

[62] Thike AA, Iqbal J, Cheok PY, et al. Triple negative breast cancer: Outcome correlation with immunohistochemical detection of basal markers. American Journal of Surgical Pathology. 2010;**34**:956-964

[63] Rakha EA, El-Sayed ME, Green AR, et al. Prognostic markers in triple-negative breast cancer. Cancer. 2007;**109**:25-32

[64] Yehia L, Boulos F, Jabbour M, et al. Expression of HIF-1α and markers of angiogenesis are not significantly different in triple negative breast cancer compared to other breast cancer molecular subtypes: Implications for future therapy. PLoS One. 2015;**10**:e0129356. DOI: 10.1371/journal. pone.0129356

4

Triple-Negative Breast Cancer, Cisplatin and Calpain-1

Shadia Al-Bahlani and Samiya Al-Jaaidi

Abstract

Chemo-resistance of breast cancer is a major obstacle for successful treatment and is mainly represented as a defect in apoptosis. The differential effects of platinum-based drugs (PBDs) were assessed on breast cancer cell ultrastructure. Three representative cells, including triple-negative breast cancer (TNBC), were treated with different concentrations and timings of cisplatin, carboplatin, and oxaliplatin. Changes on cell surface and ultrastructure were detected by scanning electron microscope (SEM) and transmission electron microscope (TEM). In addition, using advanced techniques in molecular biology, we demonstrated that calpain-1 plays an essential role in modulating breast cancer cell sensitivity to cisplatin-induced apoptosis. We also showed that the correlation of its expression to the proliferating/apoptotic index using immunohistochemical staining in TNBC tissue was variable. Exploring new pathways will help in overcoming chemoresistance in breast cancer cells.

Keywords: triple-negative breast cancer, platinum-based drugs, cisplatin, calpain-1, apoptosis

1. Introduction

Breast cancer is ranked second as one of the leading cause of deaths among women worldwide [1]. It is characterized by heterogeneity displaying a wide scope of morphological features, different immunohistochemical profiles, and unique histopathological subtypes. According to immunohistochemical phenotypes [i.e., presence or absence of estrogen receptor (ER), progesterone receptor (PgR), and epidermal growth factor receptor 2 (HER2)], breast cancer can be classified into five subtypes. These are luminal A, luminal B, HER2 overexpression, basal-like, and normal-like subtypes, each of which has distinct clinical outcomes [2]. Luminal A accounts for 50% of invasive breast cancers and are ER/PgR positive or HER2 negative. Luminal B category represents 20% of invasive breast cancers. The ER/PgR is positive, while

HER2 expression is variable (positive or negative). Luminal B tumors have higher proliferation and poorer prognosis than luminal A tumors. HER2 overexpression group accounts for 15% of all invasive breast cancers and the tumor usually tends to be ER/PR negative. The basal class is typically ER/PR negative and HER2 negative, hence the name TNBC [3]. It comprises about 15% of all invasive breast cancers and have a fairly poor prognosis. Normal-like tumors account for 7.8% of all breast cancer cases in a lymph-node negative cohort. It is positive for ER and PgR but negative for HER2 [4, 5].

Due to this heterogeneity, the treatment is complicated and the therapeutic strategies should be selected carefully. To overcome the disease, it is imperative that each patient be treated individually according to the morphological classification with molecular parameters and sensitivity to available therapy. Treatment of breast cancer includes surgery, radiation therapy, hormone-modification therapy and chemotherapy (anticancer drugs). Chemotherapy treatment has markedly reduced the risk for recurrence and mortality after primary treatment of breast cancer and have increased the 5- and 10-year survival rates [6].

One of the major modes of action of chemotherapeutic drugs may be the activation of apoptosis (programmed cell death) [7]. Hence, anticancer drugs are associated with the activation of proapoptotic genes and the suppression of antiapoptotic genes. The attenuation of proapoptotic genes and increases in antiapoptotic genes causes resistance to apoptosis [8]. Hence, in order to increase the therapeutic effect of chemotherapy, there is a need to assess the molecular mechanisms of apoptosis induced anticancer drugs. This may lead to new strategies for the enhancement of the antitumor effect against target organs.

In this chapter, we hope to summarize three attempted molecular biology studies on breast cancer that have contributed to further knowledge in this field. We have compared the effects of platinum based-chemotherapeutic drugs such as cisplatin, carboplatin and oxaliplatin on the ultrastructure of the three human breast cancer cell lines representing the most diagnosed types; MDA-MB-231, MCF-7 and BT-474 [9]. We have particularly demonstrated the role of cisplatin in inducing apoptosis in MDA-MB-231 via the endoplasmic reticulum- mediated calpain-1 pathway [10]. At the same time, we have assessed the expression of calpain-1 as a potential prognostic factor in TNBC tissues [11]. Understanding the pathways by which platinum-based drugs induce apoptosis and how these pathways are altered in chemoresistance can provide valuable information necessary to target specific cell death pathways in the treatment of clinically resistant breast cancer.

2. Platinum-based drugs and breast cancer cells

Platinum-based drugs (PBDs) are used for adjuvant chemotherapy to reduce mortality from breast cancer with reversible side-effects [12]. A key feature of platinum based drugs is that once platinum salts enter cells, they can bind to DNA to form Platinum-DNA adducts that can cause damage to the DNA. Following DNA damage, cell cycle checkpoints are activated to repair either the damaged DNA or induce apoptosis (cell death) [13, 14]. Thus, the ultimate goal in the application of platinum-based chemotherapy is to shift the dynamics away from cell growth and survival in favor of cell differentiation and apoptosis. This will in turn reduce and eliminate tumor progression and malignancy [15].

Although PBDs are initially effective, their efficacy is limited by the occurrence of resistance, which is attributed to alterations in cellular pathways such as DNA repair, drug transport, drug metabolism and apoptosis [16]. Several studies have explored the cellular and molecular pathways involved in the mechanism of PBDs resistance to breast cancer [13, 16–18]. However, only a few ultrastructural studies on the intracellular organelles of breast cancer cells have been performed to determine the effectiveness of these drugs.

2.1. Surface structure of breast cancer cells differ from normal breast cells

We used SEM to compare the surface morphology between three models of breast cancer cells, each of which is characterized with a distinct immunohistochemical profile. The MCF-7 cell line was used to represent the luminal A breast cancer [19], the BT-474 cell line, the luminal B tumor [20] and the MDA-MB-231 cell line, the basal-like subtype, TNBC [3].

Normal breast cells, MCF-10A, revealed round shape cells characterized by short lamellipodia, whereas, the breast cancer cells had a semiflattened surface structure containing microvilli with extending lamellipodia. Lamellipodia consist of protrusive filamentous actin and signaling proteins, which play a role in cell migration and cell–cell communication. These surface protrusions are important in enhancing movement and adhesion to the surrounding stroma [21]. They appeared to be lesser in number and finer in shape for both MCF-7 and BT-474 cells but higher in number and thicker for MDA-MB-231 cells. Since MDA-MB-231 cells are advanced cancer cells with metastatic characteristics, therefore it is not surprising for these cells to contain higher numbers of lamellipodia on their cell surface. This is indicative of their importance of cell shape modifications in their invasiveness process unlike the normal breast cells. These distinct features of TNBCs *in vivo* models might demonstrate their aggressiveness and give them a metastatic potential [21–23]. TEM micrographs revealed the absence of nuclei in the MDA-MB-231 cells whereas more than one nucleus were detected in MCF-7 and BT-474 cells.

2.2. Effect of PBDs on the cell membrane of breast cancer cells

Treatment with cisplatin, carboplatin and oxaliplatin, using two concentrations of 10 and 20 μm with the time period of 15 minutes, the initial response of the treated breast cancer cells started with the formation of pores on the cell membranes indicating the active process of drug influx/efflux. The pores on the surface of the MDA-MB-231 cells were deeper and wider due to the high number of lamellipodia, unlike the two cell types; MCF-7 and BT-474. Subsequently the lamellipodia retracted causing the cells to shrink and change their shape to semioval and to round shape. This was more evident to a higher extent in the MDA-MB-231 cells.

When we treated all the three types of breast cancer cells for 12 hours with the three types of PBDs, SEM revealed the early stages of apoptosis presented by convoluted membrane, membrane blebs and apoptotic bodies. The membrane blebbing is caused by deep cytoskeleton rearrangement as result of alterations in organelle distribution and cell shape, a pattern of apoptosis. Differences on the response of the cells to the three types of PBDs were detected for BT-474 and MCF-7 cells. BT-474 cells sensitivity response was maximal for Carboplatin whereas MCF-7 cells sensitivity response was maximal for cisplatin. However, MDA-MB-231 cells response was similar for all the PBDs. Hence, cell mediated drug response is dependent on the cellular characteristic and the drug action.

2.3. Effect of PBDs on the intracellular organelles of breast cancer cells

We then used TEM to gain further insight into the ultrastructural alterations induced by PBDs and to study how the drug cytotoxicity differentially caused these alterations. Other distinct morphological characteristics of apoptosis consistent with the literature were evident such as shrinkage of the cytoplasm, microvilli retraction, fragmentation and condensation of the nucleus and swelling of both the mitochondria and endoplasmic reticulum [24, 25]. Splitting of apoptotic cells characterizes the final stage of apoptosis [24]. In addition to apoptosis, TEM micrographs also revealed the necrotic type of death. Changes identified on plasma membrane shows incoherence, causing cell swelling and organelles disruption. Occasionally, apoptotic cells, *in vitro*, undergo a late process of secondary necrosis. Necrosis was considered to be a physical process of cell death that was not regulated. However, emerging evidence suggests that it is as another form of apoptosis and an independent genetically encoded cell death pathway [25, 26]. Overall, treated cells with the three types of PBDs exhibited similar ultrastructural changes exhibiting distinct features such as the increased number of vacuoles portraying as a defense mechanism for cell survival and this is consistent with other studies in other types of cancers [27–29]. PBD deposits were mainly attracted to the fat droplets of the cells suggesting an active role of cellular lipids in the potentiation of PBDs to induce apoptosis.

Few but prominent differences between the three types of breast cancer cells were detected when treated with PBDs. These included the following;

1. Carboplatin did not cause any swelling and disarrangement of the mitochondria on the BT-474 and the MDA-MB-231 cells as opposed to the MCF-7 cells.
2. Carboplatin-treated cells exhibited more lamellar bodies compared to cisplatin or oxaliplatin treated cells. Lamellar bodies are specialized lipid storage or secretory organelles, which have a core composed of multilamellar structure and can be surrounded by a membrane [30]. It is possible that PBDs induce lipidosis in cancer cells and cause accumulation of lamellar bodies.
3. Carboplatin, cisplatin and oxaliplatin caused apoptosis in all the three types of breast cancer cell lines, however, it is possible that apoptosis independent of DNA damage could have contributed to the way some of the enucleated cells of the MDA-MB-231 cells die. This will be discussed further in Section 3.

3. Cisplatin-induced calpain-1 activation by endoplasmic reticulum in TNBC cells

Cisplatin has been shown to induce apoptosis in enucleated cells [31, 32]. It does this by initially acting on the endoplasmic reticulum causing an increase in cytosolic calcium (Ca^{2+}), leading to the activation of calpain-1 [33]. Calpains belong to a family of Ca^{2+}-dependent proteases which play many roles in basic cellular processes including cell proliferation and apoptosis, through activation of the caspase pathways. Calpain-1 and calpain-2, encoded by CAPN1 and CAPN2, respectively, are the most abundant isoforms within their family [31]. Although we, and others, have shown that cisplatin-induced apoptosis occurs by way of the calpain-1 dependent pathway, [34–36]; however, information in TNBC cells is limited. This prompted us to investigate the role of the calpain-1 pathway by way of the endoplasmic reticulum in the apoptotic death of TNBC cells induced by cisplatin.

3.1. Cisplatin caused calcium release in TNBC cells

Using Von Koss staining, we were able to represent the variation of Ca^{2+} deposits between the cisplatin-treated and untreated TNBC cells. Ca^{2+} deposits in the cytoplasm increased with increasing cisplatin concentration (0, 20 and 40 μm) in the cisplatin-treated cells with no significant deposits observed in the untreated cells.

3.2. Cisplatin caused structural changes in the endoplasmic reticulum of TNBC cells

Several studies have concentrated on the investigation of non-nuclear pathways in the apoptosis of cancer cells induced by cisplatin [31, 32, 34]. Such studies contribute to the understanding of the causes of sensitivity and resistance to cisplatin [31, 37]. The endoplasmic reticulum is involved in the regulation of cellular responses to stress and alterations in Ca^{2+} homeostasis [38]. Alterations in Ca^{2+} homeostasis and accumulation of misfolded proteins in the endoplasmic reticulum caused endoplasmic reticulum stress resulting in apoptosis [39]. Using TEM, we detected the intracellular deposits of cisplatin and its structural changes on the endoplasmic reticulum in TNBC cells. TEM micrographs revealed that cisplatin induced clear structural changes in both the endoplasmic reticulum and the mitochondria. This phenomenon represented swelling of the lumen and disarrangement of their internal folding as compared to the control cells without treatment which appeared as well-defined structures. Hence, these findings were consistent with a study conducted by Mandic et al. who demonstrated that the endoplasmic reticulum is the non-nuclear target of cisplatin [31].

3.3. Location of calpain-1 in TNBC cells

Studies have reported that calpain-1 is mainly located in the cytoplasm of breast cancer cells [40, 41]. We also used immunohistochemical staining to confirm this finding. The staining intensity of calpain-1 in the cytoplasm increased with increasing concentrations (0, 20 and 40 μm) of cisplatin.

3.4. Cisplatin activated calpain-1 and induced apoptosis through the endoplasmic reticulum-mediated pathway

The results of some experiments attempted to investigate the role of calpain-1 in the apoptotic death of TNBC cells induced by cisplatin by way of the endoplasmic reticulum are summarized in **Table 1**.

Experiments			Results	
	Control (μm/nM)	Treatment after 24 hours		P value of apoptosis
Cisplatin to induce endoplasmic reticulum stress (calcium release) and activate calpain-1 was assessed as activation of endoplasmic reticulum downstream effectors; α-fodrin and caspase-12. Calpain-1, α-fodrin and caspase-12 protein content (total and cleaved) was measured by Western blotting.	Cisplatin (0 μm) Cisplatin (0 μm)	Cisplatin (20 μm) Cisplatin (40 μm)	Cisplatin activated calpain-1 as reflected in cleavage of α-fodrin and caspase-12 and induced apoptosis in TNBC cells. Although cisplatin had no effect on calpain-1 content, it significantly caused cleavage of α-fodrin and caspase-12 and induced apoptosis in a dose-dependent manner [10].	P < 0.001 vs. control P < 0.001 vs. control
Cisplatin to activate calpain-1 by way of endoplasmic reticulum using CPA treatment was assessed as activation of endoplasmic reticulum downstream effectors; GRP78, calmodulin, α-fodrin and caspase-12, were measured using immunoblotting.	Cisplatin (0 μm) + CPA (50 μm)	Cisplatin (20 μm) + CPA (50 μm)	CPA significantly enhanced upregulation of cisplatin-induced, calpain-1 activation and apoptosis compared with the controlled group [10].	P < 0.001 vs. CPA Control
Cisplatin to activate calpain-1 by way of endoplasmic reticulum using siRNA treatment was assessed as activation of α-fodrin. The effect of calpain-1 siRNA on its content and activation (indicated by α-fodrin cleavage) was measured using immunoblotting	Cisplatin (0 μm) + calpain-1 siRNA (150 nM)	Cisplatin (20 μm) + calpain-1 siRNA (150 nM)	Calpain-1 small interfering RNA (siRNA) significantly attenuated cisplatin-induced apoptosis in TNBC cells by downregulating calpain-1 in TNBC cells [10].	P < 0.01 vs. Calpain-1 siRNA Control
Apoptosis was measured by Hoechst staining using fluorescent microscopy.				

Table 1. Summary of results of experiments attempted to investigate the role of calpain-1 in the apoptotic death of TNBC cells induced by cisplatin by way of the endoplasmic reticulum.

We have shown in this study the effect of cisplatin on calpain-1 protein and its activation in TNBC cells. This has also been reported by others in other types of cancer cells [34, 35]. The finding that the increase in both calcium deposits and upregulation of endoplasmic reticulum stress indicator proteins such as GRP78 and calmodulin suggest the involvement of endoplasmic reticulum stress-dependent Ca^{2+} release in the cellular mechanism of action of cisplatin. The ability of cisplatin-induced apoptosis by way of endoplasmic reticulum stress has been shown to involve calpain-mediated activation of caspase-12 [42]. Caspase-12 is localized to the endoplasmic reticulum and may be activated by the disturbance of intracellular calcium homeostasis [43]. Cyclopiazonic acid (CPA) is a selective Ca^{2+} ATPase inhibitor, which depletes the endoplasmic reticulum (ER) of Ca^{2+} and therefore, activates Ca^{2+} – dependent proteases such calpain. For that reason, the activity of calpain-1 was enhanced by CPA through the endoplasmic reticulum-mediated pathway which further increased the TNBC cells response to cisplatin-induced apoptosis. In contrast, the sensitivity was attenuated by calpain-1 inhibition using the exogenous inhibitor, calpain-1 siRNA. These findings support the role of calpain-1 responsible for the pro-apoptotic effects of cisplatin in TNBC cells by way of endoplasmic reticulum. Hence, targeting calpain-1 activity with specific inhibitors could be a novel approach in limiting development of primary tumors and formation of metastases.

4. Calpain-1 as a potential prognostic factor in TNBC

TNBC has been reported to have a clinical and pathological aggressive pattern due to its heterogeneous characteristic [44]. The ineffectiveness of hormonal and targeted therapies and poor prognosis for this subtype requires developing alternative therapeutic strategies such as biomarkers. The expression of a number of proteins has been shown to be associated with clinical outcome in TNBC patients [40, 45, 46]. Hence, there is a need to identify additional biomarkers to allow personalized treatment for patients with TNBC. For this reason, we explored the role of calpain-1 as a potential prognostic factor for TNBC therapy. We also evaluated the proliferation and apoptotic index for their potential use as possible prognostic factors since the biological behavior of tumor growth is a result of a balance between the proliferative activity and the number of cells dying by apoptosis [47]. Thus, they are considered as dominant histopathologic features in tumors. Several studies have also shown that calpain-1 expression significantly associated with tumor grade [40], proliferation [48, 49] and apoptosis [50]. Therefore, we also assessed the association between calpain-1 expression, cell proliferation and apoptosis in TNBC tissues.

4.1. Patient characteristics

We tested calpain-1 protein expression and the proliferative/apoptotic index on paraffin-embedded tissues from a cohort of 55 patients with TNBC. The main histological type was infiltrative ductal carcinoma in 96.4% (53 of 55), infiltrative lobular carcinoma in 1.8% (1 of 55) and micropapillary carcinoma 1.8% (1 of 55). Patients were females with a median age of 47 years (19–74). A total of 34 cases (61.8%) were premenopausal with no family history of breast cancer. Based on the disease indexing system, half (50.9%) of the patients were defined as stage III or IV at the time of diagnosis. Almost half of the patients (n = 26, 47.3%)

received neoadjuvant treatment and 5 (19.2%) achieved complete pathological response. Anthracyclines and taxanes were the most commonly used chemotherapeutic agents as front-line treatment. Breast cancer related overall survival (OS) was defined as the time interval (in months) from the date of diagnosis until death from breast cancer. Similarly, recurrence-free survival (RFS) was defined as the time interval (in months) between the start of primary treatment and date of cancer relapse.

4.2. Calpain-1 expression in TNBC tissues

Immunostained tissues with calpain-1 were significantly expressed and demonstrated cytoplasmic and membranous staining with some granularity and heterogeneity between adjacent tumor cells varying from weak to intense staining in which low staining was detected in 32.7% (18 of 55), intermediate staining in 38.2% (21 of 55) and high staining in 29.6% (16 of 55) of the cases analyzed. The cut off value was determined by screening the stained tissue under light microscope where the staining intensity of calpain-1 in tumor cells was assessed as none (0), weak (1), medium (2), and strong (3) using an immunohistochemical *H*-score. The *H*-scores were calculated by multiplying the percentage area by the intensity grade (*H*-score range 0–300).

4.3. Correlation between calpain-1 expression and clinicopathological variables and outcome of TNBC patients

In order to investigate the possibility of using calpain-1 protein as a prognostic biomarker in TNBC, its expression was assessed for association with a number of clinicopathological variables. We determined that calpain-1 expression displayed a significant positive association to the lymph node status ($P = 0.02$) but not with other clinicopathological variables. Kaplan–Meier survival curves were plotted with significance determined using the log-rank test in order to determine the relationship between calpain-1 protein expression in the recurrence-free survival (RFS) and in the overall survival (OS) patients. The expression of calpain-1 in the triple-negative tissues was not significantly associated with breast cancer RFS ($P = 0.71$) or OS ($P = 0.88$) in which the median RFS was 18 months (3–77 months) and OS was 41 months (0–105 months) in the total patient cohort.

TNM classifies lymph node status as a tumor-related prognostic factor, therefore, our results suggest that calpain-1 might be used as a prognostic factor in TNBC. Calpain-1 was also found to be associated with lymph node status in other types of cancer, such as renal cell carcinoma [51]. The observation of the lack of association of calpain-1 with other clinicopathological variables is consistent with a study conducted by Storr et al. in which they demonstrated a correlation between calpain-1 expression and tumor grade but not with other clinicopathological variables [40].

The variations among the presence or absence of association with lymph node status or tumor grade which are essential in determining its prognosis can be explained by several theories; (i) the majority of patient samples were of intermediate grade tumor and therefore calpain-1 activity may have started at later stages as suggested by its correlation with the lymph node status, (ii) the lack of wide range of sample collection in regards to tumor grades may have created a diversion in the statistical analysis, (iii) the insufficiency of samples might have contributed to lack of significant correlations, (iv) the possibility of genetic differences between the populations in the current study and the ones already published may be the cause of differences on the expression of calpain-1 in breast cancer cells [40] and finally (v) the presence or absence of the hormonal receptors such as ER, PR, and HER2 that determine breast cancer behavior and thus treatment can influence the outcome. Storr *et al.* (2011) reported that there was no association between the expression of calpain-1 in HER2-positive breast cancer patients treated with trastuzumab following adjuvant chemotherapy with any of the clinicopathological variables [52]. Hence, their observation is consistent with our data but may differ in terms of the positivity of HER2.

4.4. Association between calpain-1 expression, cell proliferation and apoptosis in TNBC tissues

Calpains have been reported to be involved in the proliferation of breast cancer cells [48, 49]. However, the role of the calpain family in proliferation of TNBC cells has not been reported yet. Ki-67, a nuclear antigen is a protein encoded by Ki-67 on 10q25 and considered to be a proliferation marker for predicting tumor development [53]. It is expressed during all active phases of the cell cycle except the resting phase, thus being present only in dividing cells. Ki-67 is detected by monoclonal antibody MIB-1 which can be a useful marker of proliferation and of prognostic value [53]. The quantitative assessment of Ki-67 staining on paraffin embedded tumor sections has been reported as an accurate estimate of the proliferation index of individual tumors [53].

Therefore, proliferative fractions of paraffin embedded breast cancer tissues were determined by immunohistochemical staining for Ki-67 antibody. The cellular proliferative activity was estimated as the percentage of tumor cells stained per field ×40. Statistical analysis showed no significant correlation between calpain-1 expression and proliferation ($P = 0.29$). Possible theories of the presence and absence of the hormonal receptors, differences in the genetic makeup, and other members of calpains involvement may also influence the correlation with proliferation.

Cell proliferation along with cell death are both phenomena responsible for control of cell number in normal tissues and tumors. Since chemotherapy induces programmed cell death by apoptosis, hence, the apoptotic tumor cells can be morphologically identified using the conventional hematoxylin and eosin (H&E) method and cells are counted using light microscopy. Therefore, there has been interest in the application of the apoptotic index in malignant growths as a putative prognostic marker. The percentage of apoptotic cells in tumor sections may also be measured by a molecular-based approach, labeling of fragmented DNA breaks and calculating the apoptotic index (AI) using the terminal transferase-uridyl nick-end labeling (TUNEL) assay.

Therefore, in order to determine whether the frequency of apoptosis was related to tumorigenesis, two approaches; the conventional H&E staining method and the apoptotic TUNEL assay were both used to detect apoptotic cells and to prove that the two methods comparatively correlate with each other. H&E detects apoptosis in its degradation phase and can be subjective whereas the TUNEL assay detects apoptosis in its early phase and is more objective. Apoptotic cells were counted per 100 invasive tumor cells using ×40 objective. Apoptotic counts using either method, were significantly correlated ($P < 0.001$, $r = 0.547$). Although both assays tested apoptosis from different aspects, but the results were the same, indicating the reliability of both assays. These findings were also consistent with a previous study by Watanabe et al. [54]. In addition, the relationship between apoptosis and proliferation was investigated in TNBC tissues. For all of the patients, high apoptotic counts significantly correlated with increased cell proliferation ($P = 0.045$). The positive correlation between proliferative and apoptotic indices seen in this study is also consistent with other types of cancers such as colorectal cancers [54].

In experimental models the calpain system has been shown to influence apoptosis in breast cancer [48, 55, 56]. The relationship between calpain-1 expression and apoptosis using the two methods, H&E-based apoptotic counts and apoptotic counts derived from the apoptotic TUNEL assay was investigated in the TNBC tissues. Interestingly, the data revealed that there were no significant association between the apoptotic indices when compared to calpain-1 expression ($P = 0.710$ and 0.100), respectively. Such results suggest that the TNBC cells undergo apoptosis via other members of the calpain family such as calpain-2.

Taken together, these data have clearly demonstrated the absence of correlation between calpain-1 expression and the proliferating/apoptotic index or clinicopathological variables except with the lymph node status of TNBC patients. Hence, calpain-1 could be a useful prognostic marker in TNBC. More studies should be conducted in the future to evaluate the prognostic value of calpain-1 in TNBC.

5. Conclusion

Breast cancer is the most leading cause of cancer death in females worldwide. Although its name is based on a single tissue of origin, this cancer is heterogeneous making it a complex disease. Compared to other subtypes of breast cancer, TNBC is more biologically aggressive and has higher recurrence rate, higher frequency of metastasis and worse survival. Challenges into identifying targets and treatments have led to advances in laboratory technology and research resulting into the expansion of our knowledge of tumor biology. Though no specific therapies currently exist for TNBC except for cytotoxic chemotherapy, there is ongoing research to identify potential targets for therapy. Therefore, the understanding of breast cancer subtypes and targeted drug therapies is a key to address resistance to current targeted drugs in order to pave the way for providing personalized breast cancer care.

Author details

Shadia Al-Bahlani[1*] and Samiya Al-Jaaidi[2]

*Address all correspondence to: bahlani@squ.edu.om

1 Department of Allied Health Sciences, College of Medicine and Health Sciences, Sultan Qaboos University, Muscat, Oman

2 Department of Applied Sciences, Higher College of Technology, Muscat, Oman

References

[1] Wahba HA, El-Hadaad HA. Current approaches in treatment of triple-negative breast cancer. Cancer Biology & Medicine. 2015;**12**(2):106-116

[2] Makki J. Diversity of breast carcinoma: Histological subtypes and clinical relevance. Clinical Medicine Insights Pathology. 2015;**8**:23-31

[3] Cailleau R, Young R, Olive M, Reeves WJ Jr. Breast tumor cell lines from pleural effusions. Journal of the National Cancer Institute. 1974;**53**(3):661-674

[4] Sørlie T, Perou CM, Tibshirani R, Aas T, Geisler S, Johnsen H, et al. Gene expression patterns of breast carcinomas distinguish tumor subclasses with clinical implications. Proceedings of the National Academy of Sciences. 2001;**98**(19):10869-10874

[5] Dai X, Li T, Bai Z, Yang Y, Liu X, Zhan J, et al. Breast cancer intrinsic subtype classification, clinical use and future trends. American Journal Of Cancer Research. 2015;**5**(10):2929-2943

[6] Hortobagyi GN. Toward individualized breast cancer therapy: Translating biological concepts to the bedside. The Oncologist. 2012;**17**(4):577-5784

[7] Makin G, Hickman JA. Apoptosis and cancer chemotherapy. Cell and Tissue Research. 2000;**301**(1):143-152

[8] Kim R, Tanabe K, Uchida Y, Emi M, Inoue H, Toge T. Current status of the molecular mechanisms of anticancer drug-induced apoptosis. The contribution of molecular-level analysis to cancer chemotherapy. Cancer Chemotherapy And Pharmacology. 2002;**50**(5):343-352

[9] Al-Bahlani S, Al-Dhahli B, Al-Adawi K, Al-Nabhani A, Al-Kindi M. Platinum-based drugs differentially affect the ultrastructure of breast cancer cell types. BioMed Research International. 2017;**2017**:3178794

[10] Al-Bahlani SM, Al-Bulushi KH, Al-Alawi ZM, Al-Abri NY, Al-Hadidi ZR, Al-Rawahi SS. Cisplatin induces apoptosis through the endoplasmic reticulum-mediated, calpain 1 pathway in triple-negative breast cancer cells. Clinical Breast Cancer. 2017;**17**(3):e103-e112

[11] Al-Bahlani SM, Al-Rashdi RM, Kumar S, Al-Sinawi SS, Al-Bahri MA, Shalaby AA. Calpain-1 expression in triple-negative breast cancer: A potential prognostic factor independent of the proliferative/apoptotic index. BioMed Research International. 2017; **2017**:10

[12] Shapiro C, Recht A. Side effects of adjuvant treatment of breast cancer. The New England Journal of Medicine. 2001;**344**(26):1997-2008

[13] Jin, Jin J, Zhang W, Ji W, Yang F, Guan X. Predictive biomarkers for triple negative breast cancer treated with platinum-based chemotherapy. Cancer Biology & Therapy. 2017;**18**(6):369-378

[14] Wang D, Lippard S. Cellular processing of platinum anticancer drugs. Nature Reviews Drug Discovery. 2005;**4**(4):307-320

[15] Turkson J. Cancer drug discovery and anticancer drug development. In: Coleman WB, Tsongalis GJ, editors. The Molecular Basis of Human Cancer. New York, NY: Springer New York; 2017. pp. 695-707

[16] Galanski M. Recent developments in the field of anticancer platinum complexes. Recent Patents On Anti-Cancer Drug Discovery. 2006;**1**(2):285-295

[17] Turner NC, Tutt AN. Platinum chemotherapy for BRCA1-related breast cancer: Do we need more evidence? Breast Cancer Research. 2012;**14**(6):115

[18] Meriggi F, Di Biasi B, Zaniboni A. The renaissance of platinum-based chemotherapy for metastatic breast cancer. Journal of Chemotherapy (Florence, Italy). 2008;**20**(5):551-560

[19] Levenson AS, Jordan VC. MCF-7: The first hormone-responsive breast cancer cell line. Cancer Research. 1997;**57**(15):3071-3078

[20] Lasfargues EY, Coutinho WG, Redfield ES. Isolation of two human tumor epithelial cell lines from solid breast carcinomas. Journal of the National Cancer Institute. 1978;**61**(4):967-978

[21] Friedl P, Wolf K. Tumour-cell invasion and migration: Diversity and escape mechanisms. Nature Reviews Cancer. 2003;**3**(5):362-374

[22] Bozzuto G, Condello M, Molinari A. Migratory behaviour of tumour cells: A scanning electron microscopy study. Annali dell'Istituto superiore di sanita. 2015;**51**(2):139-147

[23] Ren J. Relationship between development of microvilli on tumor cells and growth or metastatic potential of tumor cells. [Hokkaido igaku zasshi] The Hokkaido Journal Of Medical Science. 1991;**66**(2):187-200

[24] Wong RS. Apoptosis in cancer: From pathogenesis to treatment. Journal of Experimental & Clinical Cancer Research. 2011;**30**(1):87

[25] Moela P, Motadi LR. Apoptotic molecular advances in breast cancer management. In: Ntuli TM, editor. Cell Death-Autophagy, Apoptosis and Necrosis. Rijeka: InTech; 2015. Ch. 10

[26] Portt L, Norman G, Clapp C, Greenwood M, Greenwood MT. Anti-apoptosis and cell survival: A review. Biochimica et Biophysica Acta. 2011;**1813**(1):238-259

[27] Liu D, Yang Y, Liu Q, Wang J. Inhibition of autophagy by 3-MA potentiates cisplatin-induced apoptosis in esophageal squamous cell carcinoma cells. Medical Oncology (Northwood, London, England). 2011;**28**(1):105-111

[28] Ding ZB, Hui B, Shi YH, Zhou J, Peng YF, Gu CY, et al. Autophagy activation in hepatocellular carcinoma contributes to the tolerance of oxaliplatin via reactive oxygen species modulation. Clinical Cancer Research. 2011;**17**(19):6229-6238

[29] Cho KH, Park JH, Kwon KB, Lee YR, So HS, Lee KK, et al. Autophagy induction by low-dose cisplatin: The role of p53 in autophagy. Oncology Reports. 2014;**31**(1):248-254

[30] Schmitz G, Structure MG. Function of lamellar bodies, lipid-protein complexes involved in storage and secretion of cellular lipids. Journal of Lipid Research. 1991;**32**(10):1539-1570

[31] Mandic A, Hansson J, Linder S, Shoshan MC. Cisplatin induces endoplasmic reticulum stress and nucleus-independent apoptotic signaling. The Journal of Biological Chemistry. 2003;**278**(11):9100-9106

[32] Yu F, Megyesi J, Price PM. Cytoplasmic initiation of cisplatin cytotoxicity. American Journal Of Physiology Renal Physiology. 2008;**295**(1):F44-F52

[33] Xu Y, Wang C, Su J, Xie Q, Ma L, Zeng L, et al. Tolerance to endoplasmic reticulum stress mediates cisplatin resistance in human ovarian cancer cells by maintaining endoplasmic reticulum and mitochondrial homeostasis. Oncology Reports. 2015;**34**(6):3051-3060

[34] Al-Bahlani S, Fraser M, Wong AY, Sayan BS, Bergeron R, Melino G, et al. P73 regulates cisplatin-induced apoptosis in ovarian cancer cells via a calcium/calpain-dependent mechanism. Oncogene. 2011;**30**(41):4219-4230

[35] Liu L, Xing D, Chen WR, Chen T, Pei Y, Gao X. Calpain-mediated pathway dominates cisplatin-induced apoptosis in human lung adenocarcinoma cells as determined by real-time single cell analysis. International Journal of Cancer. 2008;**122**(10):2210-2222

[36] Liu L, Xing D, Chen WR. μ-Calpain regulates caspase-dependent and apoptosis inducing factor-mediated caspase-independent apoptotic pathways in cisplatin-induced apoptosis. International Journal of Cancer. 2009;**125**(12):2757-2766

[37] Shen D-W, Pouliot LM, Hall MD, Gottesman MM. Cisplatin resistance: A cellular self-Defense mechanism resulting from multiple epigenetic and genetic changes. Pharmacological Reviews. 2012;**64**(3):706-721

[38] Kaufman RJ. Stress signaling from the lumen of the endoplasmic reticulum: Coordination of gene transcriptional and translational controls. Genes & Development. 1999;**13**(10):1211-1233

[39] Rao RV, Ellerby HM, Bredesen DE. Coupling endoplasmic reticulum stress to the cell death program. Cell Death and Differentiation. 2004;**11**(4):372-380

[40] Storr SJ, Lee KW, Woolston CM, Safuan S, Green AR, Macmillan RD, et al. Calpain system protein expression in basal-like and triple-negative invasive breast cancer. Annals of Oncology. 2012;**23**(9):2289-2296

[41] Pu X, Storr SJ, Ahmad NS, Chan SY, Moseley PM, Televantou D, et al. Calpain-1 is associated with adverse relapse free survival in breast cancer: A confirmatory study. Histopathology. 2016;**68**(7):1021-1029

[42] Nakagawa T, Yuan J. Cross-talk between two cysteine protease families. Activation of caspase-12 by calpain in apoptosis. The Journal of Cell Biology. 2000;**150**(4):887-894

[43] Nakagawa T, Zhu H, Morishima N, Li E. Xu J, Yankner BA, et al. Caspase-12 mediates endoplasmic-reticulum-specific apoptosis and cytotoxicity by amyloid-beta. Nature. 2000;**403**(6765):98-103

[44] Polyak K. Heterogeneity in breast cancer. The Journal of Clinical Investigation. 2011; **121**(10):3786-3788

[45] Alexander BM, Sprott K, Farrow DA, Wang X, D'Andrea AD, Schnitt SJ, et al. DNA repair protein biomarkers associated with time to recurrence in triple negative breast cancer. Clinical cancer research: An Official Journal of the American Association for Cancer Research. 2010;**16**(23):5796-5804

[46] Biganzoli E, Coradini D, Ambrogi F, Garibaldi JM, Lisboa P, Soria D, et al. p53 status identifies two subgroups of triple-negative breast cancers with distinct biological features. Japanese Journal of Clinical Oncology. 2011;**41**(2):172-179

[47] Liu SS, Tsang BK, Cheung ANY, Xue WC, Cheng DKL, Ng TY, et al. Anti-apoptotic proteins, apoptotic and proliferative parameters and their prognostic significance in cervical carcinoma. European Journal of Cancer. 2001;**37**(9):1104-1110

[48] Leloup L, Wells A. Calpains as potential anti-cancer targets. Expert Opinion On Therapeutic Targets. 2011;**15**(3):309-323

[49] Carragher NO. Calpain inhibition: A therapeutic strategy targeting multiple disease states. Current Pharmaceutical Design. 2006;**12**(5):615

[50] Momeni HR. Role of Calpain in apoptosis. Cell Journal (Yakhteh). 2011;**13**(2):65-72

[51] Braun C. Expression of calpain I messenger RNA in human renal cell carcinoma: Correlation with lymph node metastasis and histological type. International Journal Of Cancer. 1999;**84**(1):6

[52] Storr SJ, Woolston CM, Barros FFT, Green AR, Shehata M, Chan SY, et al. Calpain-1 expression is associated with relapse-free survival in breast cancer patients treated with trastuzumab following adjuvant chemotherapy. International Journal of Cancer. 2011;**129**(7):1773-1780

[53] Li LT, Jiang G, Chen Q, Zheng JN. Ki67 is a promising molecular target in the diagnosis of cancer (review). Molecular Medicine Reports. 2015;**11**(3):1566-1572

[54] Watanabe I. Detection of apoptotic cells in human colorectal cancer by two different in situ methods: Antibody against single-stranded DNA and terminal deoxynucleotidyl transferase-mediated dUTP-biotin nick end-labeling (TUNEL) methods. Japanese Journal Of Cancer Research. 1999;**90**(2):188

[55] Łopatniuk P. Conventional calpains and programmed cell death. Acta Biochimica Polonica. 2011;**58**(3):287

[56] Storr SJ, Carragher NO, Frame MC, Parr T, Martin SG. The calpain system and cancer. Nature Reviews Cancer. 2011;**11**(5):364-374

5

Oncoplastic Breast Surgery in the Treatment of Breast Cancer

Josie Todd

Abstract

Breast cancer is one of the commonest cancers affecting women and oncoplastic breast surgery has been firmly established as the mainstay of modern surgical treatment, replacing the traditional two-operation approach. Careful patient selection, relevance of effective communication, patient education and navigating the complex decision-making process, are some of the topics covered in this chapter. Preoperative planning, implant selection, patient marking, importance of scar placement, marking and measuring the patient preoperatively, good theatre practice, technical tips for good cosmesis, and after care; are also discussed. A brief section on revision surgery following implant reconstruction, lipomodelling and a brief overview about breast implant associated anaplastic large cell lymphoma (BIA-ALCL) and multidisciplinary approach to modern management of breast cancer. It aims to serve as a guide to surgeons on current practice and achieving the ideal balance between oncological clearance of the cancer combined with good cosmesis and high levels of patient satisfaction.

Keywords: oncoplastic breast surgery, breast cancer, scar placement, patient selection, implant reconstruction, capsular contracture

1. Introduction

Surgical management of breast cancer has undergone significant evolutionary changes since Halstead's description of radical mastectomy in 1882. Although Halstead was not credited for discovering this technique, his seminal paper published in the Annals of Surgery in 1894 demonstrated a 20% survival benefit for the first time. Not surprisingly, the Halstead mastectomy became the standard of care for the next several decades [1]. It took almost 70 years before quadrantectomy was considered a safe alternative to sacrificing the whole breast with long-term follow-up confirmed in the NSABP-B06 and Veronesi's Milan I trial [2, 3].

The term oncoplastic breast surgery (OPBS) was first coined by Werner Audretsch in the 1980s, to describe rearrangement of breast tissue to fill the defect following a partial mastectomy and recreate the breast shape, with emphasis on cosmesis. Over the last three decades, oncoplastic breast surgery has been established globally to encompass the 'quadrant-per-quadrant' approach to breast conservation advocated by Krishna Clough [4] and the Nottingham algorithm for therapeutic mammoplasty, championed by Douglas Macmillan and Stephen McCulley [5]. Introduction of biological mesh or acellular dermal matrix (ADM) in the mid-1990s defined another watershed period with increasing mastectomy rates and immediate reconstruction. Steven Kronowitz from the MD Anderson Cancer Center in Texas, USA, introduced the concept immediate-delayed reconstruction in 2002 to help women avoid the trauma of mastectomy after waking up from surgery [6].

Today, women diagnosed with a new breast cancer are offered a range of treatment options within a multidisciplinary setting [7]. Breast cancer surgery is no longer a two-operation discipline, based on cancer dimension relative to breast size or patient choice of mastectomy versus breast conservation. An oncoplastic approach to modern management of breast cancer involves careful preoperative planning with other specialists such as radiologists, pathologists and oncologists. A comprehensive breast assessment to determine the optimal breast conservation techniques is essential with emphasis on scar placement. All patients undergoing mastectomy should have a discussion around reconstruction options, where appropriate.

Good communication skills and additional time during consultation, helps safeguard patient's understanding of complex discussions around treatment. Early involvement of clinical psychologists in selected cases can help anxious patients and exclude underlying mental health concerns. Heightened anxiety at the time of diagnosis could impact decision-making and alter clinical management, with potential for decision-regret after completing treatment. Well-trained and dedicated breast care nurses are indispensable in a modern surgical breast unit [8]. Providing well designed and simple information leaflets to read outside the stressful environment of the doctor's office, can help patients navigate the complexity of the decision-making process. These combined efforts serve to demystify the various treatment options, empower women with the concept of 'patient choice' and ensure informed consent.

This chapter aims to present aspects of modern oncoplastic surgical approach in the treatment of breast cancer, with emphasis on implant-based reconstruction.

2. Oncoplastic breast surgery

Breast conserving surgery, often referred to as lumpectomy or wide local excision (WLE), is the standard treatment for the majority of early invasive and in situ breast cancer [9]. Screening programs have been established for over 60 years with early detection of small and non-palpable cancers, allowing smaller resection volumes and avoiding the need for mastectomy in most women.

2.1. Wide local excision (WLE)

Simple excision of the tumour with reasonable margins forms the basis for lumpectomy or wide local excision (WLE) and is appropriate for majority of screen-detected in situ or invasive cancer. Traditional approach of scar placement over the tumour site, without adequate mobilisation of skin or approximation of breast parenchyma and leaving the cavity to fill with seroma, was responsible for poor cosmetic outcomes in the past [10]. Volume of excision relative to breast size, location of the tumour and re-excision surgery are independent risk factors for poor cosmesis (**Figure 1**).

In a recent clinical study correlating resection volumes and tumour location with clinical photographs of patients 2 years after completing radiotherapy, was assessed by a panel and scored. Despite the small sample size, there was significant variation in the cosmetic results between oncoplastic surgeon and general breast surgeons (**Figures 2** and **3**) [11].

Oncoplastic breast surgery involves careful preoperative planning with dedicated breast radiologists in the MDT to confirm adequate clearance of the tumour from the overlying skin.

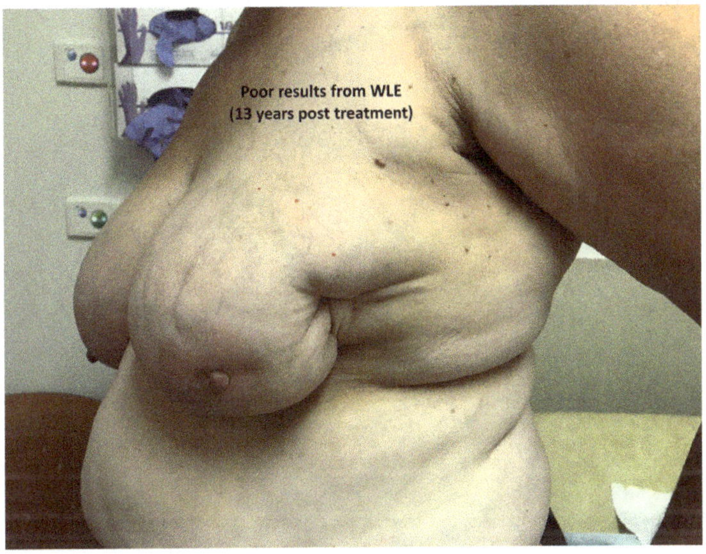

Figure 1. Poor cosmetic results from breast conserving surgery.

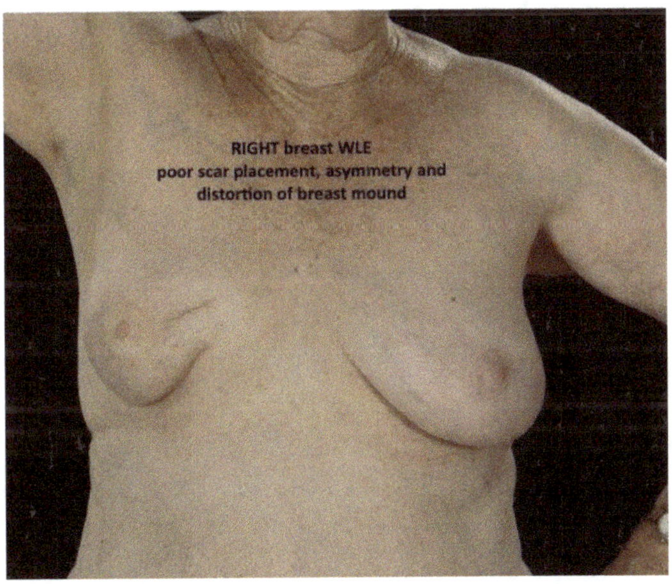

Figure 2. Clinical study results poor cosmetic outcome.

This allows aesthetically placed scars which could be remote from the tumour site and avoids disfiguring scars across the breast mound. Mobilisation and approximation of the breast parenchyma after removal of the tumour can help avoid unsightly tethering of the skin to the underlying muscle following radiotherapy (**Figure 4**). These simple measures can help ensure good cosmesis for patients whilst obtaining oncological clearance of the tumour. Almost all cases of wide local excision (WLE) are achievable via a circumareolar approach, which heals well with minimal scarring on the breast mound (**Figure 4**).

2.2. Volume displacement techniques

A number of *volume displacement* and *volume replacement* techniques in a *quadrant-per-quadrant approach* to treating breast cancer, have been described by Clough [4]. Careful assessment of the breast size, shape and density combined with preoperative estimation of resection volumes, helps determine the optimal choice of procedure. Two of the commonly used volume displacement techniques, Benelli (round block) and therapeutic mammoplasty, are discussed below.

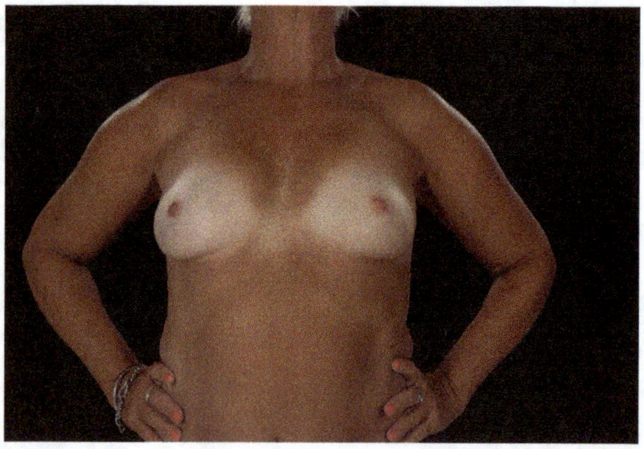

Figure 3. Clinical study results good cosmetic outcome.

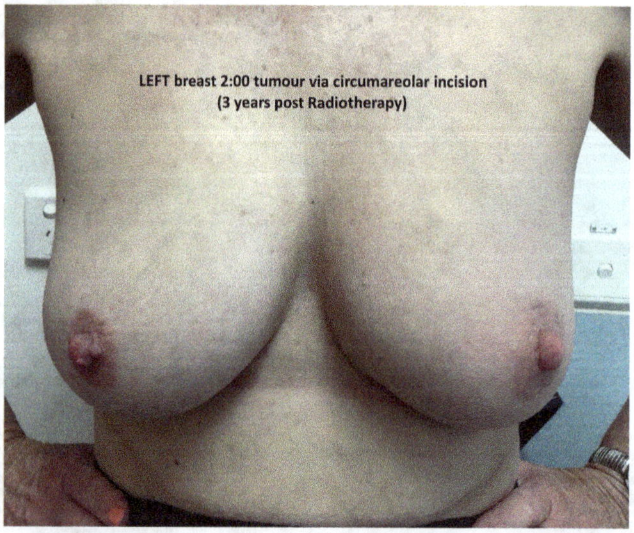

Figure 4. Wide local excision using circumareolar incision.

2.2.1. *Benelli/round-block mammoplasty*

The Benelli or round-block mammoplasty is a versatile technique used to excise tumours from various quadrants in the breast and reposition the nipple in the desired location at the end of the procedure [12]. This is essentially a variation of the *tennis racquet technique*, but without the 'handle'. The tennis racquet is a useful option if the skin overlying the tumour needs to excised and prevents the nipple from being tethered towards the index quadrant after radiotherapy and accentuating the asymmetry compared to the contralateral breast. The Benelli mammoplasty can also be used to reduce the skin envelope if required, depending on the volume of resection and the size of the patient's breasts.

Use of bilateral *round-block/Benelli mammoplasty* is illustrated in this 70-year-old patient with aged silicone implants and a new symptomatic LEFT breast cancer. The implants were more than 35 years old with MRI evidence of intra- and extracapsular rupture and silicone leakage (**Figure 5**). The tumour located in the LEFT breast at 6:00/50 mm from the nipple was excised with safe margins. Capsulectomy and removal of the aged implant was achieved through the same incision and redundant skin excised using the Benelli technique.

MRI proven ruptured aged silicone implant in the opposite breast was also removed via a similar approach with good postoperative symmetry (**Figures 6** and 7).

2.2.2. *Therapeutic mammoplasty (TM)*

Adjuvant radiotherapy in large breasted women after WLE can be difficult due to the volume of breast tissue, degree of ptosis and in some cases need to be delivered with the patient prone. *Therapeutic mammoplasty* (TM) combines breast reduction surgery and WLE to provide an opportunity for these women to achieve the desired smaller breasts, as part of their cancer treatment [13]. More importantly, breast reduction surgery after previous radiotherapy increases the risk of wound related complications and should only be undertaken by experienced plastic and oncoplastic breast surgeons. For women with large breasts, TM allows large excision volumes with excellent margins, beyond the conventional threshold for simple

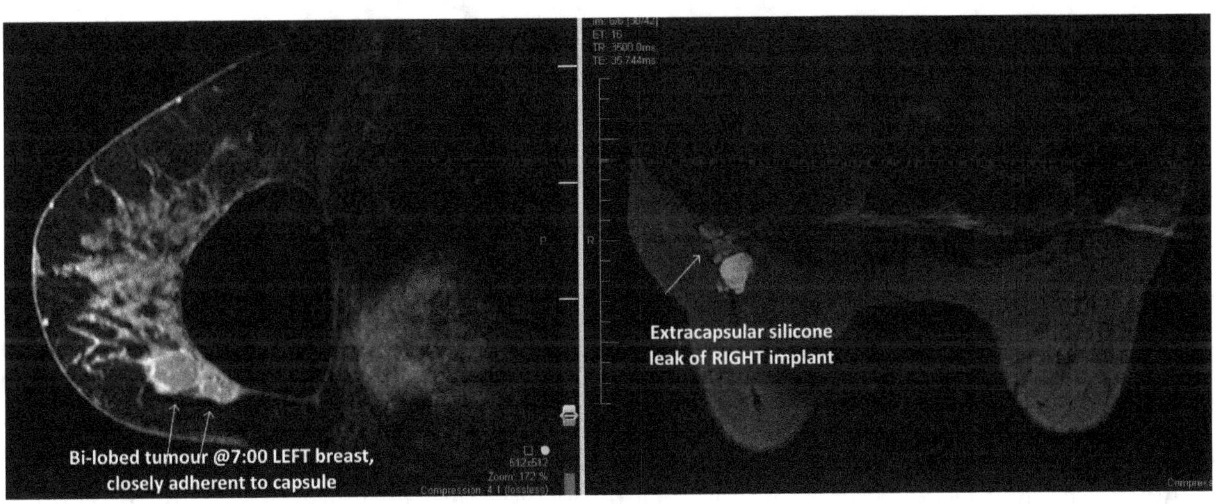

Figure 5. Pre-op MRI demonstrating tumour and silicone leak.

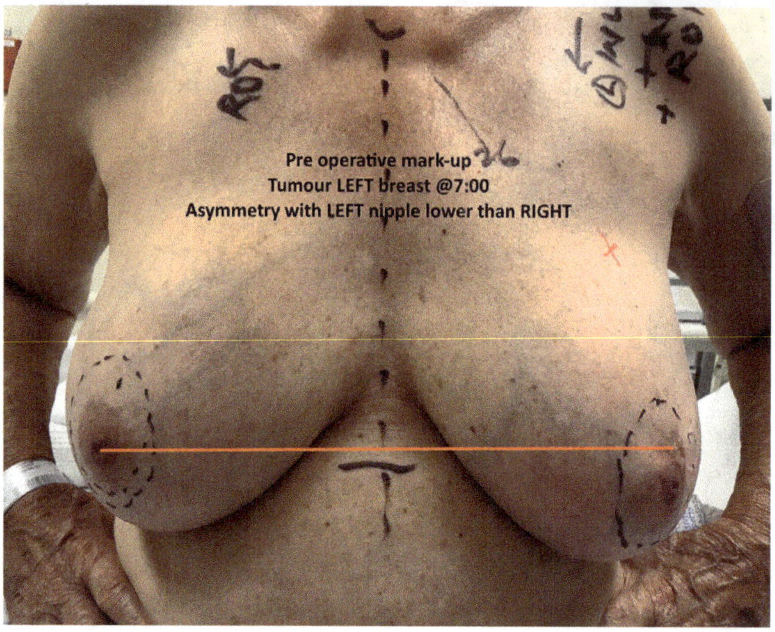

Figure 6. Pre-op capsular contracture and Benelli mammaplasty.

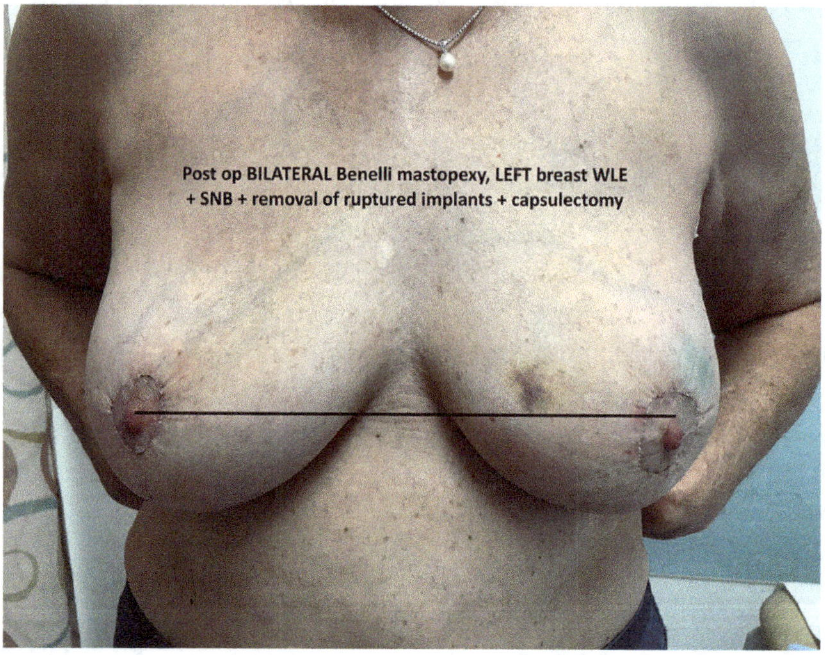

Figure 7. Post-op round block mammaplasty.

WLE. Secondary pedicles of tissue which are usually excised as part of breast reduction surgery are used to fill the WLE defect. Recovery from surgery is similar to simple mastectomy without any delay in adjuvant therapy (**Figures 8** and **9**).

The nipple-areolar complex (NAC) can be sacrificed in older patients to minimise the risk of nipple necrosis and wound complications. The NAC may also need to be removed when the tumour is located close to the nipple to ensure oncological safe margins. TM in this setting

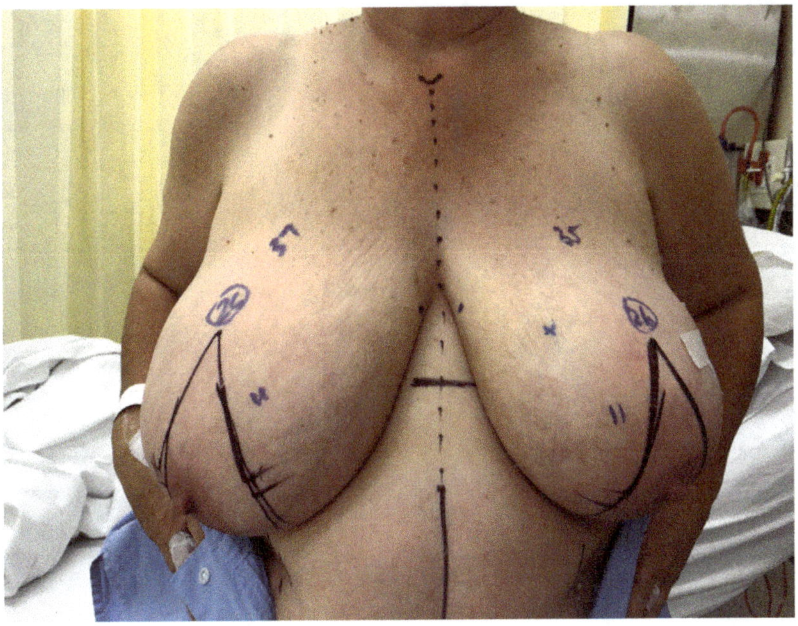

Figure 8. Pre-op therapeutic mammaplasty.

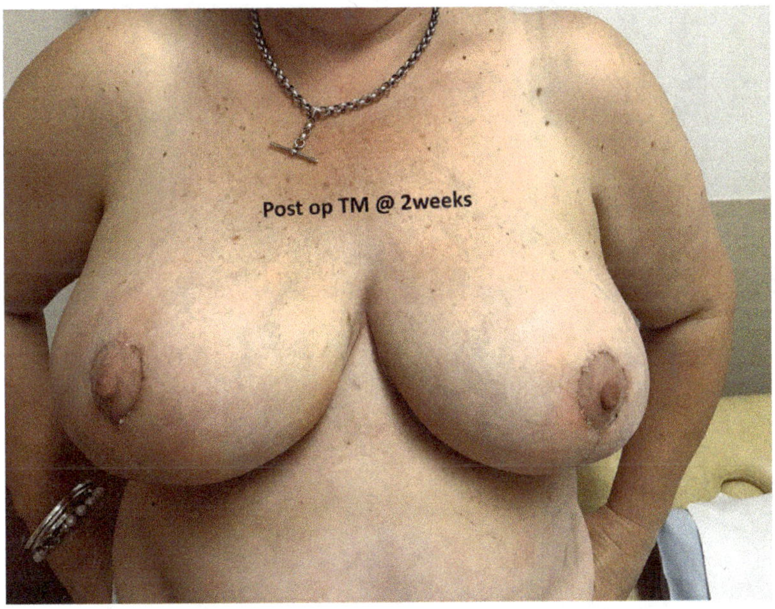

Figure 9. Post-op therapeutic mammaplasty.

provides a better alternative to mastectomy for these patients and avoids large and heavy external prosthesis to match the contralateral normal breast [14]. In this example, an 83-year-old lady with large ptotic J-cup sized breasts presented with symptomatic 45 mm RIGHT breast cancer @12:00, with associated 110 mm of suspicious calcification extending to the nipple (**Figure 10**).

Bracketed hook-wire was used preoperatively to mark the extent of calcification to ensure safe margins and confirmed on final histology (**Figure 11**). Despite the extensive nature of surgery,

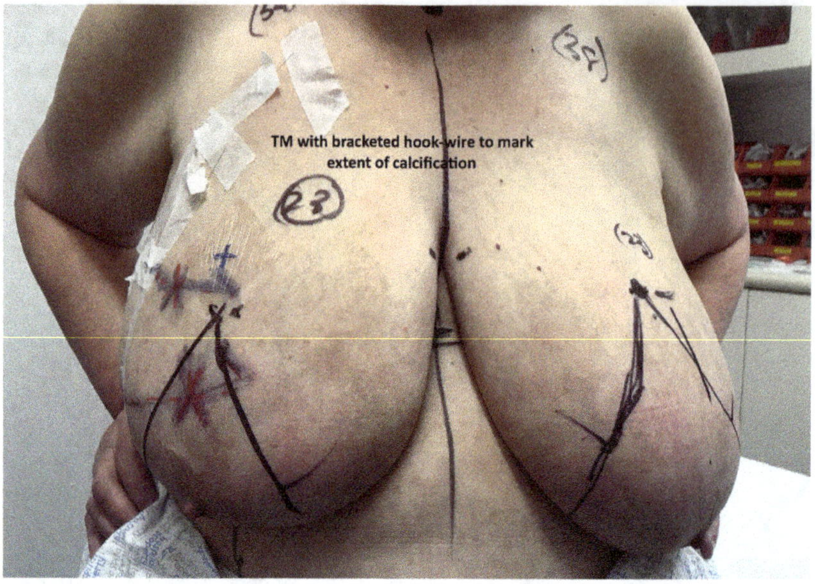

Figure 10. Pre-op hook-wire and markings for TM.

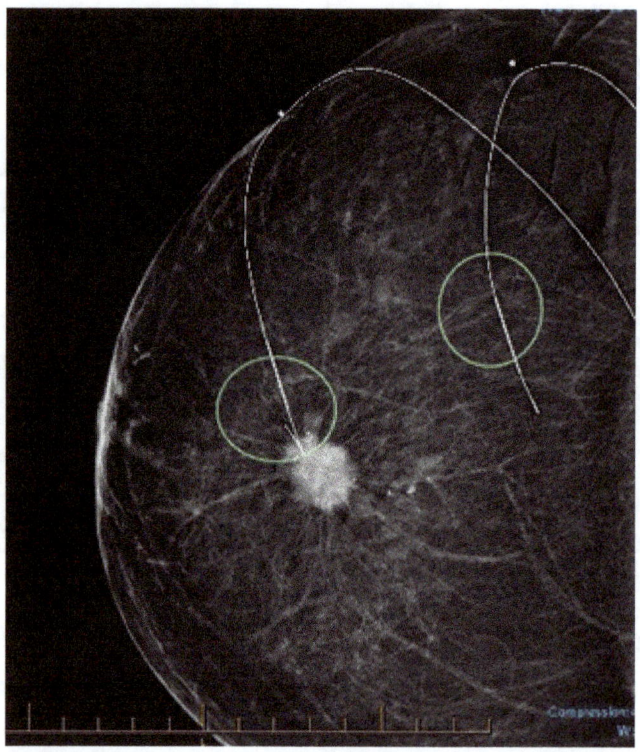

Figure 11. Bracketed hook-wire.

TM confers a high degree of patient satisfaction, without any delay in adjuvant treatment or significant morbidity; even in older patients (**Figure 12**). Well-trained breast care nurses are essential for preoperative patient education and managing complex wounds after surgery.

2.3. Volume replacement techniques

Several volume replacement techniques, such as mini-latissimus dorsi (LD), lateral thoracic artery perforator (L-TAP), intercostal artery perforators (I-CAP), serratus anterior artery perforator

(SAAP) and thoracodorsal artery perforator (T-DAP) flaps have been described to fill large defects created by WLE. Mini-LD flaps should be avoided in this setting and the latissimus dorsi muscle preserved as salvage tissue cover for complex locally advanced and recurrent disease, for lower pole support instead of mesh or as definitive reconstruction option following mastectomy.

2.3.1. *Autologous adipo-dermal perforator flaps*

The original pedicled perforator flaps described by Mustafa Hamdi in 1984 included thoracodorsal artery perforator (T-DAP), intercostal artery perforator (ICAP), serratus anterior

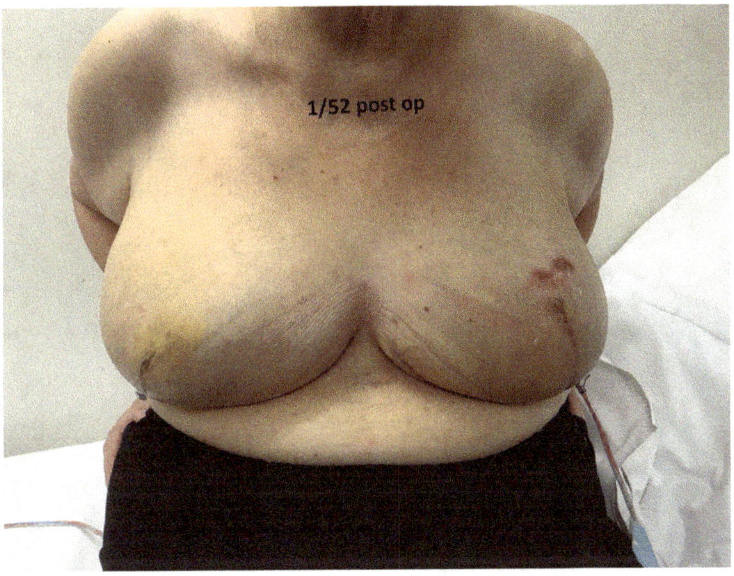

Figure 12. Post-op TM sacrificing the NAC.

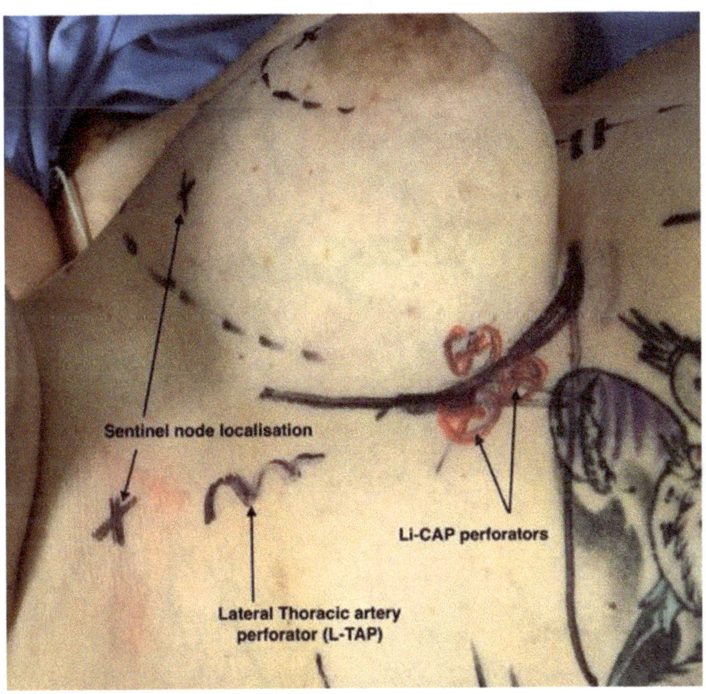

Figure 13. Pre-op marking of L-TAP and Li-CAP vessels with USS Doppler.

artery perforator (SAAP) and superior epigastric artery perforator (SEAP) flaps for immediate or delayed partial breast reconstruction or as adjuncts to implant reconstruction [15]. These versatile perforator flaps can be used to fill parenchymal defects in almost any quadrant of the breast. This technique allows large excision volumes to ensure good resection margins and the size of the flap can be adjusted to achieve good cosmesis.

The Li-CAP and T-DAP vessels are marked preoperatively with handheld Doppler's or USS colour Doppler mode prior to skin incision (**Figure 13**). These flaps utilise the skin and subcutaneous fat in the lateral chest wall and are raised on small and consistent perforator vessels (**Figure 14**).

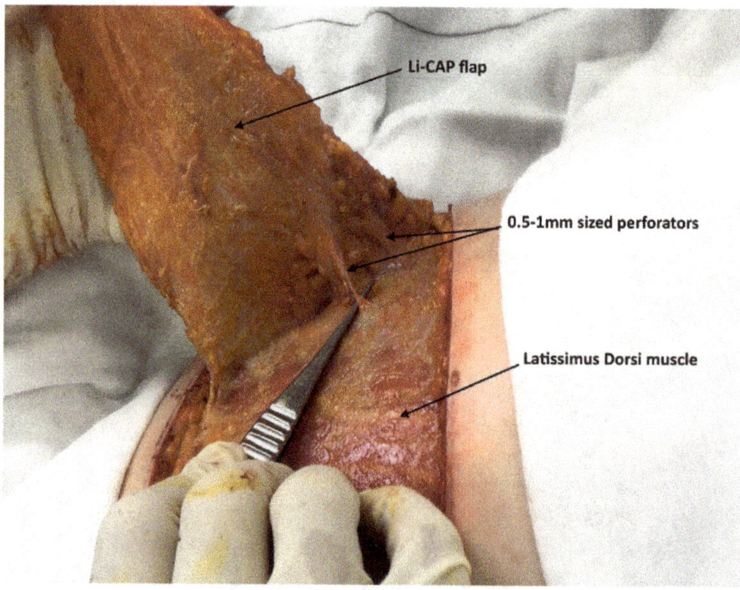

Figure 14. Perforator vessels for Li-CAP flap.

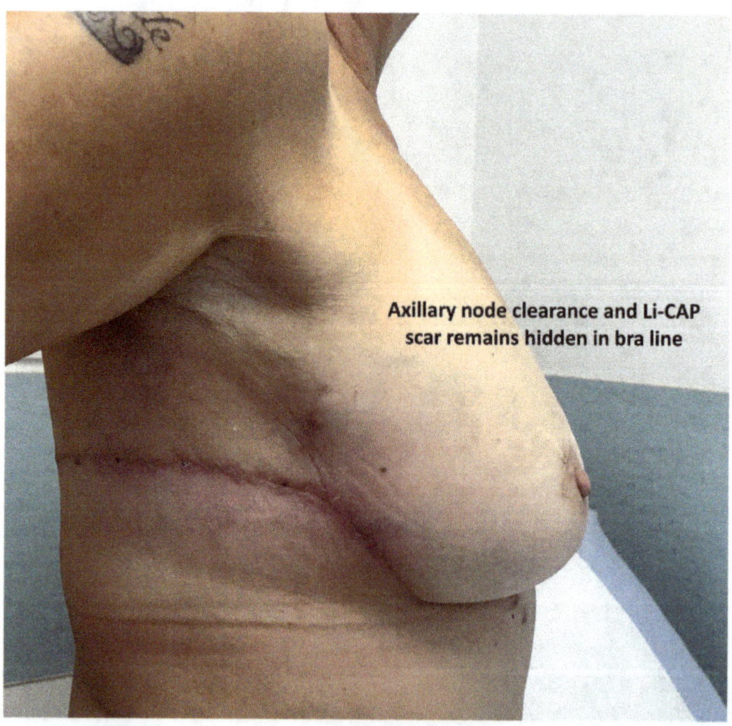

Figure 15. Lateral scar after volume replacement with Li-CAP flap.

The length of the scar is variable depending on the volume required for replacement and is mostly hidden within the bra, with less donor site morbidity compared to traditional LD flap (**Figure 15**). These autologous perforator flaps are robust and appear to tolerate radiation therapy without significant volume loss. They serve as ideal volume replacement options for high-risk patients such as diabetics, smokers and older patients, without compromising flap viability.

Two-stage procedure is recommended by the Nottingham group, particularly if the extent of disease is unclear on diagnostic imaging. WLE and axillary surgery is completed as the first stage and the cavity filled with water to keep the cavity patent. Once the histology confirms adequate margins, patients can undergo the second stage to recruit the perforator flap (**Figures 16** and **17**). If the pathology demonstrates more extensive disease than originally

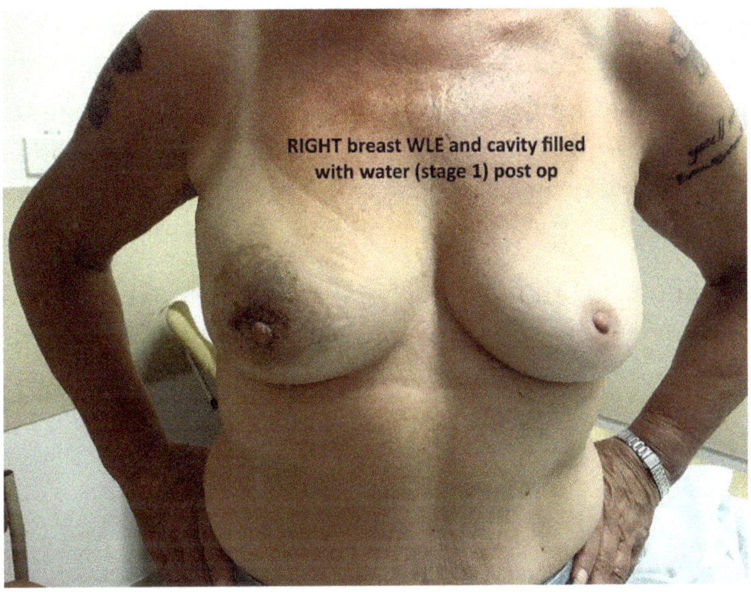

Figure 16. After first stage WLE cavity filled with water.

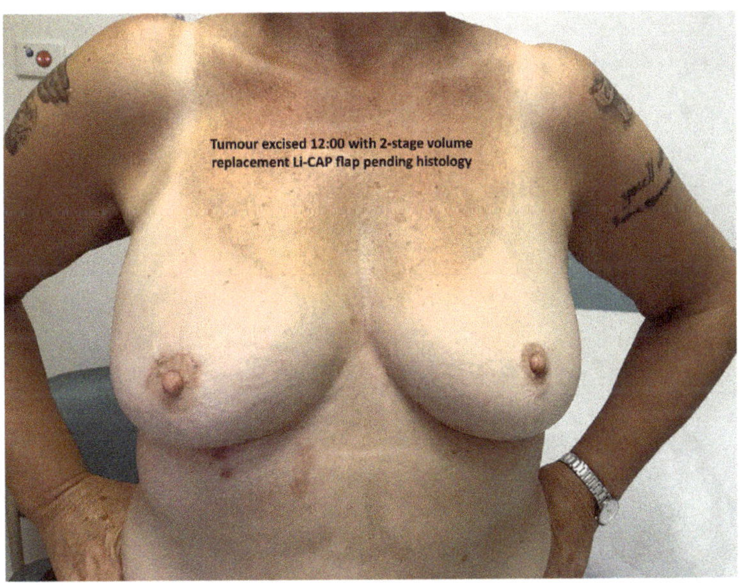

Figure 17. Post-op photo after volume replacement with Li-CAP.

anticipated, patients could be offered re-excision of margins or conversion to mastectomy. A two-stage procedure helps avoid wasting a good flap in the initial stage and serves as a bridge to definitive surgery.

3. Mastectomy and breast reconstruction

Simple mastectomy is a good surgical option for elderly patients, women living in remote areas with limited access to radiotherapy and those who do not wish to undergo immediate reconstruction (**Figure 18**). Increasing number of women is choosing to have mastectomy with immediate reconstruction instead of breast conservation [16].

'A good reconstruction starts with a good mastectomy' is an often quoted by oncoplastic breast surgeons and advocated by the Nottingham Breast Unit, UK. Historically, free-transverse rectus abdominis (TRAM) flap or deep inferior epigastric artery perforator (DIEP) flap has been regarded as the gold standard for breast reconstruction [17]. This is a significant undertaking for patients with prolonged hospital stay, delayed recovery and donor site morbidity. Not surprisingly, the incidence of these complex autologous flaps has remained static compared to the exponential increase in implant reconstruction over the past three decades [18].

Latissimus dorsi (LD) flap with implant (**Figure 19**) was a common reconstruction procedure post mastectomy in the 1980s and 1990s, due to the robust nature of the flap, consistent aesthetic results and acceptable donor site morbidity compared to TRAM flap. The incidence of LD has declined with the increasing incidence of implant reconstruction in the late 1990s and early 2000s. More recently, there appears to be a resurgence of LD flaps, according to MD Anderson data [18].

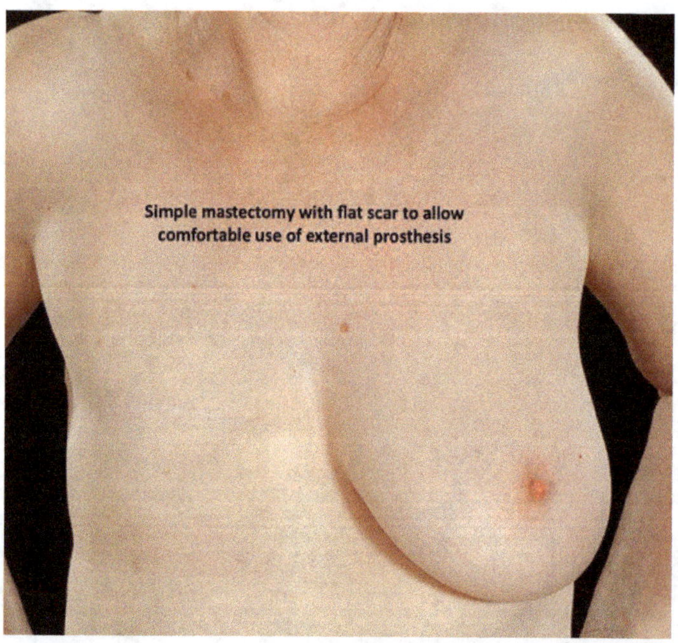

Figure 18. Right simple mastectomy.

The chest wall perforator flaps (L-TAP and Li-CAP) can also be used as complete autologous flap reconstruction following mastectomy and was first described by Losken and Hamdi in 2009 [19, 20]. This is a safe reconstruction option in the high-risk candidates, such as smokers, raised BMI, diabetics, or in patients where implant or complex autologous reconstructions are relatively contraindicated due to post-operative radiotherapy (**Figures 20** and **21**).

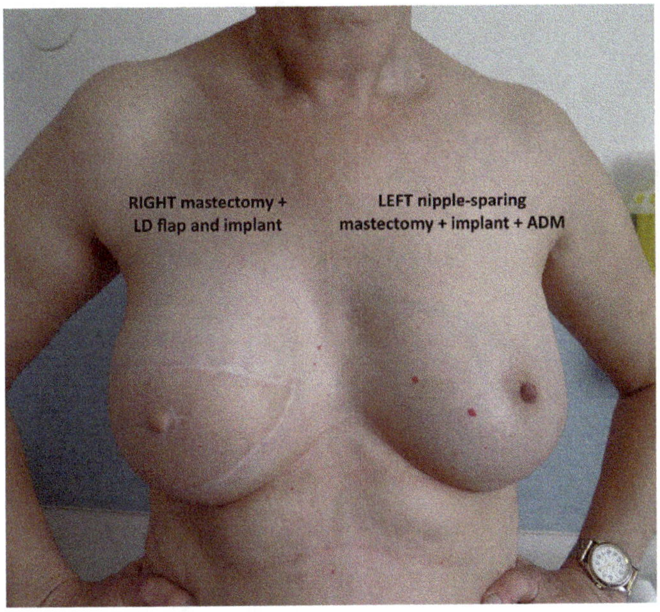

Figure 19. Right mastectomy with immediate LD flap and left mastectomy with implant reconstruction.

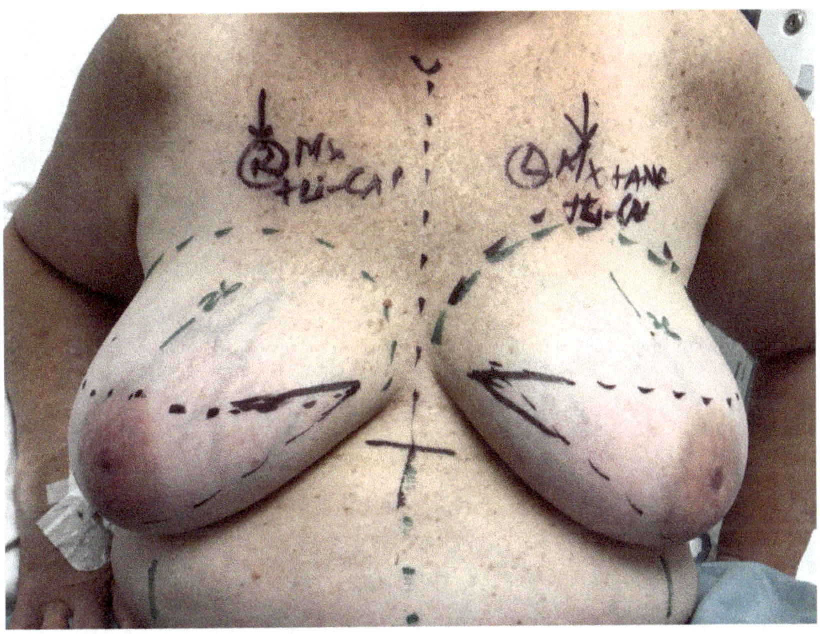

Figure 20. Pre-op marking bilateral mastectomy following neoadjuvant chemotherapy.

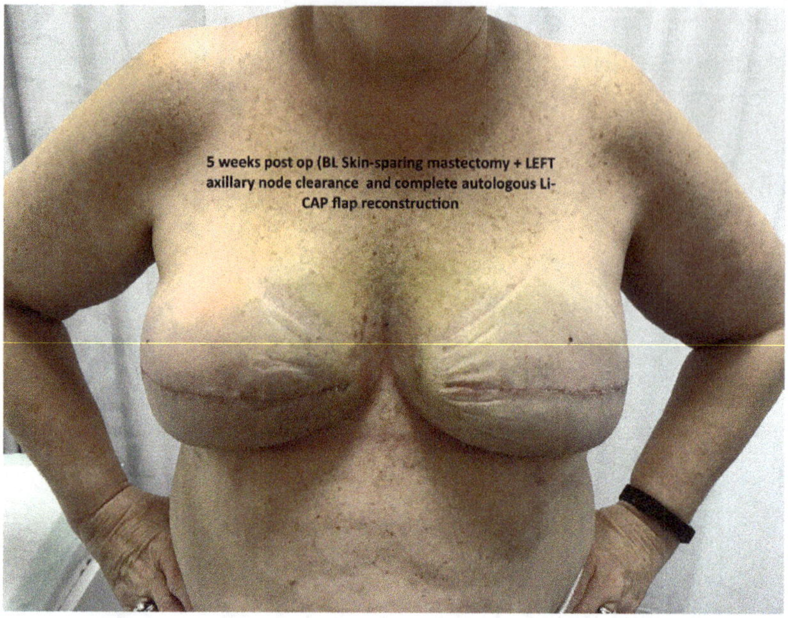

Figure 21. Post-op bilateral skin-sparing mastectomy with immediate Li-CAP flap reconstruction.

4. Mesh versus autologous tissue for lower pole support

Since its introduction in the late 1990s, the acellular dermal matrix (ADM), derived from various biological sources, has been responsible for the meteoric rise in mastectomy rates with implant and tissue expander reconstruction [21]. There is a substantial global market for ADM or biological meshes currently manufactured from porcine dermis, foetal or neonatal bovine dermis, bovine pericardium and human cadaveric skin.

Parallel to the success of ADM, there has also been an increase in synthetic mesh used for lower pole support in implant and tissue expander reconstruction (**Table 1**). The main driver for synthetic mesh has stemmed from cost associated with ADM, reports of 'red breast syndrome' (RBS) and higher seroma rates [22]. The 'red breast syndrome' (RBS) is a unique delayed hypersensitivity reaction to ADM and presents as erythematous skin overlying the mesh. Despite lack of febrile response and normal laboratory markers which characterises RBS, patients often receive increasing amounts of unnecessary antibiotics, due to concerns for the underlying implant [23].

The absorbable synthetic TIGR mesh produces a stable IMF after 18 months post-reconstruction compared to ADM with lower implant loss rates and half the volume of seroma output in the author's experience (**Figure 22**) [24].

In one of the largest reported series of TIGR mesh since May 2014, a total of 138 cases in 87 consecutive patients undergoing immediate or delayed reconstruction were recently presented in the Annual Scientific Congress of RACS (Royal Australasian College of Surgeons) in Sydney, Australia, in May 2018. There was no 90-day post-operative implant loss reported in the author's series, with three cases of delayed implant loss at 5, 12 and 28 months following radiotherapy. There were no cases of skin flap necrosis or RBS in this series [25]. These results

Mesh	ADM/synthetic	Source	Manufacturer
Strattice	ADM	Porcine	LifeCell Corp.
Permacol	ADM	Porcine	Covidien
SurgiMend	ADM	Foetal/neonatal bovine dermis	Integra LifeScience Ltd.
VERITAS	ADM	Bovine pericardium	Synovis Surgical innovations, St. Paul, MN, USA®
Alloderm	ADM	Human cadaveric skin	LifeCell Corp. Branchburg. N.J
Epiflex	ADM	Human cadaveric skin	Deutsches Institut für Zell-und Gewebeersatz [DIZG] gGmbH, Berlin, Germany
ALLOMAX™	ADM	Human cadaveric skin	Bard, Inc.
DermaMatrix®	ADM	Human cadaveric skin	Synthesis CMF/Johnson & Johnson
TIGR	Synthetic absorbable		Novus Scientific
TiLoop® Bra	Synthetic titanium coated		pfm medical, Cologne, Germany
SERAGYN BR®	Synthetic		SERAG-WIESSNER GmbH & Co. KG

Table 1. Current list of ADM and synthetic mesh used for implant and tissue expander reconstruction.

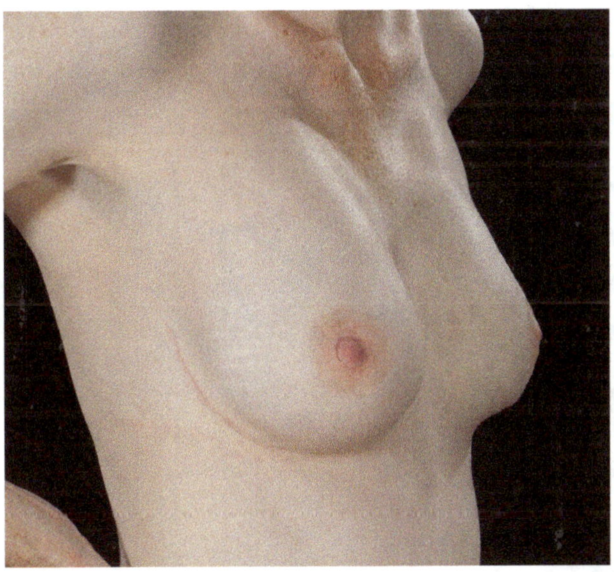

Figure 22. Nipple-sparing mastectomy via inframammary fold incision and retropectoral implant reconstruction and TIGR mesh.

are similar to a recent publication by Pompei et al., with 49 consecutive patients and 60 TIGR mesh used over a 2-year period with only 1 implant loss due to skin necrosis [26].

The following is the example of nipple-sparing mastectomy, axillary node clearance with immediate expander-implant reconstruction in a 54-year-old woman with previous breast implants and multifocal triple negative breast cancer with nodal involvement (**Figures 23–25**). Patient developed significant lymphangitis and cellulitis of the breast skin envelope 28 months after radiotherapy with explantation and request for contralateral symmetrising mastectomy.

The two-stage tissue expander (TE) reconstruction with limited mobilisation of the serratus muscle and pectoralis major was the standard procedure prior to ADM or synthetic mesh for lower pole support. The results were often inconsistent with high-riding TE and need for revision surgery. The nipple-areolar complex (NAC) and most of the redundant mastectomy skin envelope in medium to large breasted women had to be sacrificed due to limited capacity of the muscle pocket. Stable inframammary fold (IMF), preservation of the native mastectomy skin flap, retropectoral direct to implant reconstruction with predictable aesthetic results and relatively short learning curve; are some of the reasons for the exponential global uptake of biological and synthetic mesh. Shorter operative time and hospital stay, earlier recovery and return to normal function with less donor site morbidity and high patient satisfaction rates have also contributed to its popularity.

More recently, use of prepectoral implant with complete ADM coverage appears to have good outcomes with high levels of patient satisfaction [27]. 'Animation' or variable movement of the reconstructed breast when tensing the pectoral muscles is a recognised issue with retropectoral implant reconstruction (Video: https://mts.intechopen.com/download/index/process/270/authkey/a5ea41ce666a3344dd2e459c34b3d46a). The prepectoral technique circumvents the 'animation' problem and patients are able to return to physical activity without the usual restrictions of retropectoral surgery.

Any contour defect due to capsular contracture or tethering of skin to the pectoral fascia above the implant, can be addressed with fat grafting; either at the index operation or as

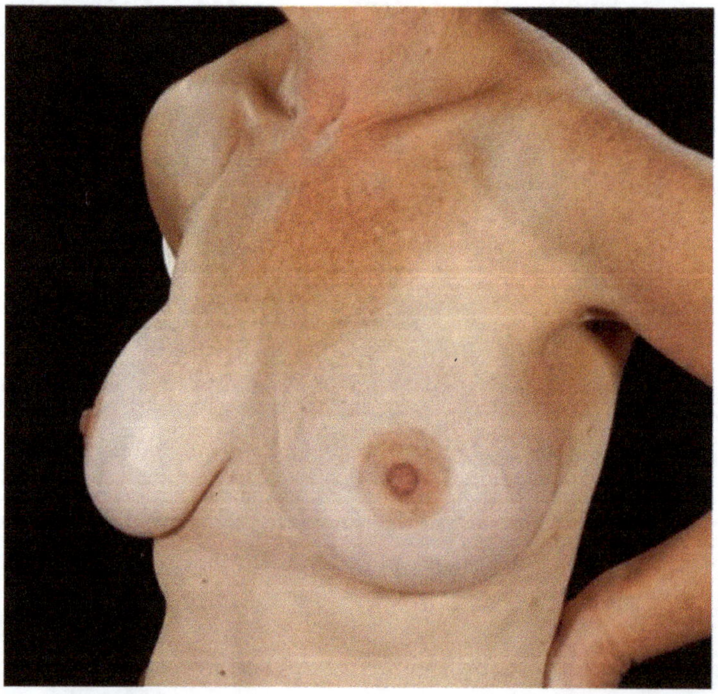

Figure 23. Left nipple-sparing mastectomy with immediate expander-implant reconstruction.

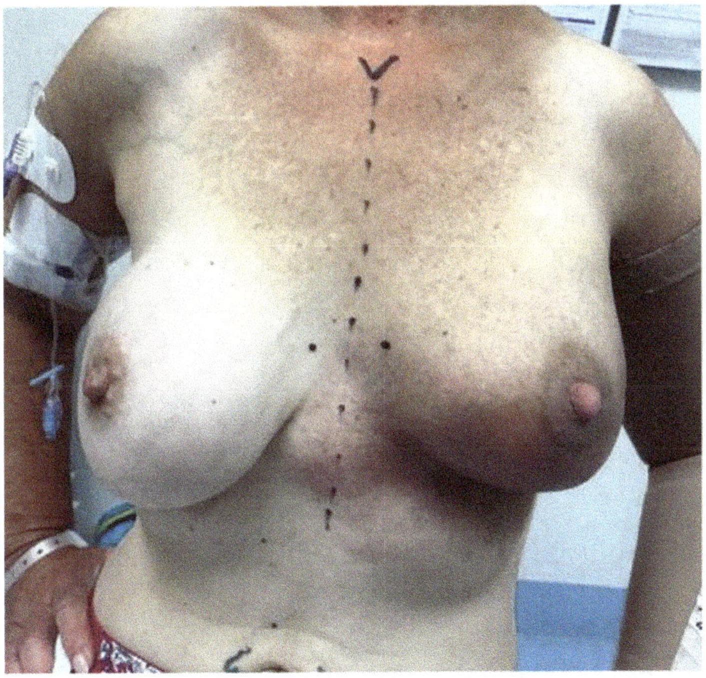

Figure 24. Cellulitis 28 months after radiotherapy.

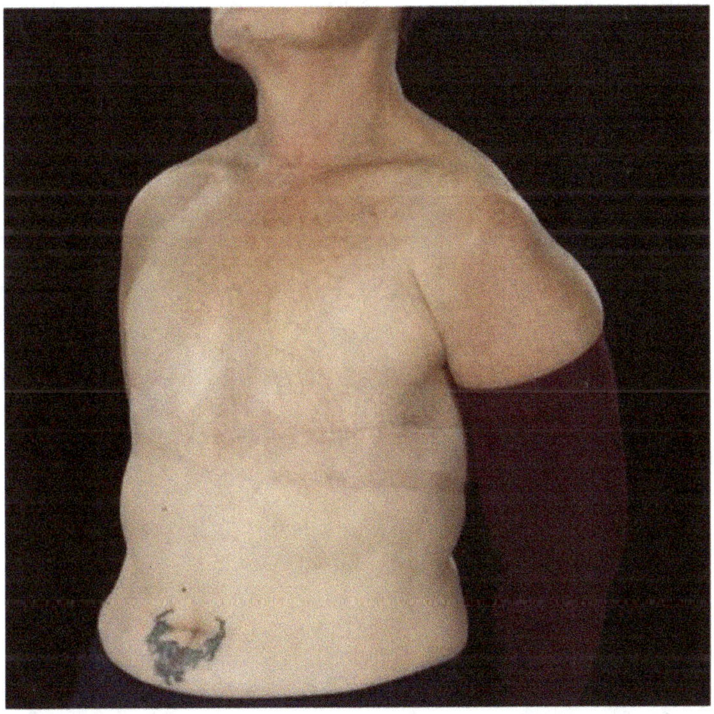

Figure 25. Bilateral mastectomy post explantation and request for delayed reconstruction.

a delayed procedure. In very slim patients without significant subcutaneous body fat, prepectoral approach may be challenging with 'ghosting' effect from the underlying implant. Braxon ADM (designed and patented by DECOmed s.r.l.) is a specially designed biological mesh, which offers complete coverage of the implant for prepectoral placement with the added convenience of suturing the mesh directly onto the chest wall.

Despite the significant global trend towards ADM and synthetic mesh-assisted implant reconstruction, recent years have also witnessed a resurgence in autologous tissue for inferior pole support, such as scar-less mini-LD flap and T-DAP flap. ADM associated 'red breast syndrome RBS', less than anticipated reduction in capsular contracture, higher seroma rates and secondary infection with implant loss; may account for this parallel rise in autologous tissue support. Some permanent synthetic meshes can result in higher rates of capsular contracture with firm tissue in the lower pole, resulting in long-term discomfort. Continued technological advances in lightweight synthetic mesh which integrate better with the host tissue, could help improve cosmetic outcomes for patients.

5. Tissue expander versus direct to implant reconstruction

The two-stage tissue expander (TE) is the standard reconstruction technique following skin-sparing or nipple-sparing mastectomy in most Western countries. TE is a safer option than direct to implant, particularly when there is uncertainty about the need for post-operative radiotherapy. Many surgeons continue to advocate the two-stage tissue expander reconstruction due to concerns about skin flap viability and risk of implant failure. Use of TE allows the mastectomy skin flap to heal without undue tension and risk of necrosis.

Two-stage tissue expander reconstruction is an option for women who wish to achieve larger cup size after breast reconstruction (**Figures 26** and **27**). The expander is replaced with a definitive implant as a second operation after completion of adjuvant therapy (such as chemotherapy). It is possible to deliver radiotherapy in women with tissue expanders or implants without compromising treatment. Patients need to be counselled about the increased risks of wound breakdown, implant infection and reconstruction failure in this setting. Use of adjustable expander-implants with a mini-remote port placed outside the radiotherapy field is helpful in reducing CT artefact during planning. There is a wide variation in the delivery of radiotherapy depending on centres.

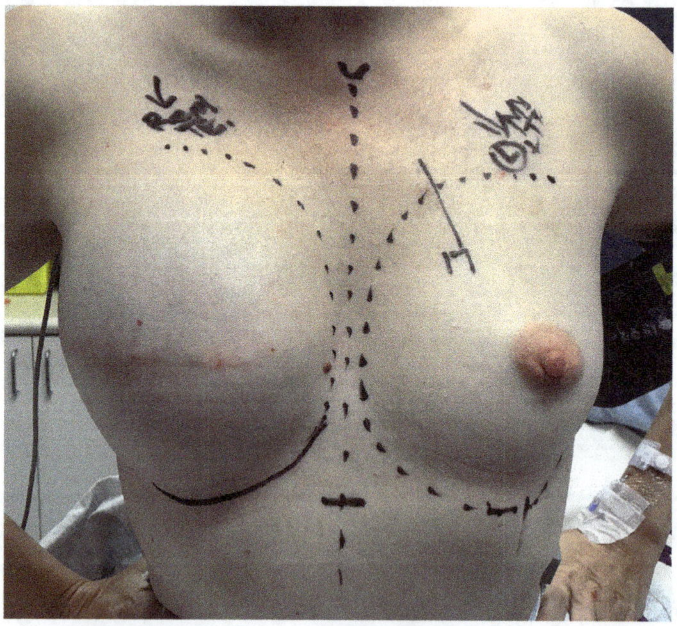

Figure 26. Right two-stage TE and left prophylactic TE reconstruction.

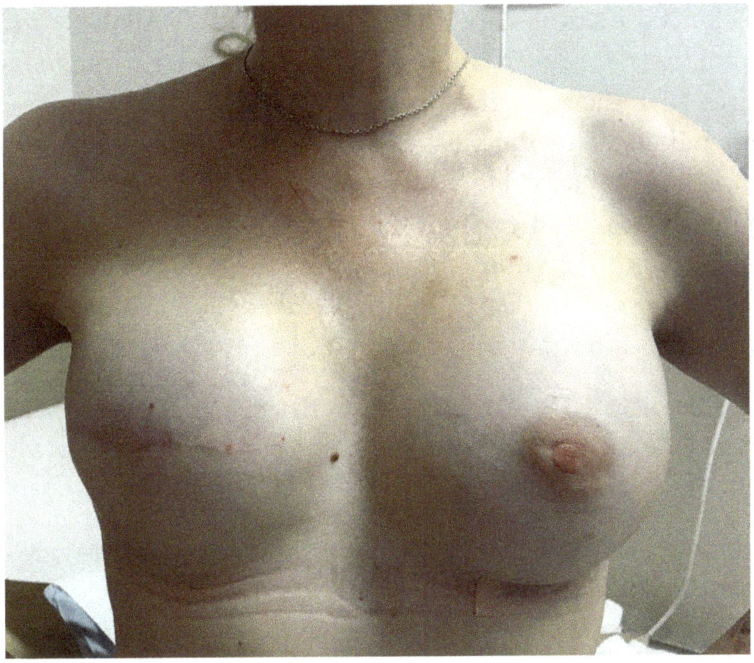

Figure 27. Final result replacement left TE with implant.

Many radiation oncologists are reluctant to deliver treatment in the presence of tissue expanders with integrated ports due to the large area of the metal backing in the port, uncertainty about treatment delivery in the area and concerns with raised temperatures and skin burn from treatment. Despite the higher risks, two-stage TE serves as a bridge to definitive reconstruction after completion of radiotherapy and helps preserve the mastectomy skin flap.

In patients who have not had radiotherapy, minor adjustments in the pocket or IMF is achievable in the second stage, but the basic footprint of the reconstruction is designed at the primary operation. Patients should be measured carefully in the clinic prior to surgery as a guide to ordering appropriate sized implants.

Newer technology such as SPY *Elite* system for intraoperative monitoring of skin flap viability and vascular supply and use of newer diathermy devices such as PlasmaBlade (Medtronic plc. ®), which ensures lower tissue temperatures during dissection, can help minimise the risk of skin flap necrosis. Basic surgical principles of gentle tissue handling, avoiding undue traction of the skin flap or use of traumatic instruments at the skin edges, keeping the patient warm perioperatively, avoiding unnecessarily thin mastectomy skin flaps, resting the flap regularly and ensuring tension-free closure of the skin over the implant reconstruction; are simple ways to avoid skin flap necrosis.

6. Nipple-sparing and skin-sparing mastectomy

The safety of nipple-sparing mastectomy, depending on tumour location, has been adequately established for both in situ and early invasive breast cancer [28]. Careful preoperative assessment to ensure adequate clearance of the skin and nipple from the tumour site helps to ensure reasonable margins and reduce the risk of recurrence.

Skin-sparing mastectomy is a simpler option in central tumours involving the NAC (**Figure 26**). This is also the commonest approach utilised by general breast surgeons when undertaking combined procedures with their plastic surgery colleagues. The volume of skin excised and scar placement is often dictated by the plastic surgeon. Upfront sentinel node biopsy is carried out as a separate operation to accurately stage the axilla, prior to any reconstruction. If the axillary nodes are involved with metastatic cancer, patients are more likely to require post-operative radiotherapy. In this situation, plastic surgeons may decline immediate implant or autologous reconstruction such as LD or DIEP flap, due to poor aesthetic outcomes and higher reconstruction failure rates after radiotherapy [29, 30].

Nipple-sparing mastectomy with direct-to-implant reconstruction in the immediate setting is a safe option in experienced hands and avoids the need for a second procedure (**Figures 28** and **29**).

The IMF incision confers adequate access for undertaking mastectomy, axillary surgery and placement of mesh for lower pole support of the implant. Temporary sizers help to determine the optimal implant size and confirm tension-free wound closure. This is an important step as the mastectomy skin envelope should drape the implant rather than stretched across it. The mastectomy skin flap relies on the fine sub-dermal capillaries for its blood supply. This could potentially be compromised with excessively large implants and tight closure of the IMF and result in skin flap necrosis.

Gentle tissue handling, avoiding excessive forceful retraction and preserving the subcutaneous fat layer during mastectomy, are some of the essential steps in preserving the integrity of the mastectomy skin flap. Poor technique is probably the commonest cause for skin flap necrosis and is often reflective of inadequate training and failure to adhere to basic principles outlined above. The product often gets blamed for inferior outcomes in some of the online publications.

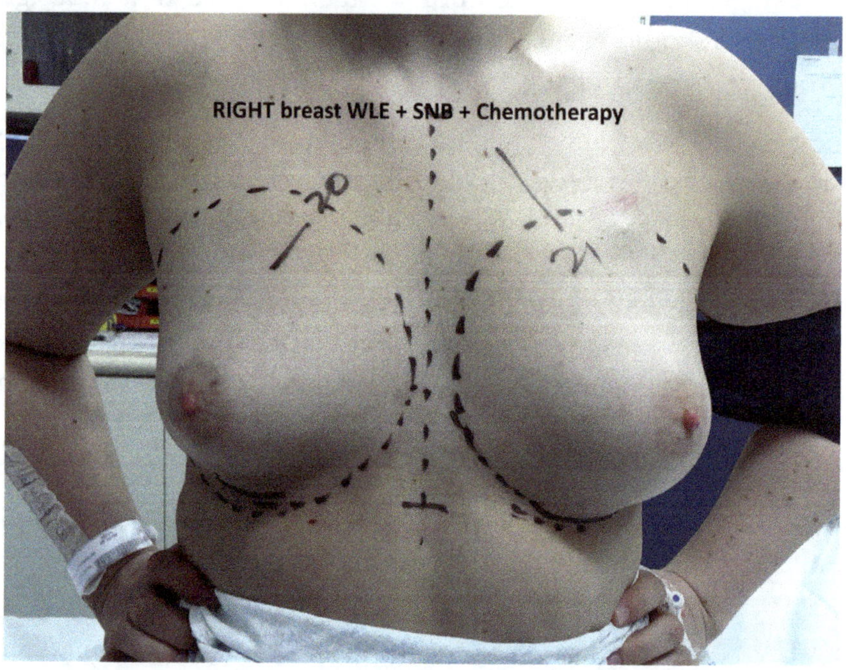

Figure 28. Post-neoadjuvant chemo BL nipple-sparing mastectomy.

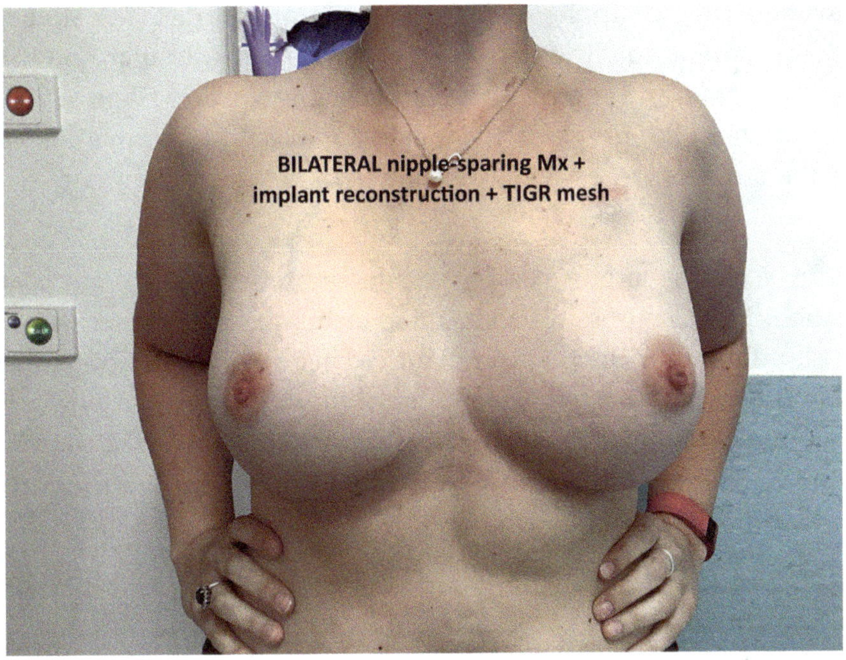

Figure 29. Six months after retropectoral implant reconstruction and TIGR mesh.

A single drain is left in the space between the skin flap and the mesh to remove the seroma following mastectomy. The drain is left in until the daily output slows down to approximately 30 ml/day. Build-up of seroma can cause additional tension along the wound edge or affect circulation of the skin flap and must be monitored carefully in the early post-operative period. Seroma formation is much lower with TIGR mesh compared to some ADM's in the author's own presented series [24].

Careful patient selection is important and direct implant reconstruction is best avoided in smokers and high-risk candidates such as diabetics and women with raised BMI. It is essential to have a well-trained, dedicated breast care nurse who is qualified in wound care management. Educating patients about postoperative recovery and precautions about physical activities in the initial months after surgery helps ensure good cosmesis and minimises the risk of wound-related complications.

7. Skin-reducing mastectomy, with or without nipple preservation

Nipple-sparing mastectomy is usually carried out via the IMF approach in small- to medium-sized breasts. It is possible to achieve nipple-sparing mastectomy in larger patients who wish to remain the similar size, via the same approach. In younger patients, some degree of skin contraction is achievable but decline in collagen levels with normal ageing process can result in redundant skin flaps.

Most large breasted women, however, are keen to achieve a smaller reconstructed breast volume and skin-reducing mastectomy techniques can be used with immediate implant reconstruction, with or without nipple preservation. Patients need to be cautioned about a higher than average risk of nipple necrosis with complex surgery. A skin reducing wise-pattern mastectomy using bi-pedicle dermal flap to maintain vascular integrity of the NAC is described by the author and recently accepted for publication (**Figures 30** and **31**). This technique is a variation of the previously published modified Letterman technique [31] and early results of the author's series were presented as poster at the Leura 8 Conference in Sydney 2016.

This technique can be used in large breasted women for immediate implant-based and autologous reconstruction. It is also possible to use this technique for revision surgery to address any redundant skin flap after previous implant reconstruction. The bi-pedicle dermal flap provides variable length for adjusting the nipple height to the desired position based on the final breast volume and maintains dual vascular supply to the NAC. The dermal flap also protects the incision site from the underlying implant and mesh and minimises risk of implant infection or reconstruction failure.

Tension-free closure of the wound helps reduce pressure on the skin flap and NAC from the underlying implant and protects the fine sub-dermal capillaries supplying the skin flap following mastectomy (**Figure 32**). Use of drains to anticipate any seroma formation and post-operative swelling also helps mitigate the additional risk at the suture line and viability of the NAC.

Goldilocks mastectomy with implant reconstruction, using a wise-pattern skin incision and dermal flap for lower pole support has been previously described. The nipple vasculature is maintained on the superior pedicle only and is best avoided in older patients or high-risk women such as smokers, diabetics and raised BMI [32].

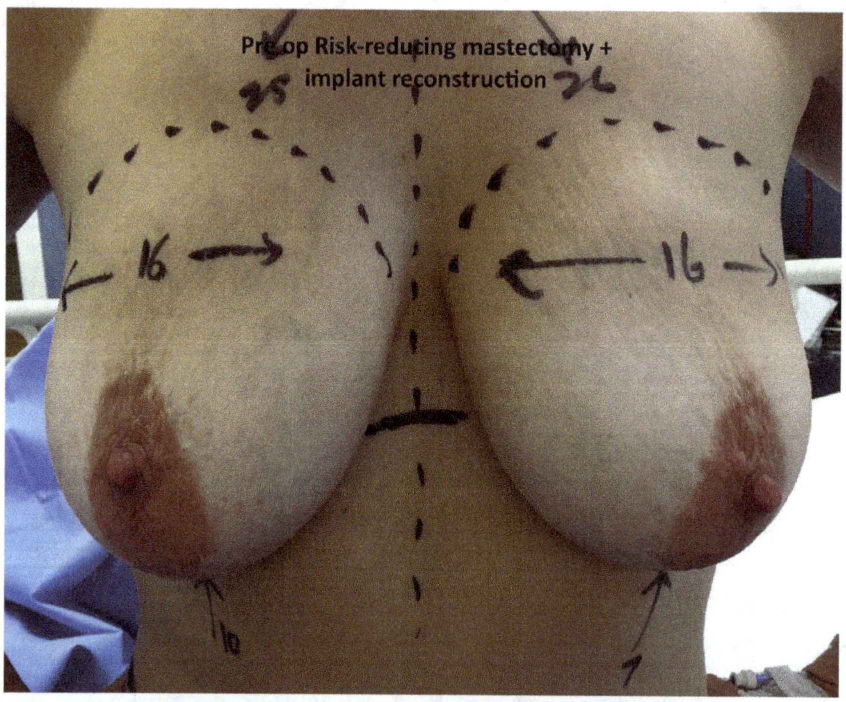

Figure 30. Pre-operative skin-reducing mastectomy.

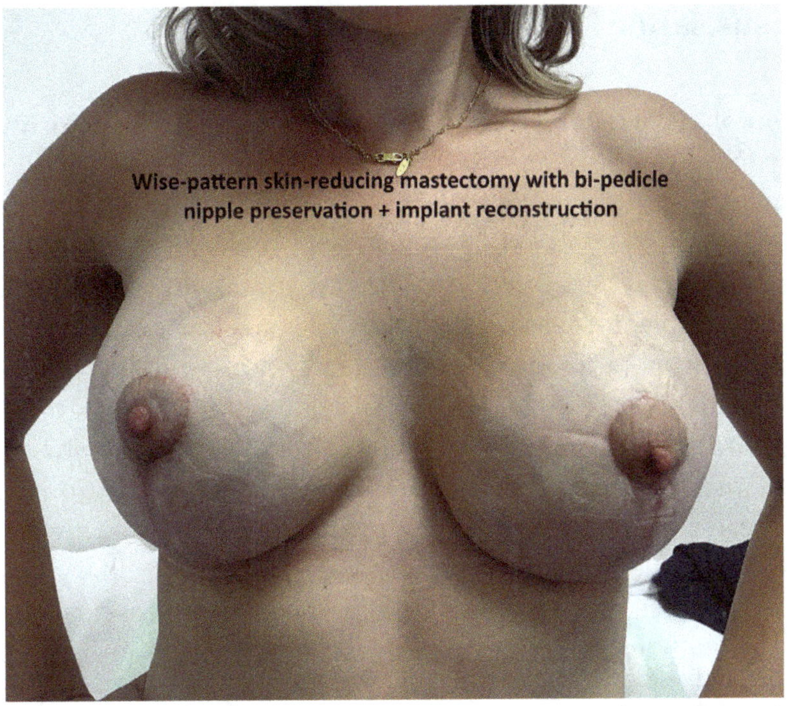

Figure 31. Wise pattern skin-reducing nipple-sparing mastectomy using bi-pedicle dermal flap and implant reconstruction with TIGR mesh.

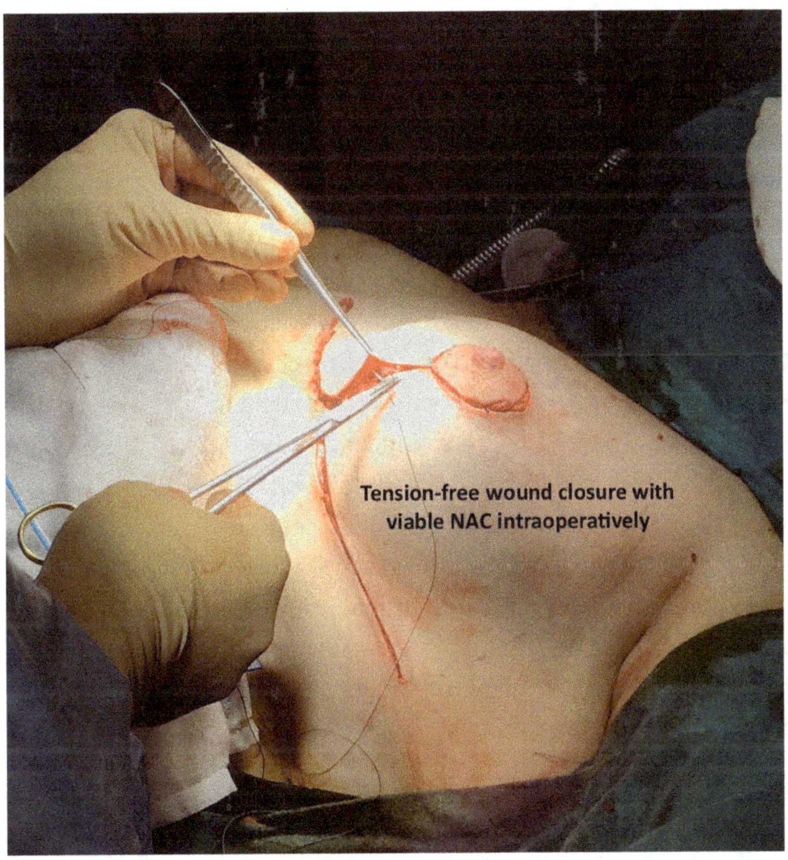

Figure 32. Viable NAC at time of skin closure.

8. Silicone versus saline implants

The first silicone implants used in breast surgery were designed in 1961 by Thomas Cronin and Frank Gerow, two American Plastic surgeons. Prior to this, a variety of products were used to fill the cavity, including the practice of injecting silicone into the breast tissue in the 1950s and 1960s. Over 50,000 women in the US who underwent this procedure ended up with silicone granuloma and hardening of the breast and many even requiring mastectomy. Early designs of these implants caused significant capsular contracture, a condition due to the host tissue creating a shell around the implant which gets progressively hard and uncomfortable. The Baker classification of grading capsular contractures from I to IV is often used as standardised measure of assessing the degree of hardness and aesthetic outcome [33]. The true incidence of capsular contracture after breast implant augmentation is quoted between 8–15%, although the incidence following breast reconstruction may be higher. The exact cause of capsular contracture is not known and range from biofilm secondary to subclinical infection and inflammatory foreign-body type reaction. The incidence of capsular contracture has been found to be less with textured implants compared to smooth implants.

Early manufacturers found the use of polyurethane foam coating on the shell of the implants helped minimise the risk of capsular contracture. This practice was discontinued due to concerns of potential health risk from 2,4-toluenediamine (TDA), a carcinogenic by-product of the chemical breakdown of polyurethane. The FDA banned the use of silicone implants in 1992 during which time saline implants were the predominant prosthetic device used in America. Coincidentally, silicone implants continued to be used across Europe and Australasia despite the FDA ban. Saline implants were first designed in France and introduced in 1964 as a medical prosthetic device but caused more wrinkling with higher rates of capsular contracture and accelerated lower pole stretch, making it less desirable as a reconstruction option post mastectomy. The FDA eventually lifted its ban in 2006 following extensive research confirming safety of silicone implants.

Silicone implants came under media scrutiny again in 2017 following reports of **Breast implant associated–Anaplastic Large Cell Lymphoma (BIA-ALCL)**. This has resulted in an almost knee-jerk response to revert back to saline implants in some centres. The actual risk of BIA-ALCL is very low and believed to be related to heavily textured implants, although few cases have been reported with smooth implants as well. As of September 2017, 409 cases of BIA-ALCL have been reported worldwide with 14 deaths. Current risk of developing BIA-ALCL with silicone implant use is quoted between 1: 30,000 and 1: 50,000. Manufacturers continue to design newer and lower textured implants in an attempt to counter the growing public concern around ALCL. The historic issues with saline implants of increased capsular contracture, rotation/flipping of the implant, rupture and migration remain with its use and could result in increased revision rates.

Decision regarding saline or silicone implants should be based on clinical indications, rather than fear of ALCL associated with textured implants. Patients should be advised about the small risk of BIA-ALCL and that the majority of cases are diagnosed early. Typical presentation is a sudden build-up of fluid around the implant and 9–13% of delayed seroma may be ALCL related. The timeframe for ALCL is usually 15 months to 5 years post implant surgery.

Ultrasound-guided aspiration of the fluid tested for CD-30 on IHC, is the definitive diagnostic test for BIA-ALCL. PET scan is recommended to stage the patient and in early stage disease, explantation with complete en-bloc capsulectomy including the posterior wall, combined with excision biopsy of lymph nodes is recommended. Due to the rarity of this condition, the Australasian Society of Plastic Surgeons (ASPS) advice that only few dedicated labs undertake the test and only specialist surgeons perform the operation to ensure good outcomes for patients. Patients should be reassured that stages I and II are completely curable. Chemotherapy in advanced cases and CD-30 targeted therapy in refractory cases have shown encouraging results. Standardised guidelines for the diagnosis and management of BIA-ALCL have been published by NCCN in 2016 [34].

Choice of anatomical versus round implants requires careful assessment of the patient's body habitus, chest wall shape and width, native breast shape and discussion regarding the desired final outcome. In a cancer setting, it is worth being cautious about having a carte blanche approach to implant options. With medium sized breasts, patients should be encouraged to remain approximately the same cup size and additional cleavage is achievable with round versus anatomical implants. Patients should be cautioned about using the appropriate implant size as determined by the mastectomy skin envelope, to avoid complications of skin flap necrosis or wound breakdown (Section 6).

It is advisable to order a range of implants to choose from at the time of surgery. Use of sizers intraoperatively can help determine ideal sized implants to ensure tension-free closure of the wound. Surgeons embarking on their career in oncoplastic breast surgery should become familiar with the range of commercially available implants in terms of height, width and profile.

9. Revision surgery and lipomodelling

Capsular contracture is a well-documented risk associated with implant reconstruction and patients should be cautioned prior to surgery. The risk of capsular contracture is higher with saline and smooth implants compared to textured or polyurethane-coated implants and in sub-muscular placement. The incidence is approximately 10–15% and is the commonest reason for revision surgery. Increasing role of lipomodelling to help reduce the risk of capsular contracture and address contour defects from previous surgery can minimise the extent or complexity of revision surgery [35, 36]. Patients should be advised that lipomodelling is different from liposuction and should not expect to achieve significant weight reduction after this procedure. There is a limited volume of lipofilling that can be achieved during revision surgery, taking care to avoid excess tension and risk of fat necrosis. Safety of fat grafting has now been adequately established and serves to improve vascularity to the thin mastectomy flaps, especially after previous radiotherapy.

It is important to set patient expectations at the outset and emphasise that the aim of oncoplastic breast surgery is not to achieve perfection, but rather obtain as close to a normal appearing breast as possible. Patients should also be cautioned that each revision surgery carries additional risks to the native skin flaps and that the aesthetic outcome may not be as good as the initial results in some cases.

10. Patient choice versus treatment options

Before the advent of oncoplastic breast surgery, limited options between WLE and simple mastectomy made surgical consultations around breast cancer treatment relatively simple. The ability to offer a wide range of surgical options does not warrant outlining the entire list to patients during their initial visit. This is particularly relevant when patients are struggling with heightened anxiety around their cancer diagnosis. There is good evidence to suggest that patients only retain a fraction of the complex discussion undertaken in a doctor's office. It requires experience and skill to navigate the complexity of information offered during the initial consultation and to gauge the patient's level of understanding.

It is important to actively enquire if the patient is satisfied with the shape and size of her breasts at the time of diagnosis, even before instigating any discussions around OPS. In this example, a 67-year-old patient with a new screen-detected 80 mm area of DCIS in the upper outer quadrant was recommended mastectomy with sentinel node biopsy by the MDT (**Figure 33**).

The patient was keen on immediate reconstruction but raised BMI with ptotic native breast and social circumstances made implant or autologous reconstruction challenging with need for symmetrising contralateral procedure (**Figure 34**). Further discussion with the patient and option for extended WLE with SNB and immediate Li-CAP autologous dermal-adipose

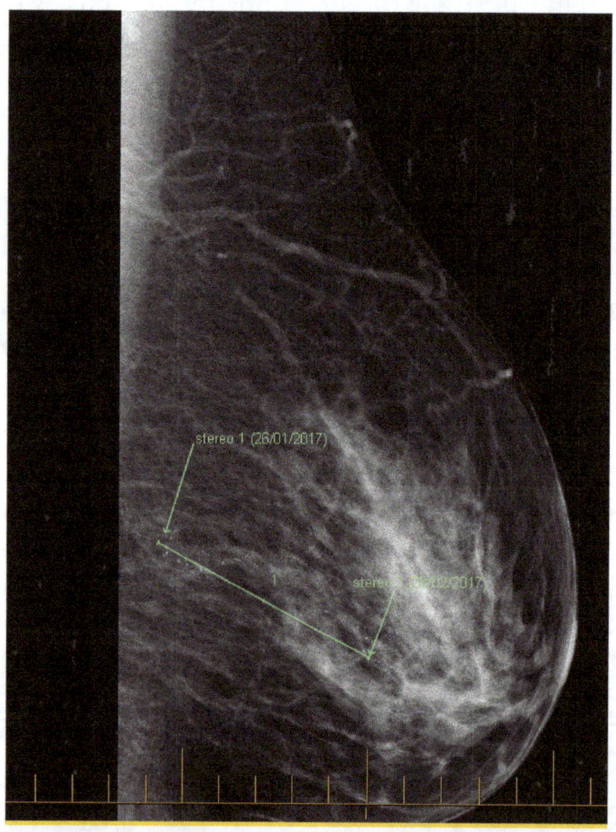

Figure 33. Mammogram with DCIS.

flap for volume replacement served as the ideal option in this patient. She was well enough to be discharged after 2 days in hospital without any delay in adjuvant radiotherapy. The lateral scar remains hidden within the bra line with good functional status, low donor site morbidity, return to normal activities and high satisfaction rates with aesthetic outcomes (**Figure 35**).

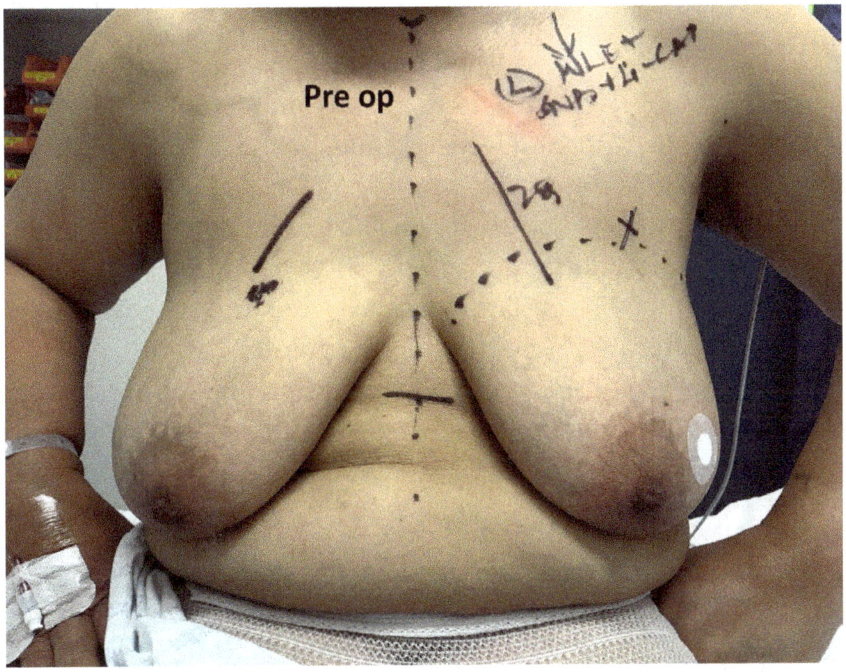

Figure 34. Pre-op left breast DCIS.

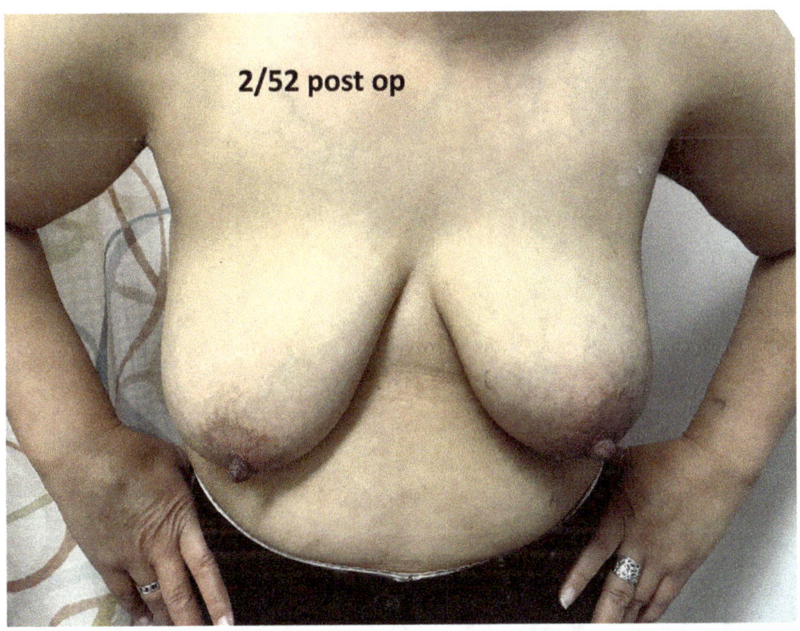

Figure 35. Post-op extended WLE with Li-CAP volume replacement.

Choice of reconstruction options may be limited by patient factors like smoking status. Implant and autologous reconstruction such as DIEP are not routinely offered to women who smoke, due to unacceptably high rates of wound complications and reconstruction failure. There are many centres where implant reconstruction is routinely offered to women who smoke, but patients need to be clearly informed about the high risk of wound related complications and implant failure. Smoking causes vasoconstriction with altered bacterial flora secondary to tissue hypoxia and is believed to be responsible for the poor wound healing (**Figure 36**). This could negatively impact on younger patients due to delays in adjuvant chemotherapy.

Raised BMI is an independent risk factor for higher seroma rates, increased wound infection and anaesthetic related issues. Implant reconstruction in larger women can be difficult due to limited choices of implants to accommodate the wide chest wall dimension. The shape of the reconstructed breast is governed by the shape and size of implant and symmetrising surgery is often required to address the large and ptotic contralateral breast. The risks for wound complications are higher if this is combined with cancer surgery and could delay adjuvant therapy. In these patients, the autologous Li-CAP perforator flap or Goldilocks mastectomy (Section 2.3.1) serves as a useful and safer alternative for immediate reconstruction after mastectomy and appears to tolerate radiotherapy well. Patients need to be cautioned about prolonged seroma formation with both these options.

There has been a global increase in the incidence of contralateral prophylactic mastectomy (CPM) in the last decade and has been often labelled the 'Angeline Jolie effect'. Over the same timeframe, a well-cited Wall Street Journal article from July 2015 has resulted in increasingly number of women taking ownership for their treatment and demanding a double mastectomy [37]. Anxiety around perceived cancer recurrence, poor diagnostic yield with standard

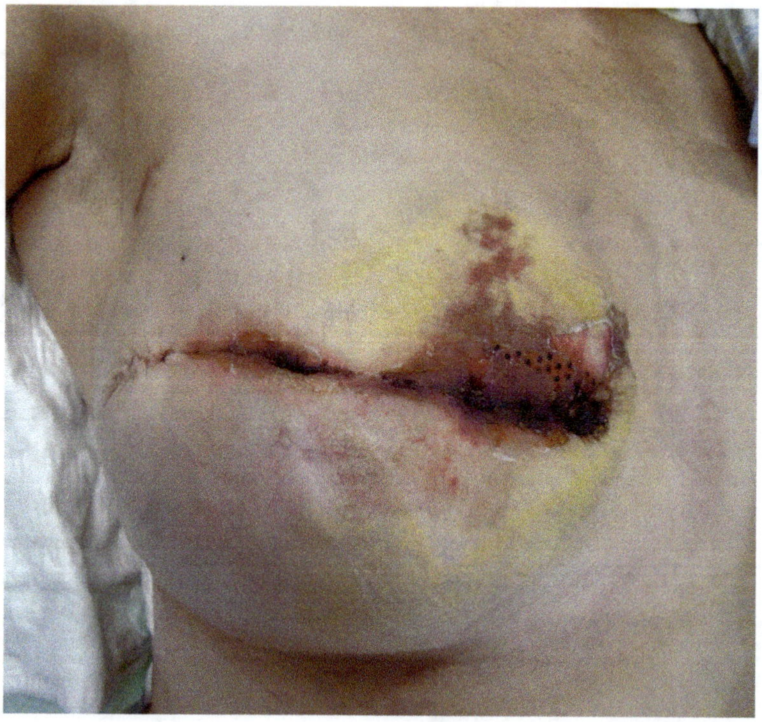

Figure 36. Smoking-related complication.

imaging in lobular cancers, family history and discomfort from multiple biopsies and repeated mammograms; are some of the reasons for women seeking CPM. More recently, the surgical community has been criticised for 'bowing down' to patient request for double mastectomy when diagnosed with a new cancer. Some women may feel strongly about undergoing one operation, which could help reduce anxiety around repeated imaging and biopsy. It is important to carefully understand the individual patient's reasons for considering CPM. There is good evidence that CPM does not confer survival benefit and risk of contralateral breast cancer for the vast majority of patients is relatively low. Patients need to be clearly explained about the higher risk of wound related complications, delayed recovery and impact on adjuvant treatment with low benefit in terms of survival and recurrence. Despite this, if they continued to feel strongly about bilateral mastectomy with or without reconstruction, it would be reasonable to offer them the option of CPM (**Figures 37** and **38**).

It is important to clearly document all aspects of preoperative discussions in the clinical records due to potential medicolegal implications.

There is potential for 'clinician bias' with even experienced surgeons which could alter the direction of the consultation. This could be due to preconceived ideations about patient body image, based on their appearance, educational background and socioeconomic status. Conversely, young women with large tumours are still subject to simple mastectomy without reconstruction in many hospitals around New Zealand and Australia; even in those with good clinical response to neoadjuvant chemotherapy. The rationale for this practice is based on historic concerns about potentially leaving disease behind, treatment delays or reduced effectiveness of adjuvant radiotherapy in the context of immediate reconstruction. This bias towards mastectomy genuinely stems from the sense of 'duty of care' with greater focus on the treatment and its outcome, rather than the psychological impact of mastectomy on

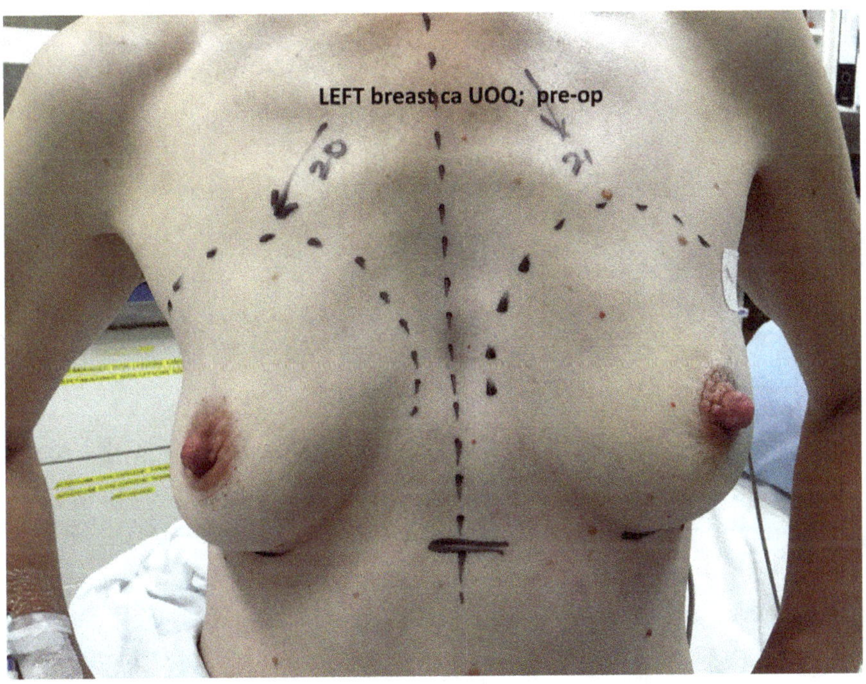

Figure 37. Pre-op left breast cancer.

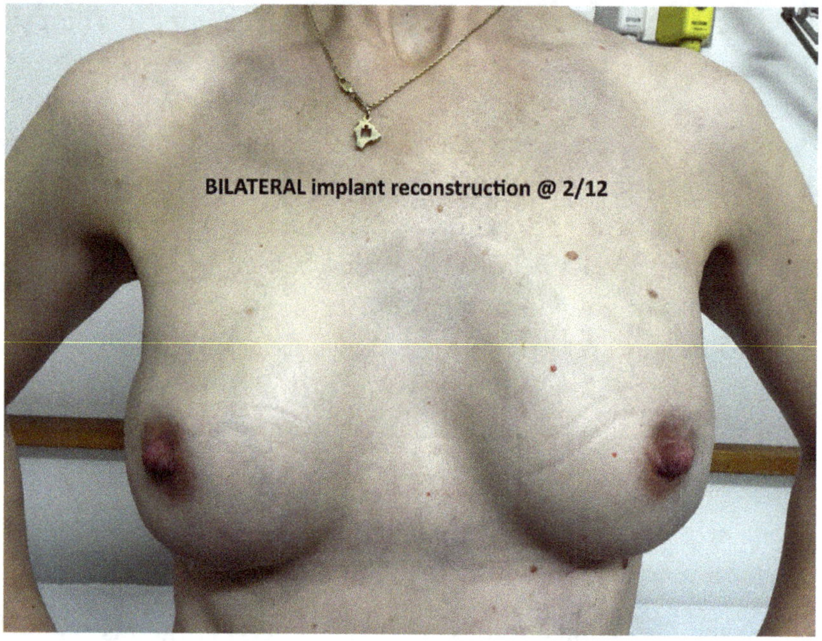

Figure 38. Left mastectomy and CPM with implant reconstruction.

a young woman. Historic data from the National Screening Unit in the UK found that 30% of women undergoing mastectomy suffered from depression after treatment; equally 30% of women undergoing breast conservation had anxiety about recurrent cancer. The emphasis therefore should not be about avoiding a mastectomy but rather considering immediate reconstruction options in those who need mastectomy. Reverse sequencing with upfront radiotherapy in young patients is a relative new concept, which allows mastectomy with immediate autologous reconstruction, such as LD flap with implant, without compromising aesthetic outcome.

Increasing use of neoadjuvant chemotherapy and neoadjuvant endocrine therapy to downstage disease, provides adequate time to plan surgery for both patients and the treating surgeon [38, 39]. This allows time to organise genetic testing when indicated and an opportunity to improve patient health status, e.g., smoking cessation, weight loss to achieve target BMI and additional sessions with the clinical psychologists. In women with normal BMI and in whom post-operative radiotherapy is indicated, use of tissue expander as an immediate-delayed reconstruction, is advocated by the MD Anderson group and serves as a bridge to definitive reconstruction whilst preserving the mastectomy skin flap. Women are able to wake up from surgery without having to deal with the trauma of mastectomy.

The traditional approach of delaying reconstruction for several months (sometimes years) after initial cancer treatment can be detrimental to the psychosocial well-being of women struggling with their cancer diagnosis. In women with raised BMI, trying to lose weight can be a challenge and many centres would not offer delayed reconstruction unless patients achieved their target weight. There are limited options viz. DIEP for delayed reconstruction in women who have had post mastectomy radiotherapy. Some plastic surgeons would consider two-stage TE reconstruction after radiotherapy, but the results are variable due to limited skin and muscle expansion with high rates of reconstruction failure.

Delayed LD flap with implant is a good option in patients who have had post mastectomy radiotherapy with less donor site morbidity compared to other forms of reconstruction. Any symmetrisation option for the native breast is probably best deferred for at least 6 months to allow the LD flap to settle and offers the opportunity to correct any contour defects with lipofilling at the time of the second procedure. Preoperative CT angiogram is recommended in the delayed setting to confirm patent thoracodorsal pedicle prior to lifting the LD flap. Simple bedside examination by getting the patient tense the latissimus dorsi muscle would suggest intact pedicle and formal imaging can help delineate the anatomy adequately. The CTA occasionally picks up occult lung metastasis in patients waiting for delayed reconstruction (**Figure 39**).

Breast reconstruction following mastectomy is a complex decision and requires detailed discussion with patients to ensure adequate understanding about the complexity of surgery. It is important to ensure patient compliance with post-operative protocols to help minimise wound-related complications and potentially poor outcome from reconstruction failure. Oncoplastic breast surgeons can offer a broad range of treatment options suitable for the individual patient based on cancer biology, proposed treatment plan and patient factors, such as breast shape and density, smoking history, BMI and other medical co-morbidities. It is recommended to have a minimum of two discussions prior to any reconstructive surgery with adequate clinic time allocated to ensure detailed discussion and patient understanding about options and operative choices. Use of detailed information leaflets to suit the organisation serves as a useful adjunct to the discussion, which patients can read at home in a less stressful environment. Additional consultations offer patients the opportunities to seek clarification about the proposed operation and the surgeon can revisit the potential risks and complications to ensure informed consent.

An experienced breast care nurse familiar with various oncoplastic procedures is invaluable in helping patients with preoperative counselling and decision-making. In some patients, this process can take a few weeks and may require input from clinical psychologists. This helps confirm patient's understanding about various treatment options available, ensure decision-making has not been unduly influenced or coerced, and minimises the risk of 'decision-regret' at a later stage.

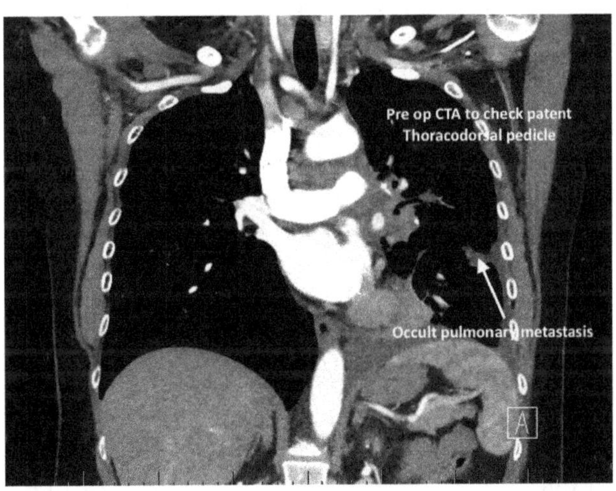

Figure 39. CTA showing occult pulmonary metastasis.

With the rapid global uptake of OPS, there remains a real danger of potentially worse patient outcome due to poor technique, improper patient selection or decision making. This is one specialty where good surgical skills are essential and inadequate training reflects on the operative outcomes with results which are glaringly obvious to both patients and clinicians.

There are well-established OPS training programmes in the UK, and post-fellowship trainees in Australasia are encouraged to undertake at least 2–3 years of additional clinical training in accredited centres. The additional training serves to up-skill their technical prowess and more importantly, learn the complex process of patient selection and the art of good communication. The rationale for oncoplastic breast surgery as an integral part of all breast cancer surgery has been eloquently detailed in a review article [40].

11. Conclusion

In summary, oncoplastic breast surgery has established a firm place in the global fight against breast cancer. Patients should be offered the appropriate range of surgical treatment options instead of the conventional two-operation strategy, prevalent for the past 40 years. Clinical discussions are therefore more complex and additional time and expertise is required to help patients with decision-making. Having a well-trained and experienced breast care nurse is invaluable in a busy oncoplastic breast practice. A multidisciplinary team approach is an integral part of modern cancer management with early contribution of clinical psychologists in selected cases. Developing an oncoplastic breast surgery practice from the ground up, can be time-consuming and challenging. It is possible to establish a modern oncoplastic breast surgical practice despite the usual constraints of a public health system and help women achieve a satisfactory cosmetic outcome combined with safe oncological treatment of their breast cancer.

Surgical residents should be trained to a high standard and accreditation of oncoplastic breast surgical training is crucial to avoid repeating the historical mistakes of the laparoscopic era. The Royal Australasian College of Surgeons has recently set up an oncoplastic breast surgery master's programme for post-fellowship trainees. This will become mandatory to help standardise clinical knowledge, technical expertise and competency levels with peer review and audit. Monash University, in Melbourne, Australia, has been tasked with monitoring all breast implants used in reconstructive surgery to ensure a national registry service for breast surgical prosthetic devices.

Whilst a detailed description of oncoplastic breast surgery has not been possible, this chapter hopes to offer a broad overview of modern surgical practice with emphasis on implant-based reconstruction.

Acknowledgements

The author wishes to acknowledge the continued dedicated efforts of Maria Winter, Oncoplastic Breast Care Nurse, Department of Surgery, Christchurch Hospital, Christchurch, New Zealand.

Her continued support and expertise has made it possible to establish Oncoplastic Breast Surgery in Christchurch since 2009. The author also would like to thank all her patients for allowing use of clinical photographs and details of their diagnosis for this book chapter.

Conflict of interest

There are no conflicts of interests to declare.

Author details

Josie Todd[1,2,3,4,5*]

*Address all correspondence to: josie.todd@cdhb.health.nz

1 Department of Surgery, CDHB, Christchurch, New Zealand

2 Royal College of Surgeons of Edinburgh, UK

3 University of Otago, New Zealand

4 Health Disability and Ethics Commission (HDEC), New Zealand

5 Accident Compensation Corporation (ACC), New Zealand

References

[1] Halsted W. The results of operations for the care of cancer of the breast performed at the Johns Hopkins hospital from June, 1889, to January, 1894. Annals of Surgery. 1894;**20**(5):497-555

[2] Fisher B, Anderson S, Bryant J, et al. Twenty-year follow-up of a randomized trial comparing total mastectomy, lumpectomy, and lumpectomy plus irradiation for the treatment of invasive breast cancer. The New England Journal of Medicine. 2002;**347**:1233-1241. [PubMed: 12393820]

[3] Veronesi U, Cascinelli N, Mariani L, et al. Twenty-year follow-up of a randomized study comparing breast-conserving surgery with radical mastectomy for early breast cancer. The New England Journal of Medicine. 2002;**347**:1227-1232. [PubMed: 12393819]

[4] Clough KS et al. Improving breast cancer surgery: A classification and quadrant per quadrant atlas for oncoplastic surgery. Annals of Surgical Oncology. 2010;**17**(5):1375-1391. DOI: 10.1245/s10434-009-0792-y

[5] McCulley S, Macmillan RD. Planning and use of therapeutic mammoplasty—Nottingham approach. British Journal of Plastic Surgery. 2005;**58**:889-901

[6] Kronowitz SJ. Delayed-immediate breast reconstruction: Technical and timing considerations. Plastic and Reconstructive Surgery. 2010;**125**(2):463-474

[7] Saini KS et al. Role of the multidisciplinary team in breast cancer management: Results from a large international survey involving 39 countries. Annals of Oncology. 2012;**23**(4): 853-859

[8] Halkett G et al. The role of the breast care nurse during treatment for early breast cancer: The patient's perspective. Contemporary Nurse. 2006;**23**(1):46-57

[9] Litiere S et al. Breast conserving therapy versus mastectomy for stage I–II breast cancer: 20-year follow-up of the EORTC 10801 phase 3 randomised trial. Lancet Oncology. 2012;**13**(4):412-419

[10] Al-Ghazal SK, Blamey RW, Stewart J, Morgan AAL. The cosmetic outcome in early breast cancer treated with breast conservation. European Journal of Surgical Oncology. 1999;**25**(6):566-570. DOI: 10.1053/ejso.1999.0707

[11] Fernando C, Todd J. Why scar placement is important for women undergoing WLE for breast cancer: Evaluating cosmetic outcome in the breast unit with use of clinical photographs and patient feedback questionnaire. ANZ Journal of Surgery. 2017;**87**(S1):6-14

[12] Benelli L. A new periareolar mammaplasty: The "round block" technique. Aesthetic Plastic Surgery. 1990;**14**(2):93-100

[13] Currie A et al. Using therapeutic mammoplasty to extend the role of breast-conserving surgery in women with larger or ptotic breasts. Annals of the Royal College of Surgeons of England. 2013;**95**(3):192-195

[14] McCulley SJ et al. Therapeutic mammaplasty for centrally located breast tumours. Plastic and Reconstructive Surgery. 2006;**117**(2):366

[15] Hamdi M, Van Landuyt K, de Frene B, Roche N, Blondeel P, Monstrey S. The versatility of the inter-costal artery perforator (ICAP) flaps. Journal of Plastic, Reconstructive & Aesthetic Surgery. 2006;**59**(6):644-652. DOI: 10.1016/j.bjps.2006.01.006

[16] More Women Choose Breast Reconstruction after Mastectomy. Medicalxpress.com> Surgery. 13 Oct 2017

[17] Schmauss D et al. Breast reconstruction after mastectomy. Frontiers in Surgery. 2015;**2**:71

[18] Yu P. Breast reconstruction at the MD Anderson Cancer Centre. Gland Surgery. 2016;**5**(4):416-421. DOI: 10.21037/gs.2016.05.03

[19] Carrasco-López C, Ibañez JFJ, et al. Anterior intercostal artery perforator flap in immediate breast reconstruction: Anatomical study and clinical application. Microsurgery. 2017;**37**(6):603-610. DOI: 10.1002/micr.30171 PMID: 28370199

[20] Hakakian CS, Lockhart RA, Kulber DA, Aronowitz JA. Lateral intercostal artery perforator flap in breast reconstruction: A simplified pedicle permits an expanded role. Annals of Plastic Surgery. 2016;**76**(Suppl 3):S184-S190

[21] Macadam SA, Lennox PA. Acellular dermal matrices: Use in reconstructive and aesthetic breast surgery. The Canadian Journal of Plastic Surgery. 2012;**20**(2):75-89

[22] Mendenhall SD, Anderson LA, Ying J, Boucher KM, Neumayer LA, Agarwal JP. The BREASTrial stage II: ADM breast reconstruction outcomes from definitive reconstruction to 3 months postoperative. Plastic and Reconstructive Surgery Global Open. 2017;**5**(1):e1209. DOI: 10.1097/GOX.0000000000001209

[23] Gaske I et al. Delayed hypersensitivity reaction to acellular dermal matrix in breast reconstruction: The red breast syndrome? Annals of Plastic Surgery. 2014;**73**(Suppl 2): S139-S143

[24] Peek K, Todd J. Does TIGR earn its stripes? – Outcomes of reconstructive breast surgery using long-term absorbable synthetic matrix (preliminary results) Poster presentation at Annual Scientific Congress, Royal Australasian College of Surgeons. ANZ Journal of Surgery. 2015;**85**(Suppl. 1):3-13

[25] Thompson B, Todd J. TIGR mesh-assisted immediate and delayed implant reconstruction following mastectomy and revision surgery: Largest single oncoplastic breast surgeon experience in a regional Centre. ANZ Journal of Surgery. 2018;**88**(Suppl 1):12

[26] Pompei S et al. The use of TIGR matrix in breast aesthetic and reconstructive surgery. Is a resorbable synthetic mesh a viable alternative to acellular dermal matrices? Clinics in Plastic Surgery. 2018;**45**:65-73

[27] Becker H et al. Immediate implant-based prepectoral breast reconstruction using vertical incision. Plastic and Reconstructive Surgery Global Open. 2015;**3**(6):e412

[28] Orzalesi L et al. Nipple-sparing mastectomy: Surgical and oncological outcomes from a national multicentric registry with 913 patients (1006 cases) over a 6 year period. Breast. 2016;**26**:75-81

[29] Fowble B et al. Rates of reconstruction failure in patients undergoing immediate reconstruction with tissue expanders and/or implants and postmastectomy radiation therapy. International Journal of Radiation Oncology, Biology, Physics. 2015;**92**(3):634-641

[30] Kronowitz S. Current status of implant-based breast reconstruction in patients receiving postmastectomy radiation therapy. Plastic and Reconstructive Surgery. 2012;**130**(4): 513e-523e. DOI: 10.1097/PRS.0b013e318262f059. PMID: 23018711

[31] Todd J. Bi-pedicle nipple-sparing mastectomy (modified Letterman technique) and TIGR mesh assisted immediate implant reconstruction, in a patient with Cowden's syndrome. Gland Surgery. 2016;**5**(3):306-311

[32] Ladizinsky DA et al. Breast reconstruction with the Bostwick autoderm technique. Plastic and Reconstructive Surgery. 2013;**132**:261-270

[33] Malahias M et al. A literature review and summary of capsular contracture: An ongoing challenge to breast surgeons and their patients. International Journal of Surgery Open. 2016;**3**:1-7

[34] Clemens M et al. NCCN consensus guidelines for the diagnosis and management of breast implant-associated anaplastic large cell lymphoma. Aesthetic Surgery Journal. 2017;**37**(3):285-289

[35] Breast Reconstruction using Lipomodelling after Breast Cancer Treatment. NICE Interventional Procedures Guidance [IPG417]. Published date: January 2012

[36] Chan CW, McCulley SJ, Macmillan RD. Autologous fat transfer—A review of the literature with a focus on breast cancer surgery. Journal of Plastic, Reconstructive & Aesthetic Surgery. 2008;**61**:1438-1448

[37] Lagnado L, Doctors D. More women with breast cancer choose double mastectomies. Wall Street Journal. 10 July, 2015

[38] EBCTCG. Long-term outcomes for neoadjuvant versus adjuvant chemotherapy in early breast cancer: Meta-analysis of individual patient data from ten randomised trials. The Lancet Oncology. 2018;**19**:27-39

[39] Cain H et al. Neoadjuvant therapy in early breast cancer: Treatment considerations and common debates in practice. Clinical Oncology. 2017;**29**:642-652

[40] Macmillan RD, McCulley SJ. Oncoplastic breast surgery: What, when and for whom? Current Breast Cancer Reports. 2016;**8**:112-117

6

Photodynamic Therapy, a Potential Therapy to Improve Cancer Management

Heidi Abrahamse and Ivan Sosthene Mfouo Tynga

Abstract

Cancer is a mass of abnormal and detrimental cells in a given part of the body. The main elucidated cause is the uncontrolled growth and proliferation of those cells after the corruption of the physiological processes responsible for normal development and functioning. The advantage of adjuvant therapy, therapy done after surgery, is to prevent the occurring of symptoms and not necessarily to make sure of the integrity of mechanisms that are crucial in preventing abnormal cell proliferation such cell cycle regulation, cell death, which include autophagy, necrosis, and apoptosis. The understanding of dysregulated cell death mechanisms combined with suitable alternative cancer therapies could lead to novel treatment modalities for cancer. Currently, breast cancer is the leading occurring cancer in sub-Saharan women after that of the cervix. This potentially curable condition kills more than half of the diagnosed group, which consists mainly of females aged between 35 and 49 years and with 77% being in stages III and IV. The social economic status of populations coupled with the limited access to proper control strategies and infrastructures in sub-Saharan regions accentuate the burden of the disease. Photodynamic therapy (PDT) has shown great potential in treating breast cancer and even greater therapeutic outcomes can be obtained when combining PDT with other therapies such as immunotherapy or nanomedicine.

Keywords: cancer, breast cancer, current treatment, photodynamic therapy, photosensitizers, photochemical reactions, cell death immunotherapy, nanomedicine

1. Introduction

The unregulated growth and proliferation of abnormal cells to form solid or liquid tumor in a given part of the body is referred as cancer. Currently, the condition denotes a collection of related diseases with more than 100 types of cancer have been identified and named after the organs or tissues of origin [1]. Carcinoma is a common category that affects the inner and outer surfaces of the body and the subcategories include basal cell, squamous cell, transitional cell and adenocarcinoma. Sarcoma affects the cells in bones and smooth tissues, leukemia and lymphoma that of the blood and lymphocytes, respectively [1]. Due to the nature of the condition, the detection has to be as early as possible, followed by appropriate managerial approach based on the type of cancer to insure the survival of cancer patients. Early detection and treatment have increased the lifespan of patients diagnosed with cancers, and the survival rate is thrice higher than that observed in postponed intervention scenarios [2, 3]. Cancer has become a major health problem and foremost cause of death, claiming more than 8.8 million deaths in 2015, and 8.2 million deaths with 14 million new cases been diagnosed in 2012 [4–6]. The lifestyle plays a decisive role in determining cancer incidence and mortality rates, for example, the consumption of tobacco alone is one of the deadliest causes and accounts for 22% of the global cancer related deaths [5]. In developing countries, about a quarter of the incidence rate is infection-dependent, such as Hepatitis and Human Papilloma Virus (HPV) are known to facilitate carcinogenesis. While more than 90% of proper facilities and services for cancer management are reportedly available in the developed parts of the globe, less than 30% of those are in the low and middle countries. It has been established that the cancer mortality rate is proportionate to the regional dietary behavior and a third of the global cancer related deaths could be avoided as it is associated with obesity, high both tobacco and alcohol consumption, both low vegetable and fruit consumption, and physical inactivity [7, 8].

When a cancer develops and originates from the lobular or ductal tissues in the breast, it is commonly known as breast cancer, one of the most deadly cancers and the most common womanlike cancers globally [9, 10]. This carcinoma can be either recurrent, metastatic, invasive (or not) and seldom originates in the connective tissues of muscles, fat and blood vessels. A well developed breast is a tear-shaped milk producing gland and breast cancer is classified according to level of differentiation, from well differentiated in normal breast to moderately and poorly differentiated glands in breast cancer. Additionally, the size of the tumor, the possible invasion to lymph nodes in the armpits and metastatic ability help oncologists to stage breast cancer from the small ductal/lobular precancerous stage (stage 0) to medium sized in breast and lymph nodal regions (stage 1–3) and large metastatic phase (stage 4), the latter is usually associated with worse prognosis [10, 11]. Better prediction of prognosis is facilitated by the presence or not of certain receptors and the human epidermal growth factor receptor-2 (HER2) together with hormone receptors (HR, estrogen and progesterone) are usually considered. The luminal A type (HR+/HER2-) of breast cancer has the best prognosis, the luminal B type (HR+/HER2+) and the HER2-enriched type (HR−/HER2+) have moderate prognosis and the worst scenario is observed with the triple negative type (HR−/HER2+) [12–15].

The management approach of any kind of breast cancer mainly depends on the stage and the predicted prognosis; with the more hostile treatments administrated to patients, whose conditions have predicted poor prognosis and elevated probability of recurrence after intervention. Although the occasional and circumscribed effectiveness, surgery remains the main treatment modality for breast cancer, including entire (mastectomy), partial (quadrantectomy) or minute (lumpectomy) removal of the breast. The multidisciplinary approach is often preferred and necessitates the accompaniment of chemotherapy or radiation therapy, or both for improved results [16]. Generally, hormone-blocking agents act as effectors for treatment of luminal (HR+) types and immune-modulators are favored for certain metastatic and late-staged breast cancer [17–19].

Photodynamic therapy is an unconventional treatment modality for neoplastic conditions and a promising treatment for recurrent cancers, depending on photochemical reactions and subsequent damage, and leading to cancer cell death [20, 21]. Experimental data from a diverse pool of research reports proved Photodynamic therapy to be a good treatment option for numerous cancers, offering reduced long-term mobility, very limited side-effects, better cancer-specificity over surgery, chemotherapy or radiotherapy [20, 22–23]. The radiotherapy causes loss of oxygen while oxygen is required during the Photodynamic therapy, therefore the two approaches should not be considered for a combined therapy. Furthermore, combination with conventional chemotherapeutic agents should be avoided as it would forfeit the cancer control and selectivity benefits of Photodynamic therapy. A superior targeting and eradication of breast cancer cells was achieved with photodynamic therapy, which is appealing and leaving normal-like cells such as breast epithelium and fibroblast unaffected, thus satisfying a safe usage norms. This emphasizes the edge of photodynamic therapy over other therapeutic methods; limited to none side-effects to patients. Photosensitivity is the usually side-effect observed and involves skin redness, tingling or burning sensation up to 24 hours post Photodynamic therapy, which can only treat tumors where light can reach and [21–25].

2. Fundamentals of photodynamic therapy

Photodynamic therapy was discovered more than a century ago and now is a minimally invasive and clinically approved therapeutic modality for neoplastic conditions. It involves the administration of photochemotherapeutic agents, known as photosensitizers, followed by the irradiation of the agents at a wavelength that matches their absorption properties. When this occurs in the presence of molecular oxygen, a sequence of reactions that lead to the tumor microvasculature damage, cytotoxicity and subsequent tumor cell death (**Figure 1**) [21, 26, 27]. Photosensitizers have evolved over time and are nontoxic, light absorbing dyes, able to undergo photochemical changes and transitions between the ground state and first or higher excited states. The deactivation can happen by heat-release (nonradioactive decay), emission as fluorescence or undergoing intersystem crossing (ISC). Ideal photosensitizers are readily able to be excited by appropriate photons, available in simple chemical formulation, easily synthesized from their precursors, stable and soluble in physiological environments, easily delivered into the body (injection or other means), and excreted from the body upon completion of therapy. They have high singlet oxygen quantum yield with strong absorption in the red region of the visible spectrum (680–800 nm) and high extinction coefficient, and effective accumulation in tumor tissues and low dark toxicity [28].

The third generation of photosensitizers are currently being developed from conjugating previous ones with organic and inorganic polymers, immunologic agents and nanoparticles. The first generation of photosensitizers include the members of Photofrin and hematoporphyrin

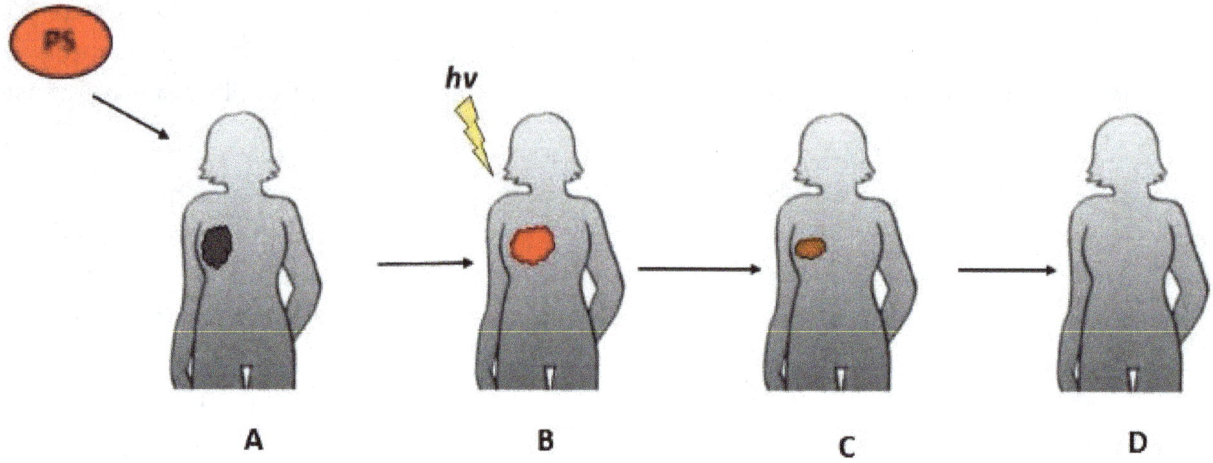

Figure 1. Elementary chronological events during photodynamic therapy. (A) Intravenous administration of photosensitizer(PS) to cancer patient. (B) Irradiation and activation of photosensitizer, which is localized in the cancer site. (C) Induction of cancer destruction mechanisms. (D)cancer-free patient after successful photodynamic therapy.

derivatives. They are complex mixtures of simple macrostructured hematoporphyrin and absorb light weakly at 630 nm, which resulted in their limited photodynamic effects. They were mostly used for surface tumors as at this wavelength of 630 nm the tissue penetration of light cannot exceed 4 mm and the major inconvenient was the extended light sensitivity period after the treatment. However, members of the first generation were efficient in generation of singlet oxygen per photon absorbed and met the standard for approval usage for clinical trials [28–31]. The development of second generation photosensitizers aimed to overcome the shortcomings of their predecessors naming low absorption in the near infrared region of the visible spectrum, prolonged light sensitivity and skin photo toxicity, and synthesizing method. From the porphyrin, many second generations were developed and included meta-tetra (hydroxyphenyl) porphyrin (m-THPP), 5,10,15,20-tetrakis(4-sulfanatophenyl)-21H,23H-porphyrn (TTPS4), 1,5-aminolevulinic acid (ALA) and numerous derivatives, the chlorin family derivatives, pheophorbides, bacteriopheophorides, texaphyrins, phthalocyanines. The members of the phthalocyanine family have great photodynamic actions and intersystem crossing capabilities due to the incorporation and formation of metal complexes in their core areas [32–36]. Some non-porphyrinoid photosensitizers exhibit photodynamic activity and include the anthraquinones, phenothizanies, xanthenes, cyanines and curcuminoids [37–39]. The development of third generation of photosensitizers is motivated by the fact that solubility remains poor with second generation photosensitizers, especially in aqueous environments at physiological condition, thus preventing intravenous delivery into the bloodstream. Currently, the research endeavors focus on developing delivery systems to facilitate the transportation to the target areas and to achieve greater selectivity and specificity of the third generation photosensitizers in order to increase their cellular uptake [40].

Light plays pivotal role for the successful activation of photosensitizers and subsequent outcomes of photodynamic cancer therapy. In ancient Egyptian, Indian, Greek and Chinese civilizations, light had a long track record in medical applications and the most usage being the remarkable efficacy in treat skin conditions [41]. Current applications use specific light sources to irradiate targeted tumor tissues. The optical power, wavelength matching the absorption spectrum of used photosensitizers and the depth of tissue penetration are among the priorities to be considered. The best tissue penetration of light is achieved in the therapeutic window, and most currently used photosensitizers absorb light maximally around that region of the spectrum, which is also known as the near infrared region (**Figure 2**) [42, 43]. Various types of light sources exist and the most commonly used in Photodynamic therapy applications are lasers, filtered lamps and light emitting diodes (LEDs). Lasers were the first to be utilized and offer high power coherent light in a narrow wavelength bandwidth but high manufactured skills and high cost are associated with them. Filtered lamps are the second and also the most flexible as they can be adapted, allowing their filters to be changed according to the properties of photosensitizers used but require an endoscope, which limits the efficiency, especially when using optical fibers. The most recent, LEDs are commonly used in Photodynamic applications and offer enhanced optical power [44, 45].

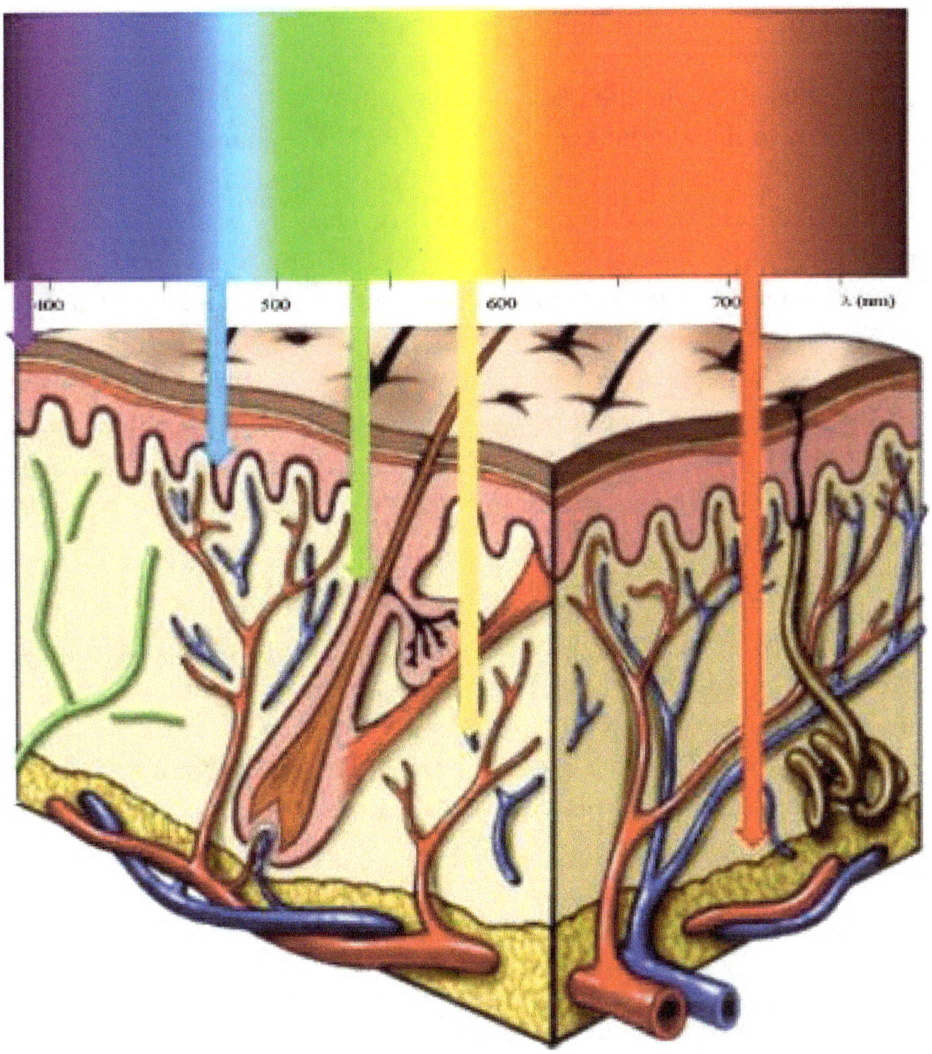

Figure 2. Light wave length and tissue penetration. Light penetration is proportional to the length of the wavelength used, the longer the wavelength, the deeper light penetrates into tissues.

The final objective of a photosensitizer is to successful transfer energy to molecular oxygen ($^3O_2$) or direct transfer of energy and production of reactive oxygen species. In photodynamic reactions, one of the most cytotoxic agent is the singlet oxygen ($^1O_2$), produced after the active interaction with a triplet state photosensitizer, and can be determined by measuring the weak near infrared luminescence of $^1O_2$, possible in both cells *in vitro* and tissues *in vivo*. In all of the cases, the treatment efficacy and cell eradication correlate strongly with the cumulative $^1O_2$ luminescence [46]. The amount of different forms of oxygen present in targeted tissues appear as an important factor to be considered for prognosis. The efficacy of Photodynamic therapy depends on the interaction of light, photosensitizers and oxygen, all in appropriate dose, and three dosimetry methods have emerged including explicit dosimetry to measure different treatment parameters and predict the outcomes, implicit dosimetry to measure biological intermediates and damage (photo bleaching) and adjust to effective dosage, and direct dosimetry to measure the critical photobiological toxins and avoid limitations seen with the previous two [46, 47].

2.1. Mechanisms of photodynamic therapy

Photodynamic therapy involves the use of light exposures to excite a photosensitizer from the ground state (PS) to the singlet excited state ($^1PS^*$). The stability of the photosensitizer in the excited state determines the occurrence of the intersystem crossing to the triplet and long-lived excited state ($^3PS^*$). Many physical pathways may be involved during intersystem crossing, converting the excited singlet state to the long-lived and excited triplet state photosensitizer. The triplet state has the ability to undergo photochemical processes and interact with triplet state molecules such as molecular oxygen. At this point, two possible photoreactions are envisaged, type I or type II reactions, involving molecular oxygen (**Figure 3**). In a type I reaction, electrons are transferred from the excited triplet state photosensitizer to molecular oxygen, when in the presence of a suitable reducing agent, to produce reactive oxygen species such as superoxide anion, hydrogen peroxide, hydroxyl radical and hydroxide ions [9].

The second reaction, Type II, energy or electrons from the excited triplet state photosensitizer are directly transferred to molecular oxygen ($^3O_2$), promoting it to an excited state singlet oxygen ($^1O_2$). Energy transfer to $^3O_2$ can occur only if both photosensitizer and oxygen (Triplet ground state) are in the same triplet state. Both type I and type II reactions generate reactive oxygen species, which are responsible for the cytodamage observed during Photodynamic therapy and type II reactions occur more frequently in photodynamic reactions (**Figure 4**) [9].

2.2. Photodynamic therapy, a localized therapy

Photosensitizers are tumor-localizing nontoxic agent, they selectively accumulate in neoplastic tissues, making Photodynamic therapy a restricted therapy. The irradiation of tumor tissues with visible light in the presence of oxygen, activates photosensitizers to generation reactive oxygen species into the tumor cells and thus induces tumor death and tissue destruction, preventing side-effects to health tissues [47]. Although the photosensitizers will effectively localize in all tumors, Photodynamic therapy is more suitable for localized diseases as

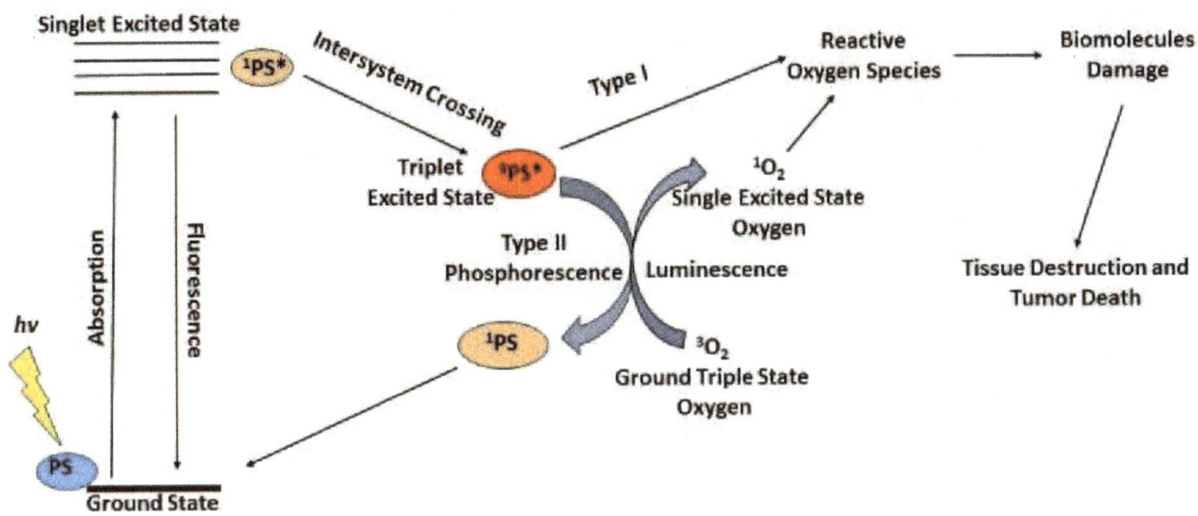

Figure 3. Schematic representation of type I and type II photoreactions following photo dynamic therapy (Jablonski Diagram). When the photosensitizer(PS) absorb a photon of light, it is elevated from the ground to the singlet excited state, it can either return back to the initial ground state by fluorescence or undergo intersystem crossing into the long triplet excited state. The photosensitizer in the triplet excitable state can transfer energy to an oxygen molecule forming reactive oxygen species (type I) or to the highly reactive triplet state (type II). There active oxygen species are responsible for the subsequent damage to biomolecules(nucleic acids, lipids and proteins) and the resulting cell death events.

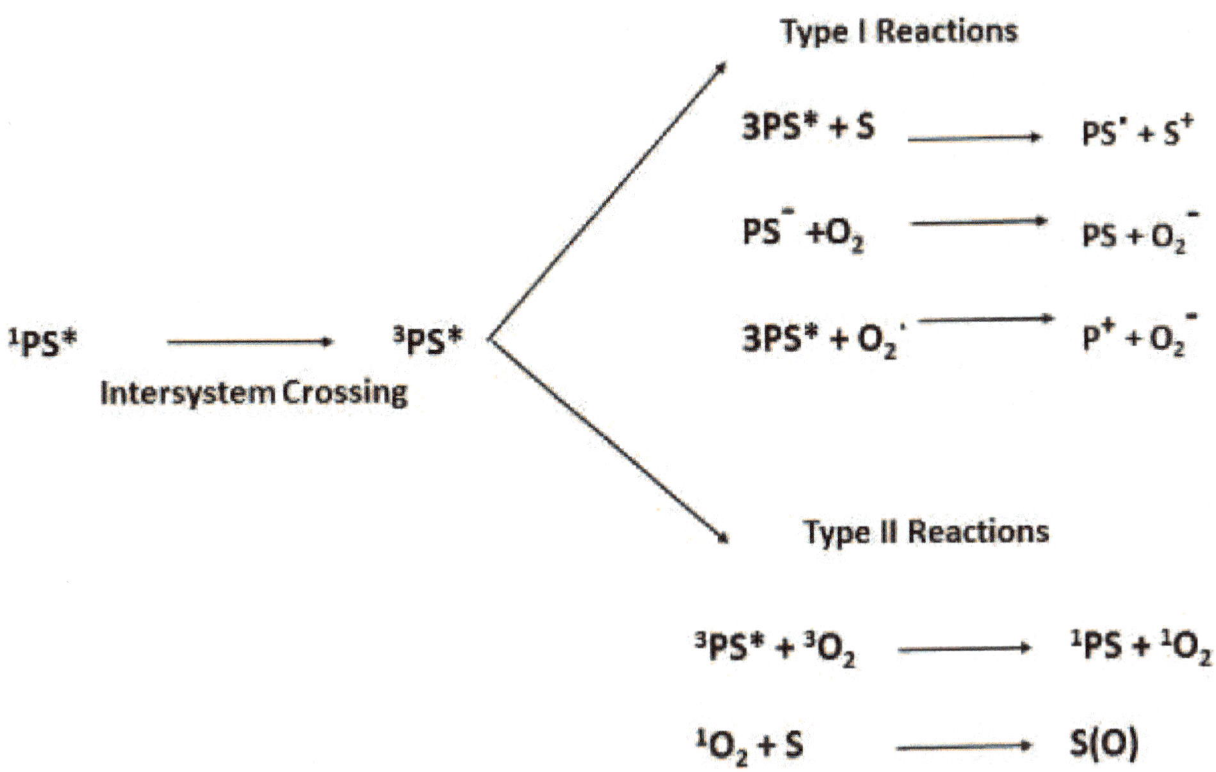

Figure 4. Possible photochemical reactions of photosensitizer (PS) in the triple excited state.

the irradiation is more feasible and efficient than in metastatic diseases. Most photosensitizers interconnect with tumor cells though their numerous low density lipoprotein receptors, facilitating the uptake of photosensitizers. Once inside the cells, the photosensitizers tend to selective accumulate in some organelles, include in the mitochondria, lysosomes and those near the nuclear areas. Mitochondria are consistent and preferential sites of accumulation of photosensitizers and the efficiency of Photodynamic therapy is not always affect by differential localization patterns between various cells. However, all Photodynamic therapy-treated cells exhibit significant mitochondrial disruption, leading to decreased mitochondrial activity and adenosine triphosphate production. Most cationic photosensitizers have stronger water solubility properties and localize in mitochondria, yielding enhanced photodynamic activities [48, 49]. Most of the photosensitizers that localize in mitochondria of certain kind of cancer cells, including breast cancer cells, show relatively high co-localization level in near nuclear areas such as endoplasmic reticulum, and are believed to be good candidates for photodiagnosis and photodynamic therapy [50, 51]. Reduced mitochondrial oxygen consumption, decreased mitochondrial membrane potential and inhibited activity of complexes (I to IV) are all often seen after photodynamic therapy-mediated by mitochondrial localizing photosensitizers, which have apoptosis-inducing capabilities [52, 49–51]. Some lysosomal-localizing photosensitizers are hydrophilic and show excellent tumor destruction, they are usually associated with the induction of both apoptotic and necrotic responses following photodynamic therapy [53–55].

2.3. Photodynamic therapy and the induction of cell death

Cellular uptake of the photosensitizers can assist in predicting the mode of cell death as reactive oxygen species accumulated first in the organelles where photosensitizers are localized [56]. Photosensitizers that favorably localize in mitochondria seem to have the predisposition of inducing apoptosis. Damage to mitochondria following photodynamic actions, would lead to mitochondrial leakage and apoptotic response as mitochondria are well known to play critical roles in most apoptotic pathways [57, 58]. Apoptosis is a highly regulated and programmed cell death response that comprises interdependent and synchronized pathways [58, 59]. Photodamage-mediated permeabilized mitochondrial membranes induce leakage of apoptogenic proteins, such as cytochrome C. In return, the released apoptogenic proteins activate the caspase mediated apoptotic pathway [60, 61]. Photodamage may also lead to the induction of other apoptotic pathways [62, 63].

With high dose of photodynamic therapy, cellular components that are essential for the induction of an apoptotic response, become damaged in the process leading to a necrotic type of response [64]. Necrosis is a cell death response associated with the pathological processes and irreversible cellular injury [65]. Sometimes, necrosis is accompanied by an inflammatory reaction accompanies, which is caused by the direct release of intracellular components into the cell environment [66]. Successful induction of the necrotic cell death response after photodynamic therapy had been reported, especially as a result of photosensitizers accumulating maximally in the plasma membranes [67]. Photosensitizers that localize in plasma membranes showed co-localization in mitochondria and slightly in lysosomes, and the observed post treatment changes at different incubation intervals included cell membrane damage, initiated cell repair, irreversible damage, induction of apoptotic-like response, and cell cycle S phase arrest [68].

Autophagy is a cytoprotective and recycling mechanism responsible to deal with cellular organelles and cytoplasmic components after damage. The main effector of this function is the autophagosome, a temporally doubled membrane structure, with the ability to engulf cell debris and fuse with lysosomes for complete degradation of its contents [69]. Photosensitizers that localize in mitochondria and endoplasmic reticulum stimulate a prosurvival autophagic response while the lysosomal-localized photosensitizers trigger an inhibitory autophagy response [55, 70]. Furthermore, low doses of photodynamic therapy lead to the induction of a cytoprotective autophagic mechanism, and autophagic cell death mechanism is induced with the high doses [71]. When an apoptotic response is undergoing, the autophagic cell death complements it and when absent, autophagy stands as the main cell death mechanism induced after photodynamic therapy [72, 73]. Such observation indicates that photodynamic treatment gives a concurrent occurrence of various cellular responses, which all depend on the treatment parameters (types of photosensitizers, cellular localization, dose, light sources, dose, and incubation time).

2.4. Cancer recurrence and photodynamic therapy

After remaining undetected for a period following treatment, cancer can recur and according to the localization; a local, regional or distant recurrence needs to be dealt with. Surgery and other conventional cancer treatments are not suitable for advanced stage and metastatic tumors, and leaving room for development of drug-resistant cancer, which is often associated with cancer stem cells [74]. Cancer stem cells are normal stem cells, with special ability to give rise to all types of cells found in a particular cancer sample, so making them able to generate tumors through the stem cell processes of self-renewal and differentiation [75, 76]. The development of treatment modalities that target both primary and secondary and cancer stem cells becomes more than required, due to the selectivity of photosensitizers, Photodynamic therapy appears as a promising therapy for drug-resistant cancer stem cells with the photosensitizer-targeted delivery to cancer and particularly cancer stem cells [77]. For this reason, the capabilities of photosensitizers are being upgraded with prospective approaches based on nanoscience and nanotechnology for conjugating nanoparticles to photosensitizers to achieve nano-photosensitzers targeted delivery in the photodynamic treatment of cancer and cancer stem cells [78]. The use of nanoparticles makes it able to explore the poor lymphatic drainage and ensure that the photosensitizers is much more easily retained in cancer-like tissues than in normal tissues, a phenomena known as enhanced permeability and retention effect [79]. The conjugation of anticancer photosensitizers and water-dispersible nanoparticles with specific affinity for cancer stem cells yields a systemic self-deliverable photodynamic therapy, which maintains the pharmacological efficacy while improving the safety and delivery profiles [78, 80]. The nanocarriers are known to achieve both passive and active targeting delivery, which is an additional benefit to increase the therapeutic effects and reduce the side-effects [81]. With such development, the burden of enduring several drugs as currently accomplished in clinical treatment will be alleviated with the development of multifunctional nanocarriers. Another potential active targeting delivery approach will be conjugation with monoclonal antibodies specific to cancer and cancer stem cells. Multifunctional carriers of antibodies targeted against HER2 or estrogen or any other steroid hormone receptors that are overexpressed in breast cancer and cancer stem cells could be exploited to achieve better targeting, uptake and therapeutic outcomes both *in vivo* and *in vitro*. Multifunctional drug delivery carriers containing antibodies tend to show enhanced eradication of cancer and cancer stem cells, prospect targeting drug delivery systems depend on the discovery of cancer stem cell interacting mediators [81–83].

Novel types of targeted cancer therapy like the multifunctional complexes-mediated photodynamic therapy are currently being considered along with other treatments including cancer vaccines, oncolytic virotherapy and immunotherapy [84–85]. The transcription factors that regulate cell mobility, invasion and migration during metastatic tumor stages of breast cancer are becoming attractive and constitute essential molecular targets for future treatment modalities [86, 87]. Hormone receptors remain the most currently used markers in clinical trials and the usage of breast cancer markers BRCA1 and BRCA2 is increasing as seen by numerous report studies [88, 89]. Most of the preclinical studies are performed with cell lines derived from breast cancers, and MCF-7, T-47D and MDA-MB-231 are among the most commonly used [90].

3. Conclusion

Cancer, an uncontrolled cell proliferation condition, has become a major health challenge and global killer. The incidence and related treatment facilities are unfortunately determined by the lifestyles and geographic locations of cancer patients. Breast cancer is a common carcinoma that affects the tear-shaped milk glands in women and its classification is been facilitated by the presence or not of certain receptors (HER-2 and HR), which are also to predict the prognosis. Photodynamic therapy is a promising cancer treatment and offers better specific targeting of cancer and limited side-effects, when compared to conventional therapy. Mitochondria, lysosomes and perinuclear areas are reported as the most frequent localization sites for third generations of photosensitizers. The treatment efficiency depends upon the successful light-activation and intersystem conversion into the excited triplet state, only then photosensitizers interact with molecular oxygen to produce reactive oxygen species, toxins responsible for cytodestruction and cell death. If required, Photodynamic can be repeated but the contribution of nanoparticles in combination therapy for cancer and particularly breast cancer, has permitted the successful delivery of therapeutic agents to the targeted tumor site and enhancement of therapeutic effects. When conjugated, they facilitate the delivery of hydrophobic drugs into biological environments, ensure the preservation of the pharmacologic properties of the drugs, and enhance selective targeting to cancer cells through their large surfaces, which can be functionalized with a various kind of components. The use of photodynamic therapy offers controlled conditions with high selectivity to cancer, hence reducing the undesired side-effects seen with conventional treatments. Whether used as main or adjuvant therapy, the aim of combination cancer therapy using photodynamic therapy is to selectively and completely eradicate cancer by targeting and killing both cancer and cancer stem cells.

Acknowledgements

The work was conducted at the Laser Research Centre, Faculty of Health Sciences, University of Johannesburg, South Africa. The study was supported by the University Research Council of the University of Johannesburg. This work is based on the research supported by the South African Research Chairs Initiative of the Department of Science and Technology and National Research Foundation of South Africa (Grant No 98337), and the African Laser Centre.

Conflict of interest

The authors report no conflict of interest in this work.

Author details

Heidi Abrahamse* and Ivan Sosthene Mfouo Tynga

*Address all correspondence to: habrahamse@uj.ac.za

Laser Research Centre, Faculty of Health Sciences, University of Johannesburg, Doornfontein, South Africa

References

[1] National Cancer Institute. What is cancer? [Internet]. 2015. Available from: https://www.cancer.gov/about-cancer/understanding/what-is-cancer [Accessed: 2017-11-30]

[2] Roope R. Cancer survival rates three times higher with early diagnosis, The Guardian [Internet]. 2017. Available from: https://www.theguardian.com/society/2015/aug/10/cancer-survival-rates-higher-early-diagnosis [Accessed: 2017-11-30]

[3] Cancer Research UK. Let's be cancer sooner. [Internet]. 2017. https://www.cancerresearchuk.org/ [Accessed Retrieved 2017-11-30]

[4] Siegel RL, Miller KD, Jemal A. Mint: Cancer statistics. CA: a Cancer Journal for Clinicians. 2017;**67**:7-30. DOI: 10.3322/caac.21387

[5] GBD 2015 Risk Factors Collaborators. Global, regional, and national comparative risk assessment of 79 behavioural, environmental and occupational, and metabolic risks or clusters of risks, 1990-2015: A systematic analysis for the global burden of disease study 2015. Lancet. 2016;**388**(10053):1659-1724

[6] Ferlay J, Soerjomataram I, Ervik M, Dikshit R, Eser S, Mathers C et al. GLOBOCAN 2012 v1.0, Cancer Incidence and Mortality Worldwide: IARC CancerBase No. 11

[7] Plummer M, de Martel C, Vignat J, Ferlay J, Bray F, Franceschi S. Mint: Global burden of cancers attributable to infections in 2012: A synthetic analysis. The Lancet Global Health. 2016;**4**(9):e609-e616. DOI: 10.1016/S2214-109X(16)30143-7

[8] Stewart BW, Wild CP, editors. World Cancer Report 2014. Lyon: International Agency for Research on Cancer; 2014

[9] Ferlay J, Héry C, Autier P, Sankaranarayanan R. Global burden of breast cancer. In: Li C, editor. Breast Cancer Epidemiology. New York, NY: Springer; 2010. DOI: 10.1007/978-1-4419-0685-4_1

[10] Fragomeni SM, Sciallis A, Jeruss JS. Molecular subtypes and local-regional control of breast cancer. Surgical Oncology Clinics of North America. 2018;**27**(1):95-120. DOI: 10.1016/j.soc.2017.08.005

[11] Carlson RW, Allred DC, Anderson BO, Burstein HJ, Carter WB, Edge SB, Erban JK, Farrar WB, Goldstein LJ, Gradishar WJ, Hayes DF, Hudis CA, Jahanzeb M, Kiel K, Ljung BM, Marcom PK, Mayer IA, McCormick B, Nabell LM, Pierce LJ, Reed EC, Smith ML, Somlo G, Theriault RL, Topham NS, Ward JH, Winer EP, Wolff AC. Mint: Breast cancer. Clinical practice guidelines in oncology. Journal of the National Comprehensive Cancer Network. 2009;**7**(2):122-192. PMID 19200416

[12] Triple Negative Breast Cancer Foundation. Annual Breast Cancer Report by Subtype [Internet]. 2015. http://forum.tnbcfoundation.org/annual-breast-cancer-report-by-subtype_topic12465.html [Accessed: 2017-12-01]

[13] Romond EH, Perez EA, Bryant J, Suman VJ, Geyer CE, Davidson NE, Tan-Chiu E, Martino S, Paik S, Kaufman PA, Swain SM, Pisansky TM, Fehrenbacher L, Kutteh LA, Vogel VG, Visscher DW, Yothers G, Jenkins RB, Brown AM, Dakhil SR, Mamounas EP, Lingle WL, Klein PM, Ingle JN, Wolmark N. Mint: Trastuzumab plus adjuvant chemotherapy for operable HER2-positive breast cancer. New England Journal of Medicine. 2005;**353**(16):1673-1684. DOI: 10.1056/NEJMoa052122

[14] Sotiriou C, Pusztai L. Mint: Gene-expression signatures in breast cancer. New England Journal of Medicine. 2009;**360**(8):790-800. DOI: 10.1056/NEJMra0801289

[15] Kumar V, Abbas A. Robbins and Cotran Pathologic Basis of Disease. Philadelphia: Saunders, an imprint of Elsevier inc; 2010. p. 1090. ISBN: 978-1-4160-3121-5

[16] Saini KS, Taylor C, Ramirez AJ, Palmieri C, Gunnarsson U, Schmoll HJ, Dolci SM, Ghenne C, Metzger-Filho O, Skrzypski M, Paesmans M, Ameye L, Piccart-Gebhart MJ, de Azambuja E. Mint: Role of the multidisciplinary team in breast cancer management: Results from a large international survey involving 39 countries. Annals of Oncology. 2011;**23**(4):853-859. DOI: 10.1093/annonc/mdr352

[17] Kaur S, Elkahloun AG, Singh SP, Arakelyan A, Roberts DD. Mint: A function-blocking CD47 antibody modulates extracellular vesicle-mediated intercellular signaling between breast carcinoma cells and endothelial cells. Journal of cell communication and signaling International CCN Society. 2017. DOI: 10.1007/s12079-017-0428-0

[18] Pessina F, Navarria P, Cozzi L, Franceschini D, Tomatis S, Clerici E, Ascolese AM, DE Rose F, Bello L, Masci G, Santoro A, Scorsetti M. Mint: Outcome evaluation of HER2 breast cancer patients with limited brain metastasis. Anticancer Research. 2017;**37**(12):7057-7062. DOI: 10.21873/anticanres.12177

[19] Burstein HJ, Temin S, Anderson H, Buchholz TA, Davidson NE, Gelmon KE, Giordano SH, Hudis CA, Rowden D, Solky AJ, Stearns V, Winer EP, Griggs JJ. Mint: Adjuvant endocrine therapy for women with hormone receptor-positive breast cancer: American Society of Clinical Oncology clinical practice guideline focused update. Journal of Clinical Oncology. 2014;**32**(21):2255-2269

[20] Acedo P, Stockert JC, Cañete M, Villanueva A. Mint: Two combined photosensitizers: A goal for more effective photodynamic therapy of cancer. Cell Death & Disease. 2014;**5**: e1122. DOI: 10.1038/cddis.2014.77

[21] dos Santos AF, Terra LF, Wailemann RAM, Oliveira TC, de Morais Gomes V, Mineiro MF, Meotti FC, Bruni-Cardoso A, Baptista MS, Labriola L. Mint: Methylene blue photodynamic therapy induces selective and massive cell death in human breast cancer cells. BMC Cancer. 2017;**17**:194-209. DOI: 10.1186/s12885-017-3179-7

[22] Agostinis P, Berg K, Cengel KA, Foster TH, Girotti AW, Gollnick SO, Hahn SM, Hamblin MR, Juzeniene A, Kessel D, Korbelik M, Moan J, Mroz P, Nowiz D, Piette J, Willson BC, Golab J. Mint: Photodynamic therapy of cancer: An update. American Cancer Society. 2011;**61**:250-281. DOI: 10.3322/caac.20114

[23] Simone CB, Friedberg JS, Glatstein E, Stevenson JP, Sterman DH, Stephen M, Cengel KA. Mint: Photodynamic therapy for the treatment of non-small cell lung cancer. Journal of Thoracic Disease. 2012;**4**(1):63-75. DOI: 10.3978/j.issn.2072-1439.2011.11.05

[24] Mfouo-Tynga I, Nicolette N, Houreld NN, Heidi Abrahamse H. Mint: Characterization of a multiple particle delivery complex and determination of cellular photodamage in skin fibroblast and breast cancer cell lines. Journal of Biophotonics. 2017. DOI: 10.1002/jbio.201700077

[25] Banerjee SM, MacRobert AJ, Mosse CA, Periera B, Bown SG, Keshtgar MRS. Mint: Photodynamic therapy: Inception to application in breast cancer. The Breast. 2017;**31**:105-113. DOI: 10.1016/j.breast.2016.09.016

[26] George BP, Abrahamse H. A review on novel breast cancer therapies: Photodynamic therapy and plant derived agent induced cell death mechanisms. Anti-Cancer Agents in Medicinal Chemistry. 2016;**16**(7):793-801. DOI: 10.2174/1871520615666151026094028

[27] Bonnett R. Mint: Photosensitizers of the porphyrin and phthalocyanine series for photodynamic therapy. Chemical Society Reviews. 1995;**24**:19-33. DOI: 10.1039/CS9952400019

[28] Pushpan SK, Venkatraman S, Anand VG, Sankar J, Parmeswaran D, Ganesan S, Chandrashekar TK. Mint: Porphyrins in photodynamic therapy—A search for ideal photosensitizers. Current Medicinal Chemistry. Anti-Cancer Agents. 2002;**2**:187-207. DOI: 10.2174/1568011023354137

[29] Ormond AB, Harold S, Freeman HS. Mint: Dye sensitizers for photodynamic therapy. Materials. 2013;**6**:817-840. DOI: 10.3390/ma6030817

[30] Trindade FZ, Pavarina AC, Ribeiro APD, Bagnato VS, Vergani CE, Souza Costa CA. Mint: Toxicity of photodynamic therapy with LED associated to Photogem®: An in vivo study. Lasers in Medical Science. 2012;**27**:403-411. DOI: 10.1007/s10103-011-0909

[31] Hage R, Ferreira J, Bagnato VS, Vollet-Filho JD, Plapler H. Mint: Pharmacokinetics of photogem using fluorescence spectroscopy in dimethylhydrazine-inducedmurine colorectal carcinoma. International Journal of Photoenergy. 2012:1-8. DOI: 10.1155/2012/615259

[32] Chevalier S, Anidjar M, Scarlata E, Hamel L, Scherz A, Ficheux H, Borenstein N, Fiette L, Elhilali M. Mint: Preclinical study of the novel vascular occluding agent, WST11, for photodynamic therapy of the canine prostate. Journal of Urology. 2011;**196**:302-309. DOI: 10.1016/j.juro.2011.03.039

[33] Furre IE, Shahzidi S, Luksiene Z, Moller MTN, Borgen E, Morgan J, Tkacz-Stachowska K, Nesland JM, Peng Q. Mint: Targeting PBR by hexaminolevulinate-mediated photodynamic therapy induces apoptosis through translocation of apoptosis-inducing factor in human leukemia cells. Cancer Research. 2005;**65**:11051-11060. DOI: 10.1158/0008-5472.CAN-05-0510

[34] Kobayashi W, Liu Q, Nakagawa H, Sakaki H, Teh B, Matsumiya T, Yoshida H, Imaizumi T, Satoh K, Kimura H. Mint: Photodynamic therapy with mono-L-aspartyl chlorin e6 can cause necrosis of squamous cell carcinoma of tongue: Experimental study on an animal model of nude mouse. Oral Oncology. 2006;**42**:46-50. DOI: doi.org/10.1016/j.oraloncology.2005.05.009

[35] Gilchrest BA. Photodynamic therapy and selected off-label uses. In: Tuleya S, editor. Proceedings of the Winter Clinical Dermatology Conference. Kohala Coast, HI, USA: HMP Communications, LLC; 2010. pp. 10-12

[36] Triesscheijn M, Ruevekamp M, Aalders M, Baas P, Stewart FA. Mint: Outcome of mTHPC mediated photodynamic therapy is primarily determined by the vascular response. Photochemistry and Photobiology. 2005;**81**:1161-1167. DOI: 10.1562/2005-04-04-RA-474

[37] Dovigo LN, Pavarina AC, Ribeiro APD, Brunetti IL, Costa CADS, Jacomassi DP, Bagnato VS, Kurachi C. Mint: Investigation of the photodynamic effects of curcumin agains *Candida albicans*. Photochemistry and Photobiology. 2011;**87**:895-903. DOI: 10.1111/j.1751-1097.2011.00937

[38] Mousavi SH, Tavakkol-Afshari J, Brook A, Jafari-Anarkooli I. Mint: Direct toxicity of rose Bengal in MCF-7 cell line: Role of apoptosis. Food and Chemical Toxicology. 2009;**47**:855-859

[39] Chen Y, Zheng W, Li Y, Zhong J, Ji J, Shen P. Mint: Apoptosis induced by methylene-blue-mediated photodynamic therapy in melanolmas and the involvement of mitochondrial dysfunction revealed by proteomics. Cancer Science. 2008;**99**:2019-2027. DOI: 10.1111/j.1349-7006.2008.00910.x

[40] Josefsen LB, Boyle RW. Mint: Unique diagnostic and therapeutic roles of porphyrins and phthalocyanines in photodynamic therapy, imaging and theranostics. Theranostics. 2012;**2**(9):916-966. DOI: 10.7150/thno.4571

[41] Moan J, Peng Q. Mint: An outline of the hundred-year history of PDT. Anticancer Research. 2003;**23**(5A):3591-3600

[42] Gold MH, Goldman MP. Mint: 5-Aminolevulinic acid photodynamic therapy: Where we have been and where we are going. Dermatologic Surgery. 2004;**30**:1077-1084. DOI: 10.1111/j.1524-4725.2004.30331.x

[43] Vo-Dihn T. Biomedical Photonics Handbook. USA: CRC Press LCL; 2003

[44] Dong-Sheng Y. Digital closed-loop fiber optic gyroscope design based on the FPGA, Solid-State and Integrated Circuit Technology (ICSICT) 2016 13th IEEE International Conference on. pp. 1164-1166

[45] Wilson BC, Patterson MS. Mint: The physics, biophysics and technology of photodynamic therapy. Physics in Medicine and Biology. 2008;**53**:61-109. DOI: 10.1088/0031-9155/53/9/R01

[46] Niedre MJ, Secord AJ, Patterson MS, Wilson BC. Mint: In vitro tests of the validity of singlet oxygen luminescence measurements as a dose metric in photodynamic therapy. Cancer Research. 2003;**63**(22):7986-7994

[47] van Straten D, Mashayekhi V, de Bruijn HS, Oliveira S and Robinson DJ: Mint: Oncologic photodynamic therapy: Basic principles, current clinical status and future directions. Cancers (Basel) 2017;9(2):19. DOI: 10.3390/cancers9020019

[48] Horne TK, Cronjé MJ. Mint: Novel carbohydrate-substituted metallo-porphyrazine comparison for cancer tissue-type specificity during PDT. Journal of Photochemistry and Photobiology, B: Biology. 2017;**173**:412-422. DOI: 10.1016/j.jphotobiol.2017.06.013

[49] Hammerer F, Poyer F, Fourmois L, Chen S, Garcia G, Teulade-Fichou MP, Maillard P, Mahuteau-Betzer F. Mint: Mitochondria-targeted cationic porphyrin-triphenylamine hybrids for enhanced two-photon photodynamic therapy. Bioorganic and Medicinal Chemistry. 2017;**S0968-0896**(17):31795-31799. DOI: 10.1016/j.bmc.2017.11.024

[50] Leandro FZ, Martins J, Fontes AM, Tedesco AC. Mint: Evaluation of theranostic nanocarriers for near-infrared imaging and photodynamic therapy on human prostate cancer cells. Colloids and Surfaces. B, Biointerfaces. 2017;**154**:341-349. DOI: 10.1016/j.colsurfb.2017.03.042

[51] Wu J, Xiao Q, Zhang N, Xue C, Leung AW, Zhang H, Tang QJ, Xu C. Mint: Palmatine hydrochloride mediated photodynamic inactivation of breast cancer MCF-7 cells: Effectiveness and mechanism of action. Photodiagnosis and Photodynamic Therapy. 2016;**15**: 133-138. DOI: 10.1016/j.pdpdt.2016.07.006

[52] Quayle LA, Pereira MG, Scheper G, Wiltshire T, Peake RE, Hussain I, Rea CA, Bates TE. Mint: Anti-angiogenic drugs: Direct anti-cancer agents with mitochondrial mechanisms of action. Oncotarget. 2017;**8**(51):88670-88688. DOI: 10.18632/oncotarget.20858

[53] Huang H, Yu B, Zhang P, Huang J, Chen Y, Gasser G, Ji L, Chao H. Mint: Highly charged ruthenium (II) Polypyridyl complexes as lysosome-localized photosensitizers for two-photon photodynamic therapy. Angewandte Chemie International Edition in English. 2015;**54**(47):14049-14052. DOI: 10.1002/anie.201507800

[54] Nishie H, Kataoka H, Yano S, Kikuchi JI, Hayashi N, Narumi A, Nomoto A, Kubota E, Joh T. Mint: A next-generation bifunctional photosensitizer with improved water-solubility for photodynamic therapy and diagnosis. Oncotarget. 2016;**7**(45):74259-74268. DOI: 10.18632/oncotarget.12366

[55] Berndt-Paetz M, Weimann A, Sieger N, Schastak S, Riyad YM, Griebel J, Arthanareeswaran VKA, Stolzenburg JU, Neuhaus J. Mint: Tetrahydroporphyrin-tetratosylat (THPTS): A near-infrared photosensitizer for targeted and efficient photodynamic therapy (PDT) of human bladder carcinoma. An in vitro study. Photodiagnosis and Photodynamic Therapy. 2017;**18**:244-251. DOI: 10.1016/j.pdpdt.2017.02.017

[56] Sekhejane PR, Houreld NN, Abrahamse H. Mint: Multiorganelle localization of Metal-lated Phthalocyanine photosensitizer in colorectal cancer cells (DLD-1 and CaCo-2) enhances efficacy of photodynamic therapy. International Journal of Photoenergy. 2014;**2014**: ID 383027:10. DOI: 10.1155/2014/383027

[57] Kessel D, Reiners JJ Jr. Mint: Apoptosis and autophagy after mitochondrial or endoplasmic reticulum photodamage. Photochemistry and Photobiology. 2007;**83**:1024-1028. DOI: 10.1111/j.1751-1097.2007.00088.x

[58] Oleinick NL, Morris RL, Belichenko I. Mint: The role of apoptosis in response to photodynamic therapy: What, where, why, and how. Photochemistry and Photobiology Sciences. 2002;**Sci. 1**:1-21

[59] Igney FH, Krammer PH. Mint: Death and anti-death: Tumour resistance to apoptosis. Nature Reviews Cancer. 2002;**2**:277-288. DOI: 10.1038/nrc776

[60] Mfouo-Tynga I, Abrahamse H. Mint: Cell death pathways and Phthalocyanine as an effective agent for photodynamic cancer therapy. Status: Published by International Journal of Molecular Science. 2015;**16**:10228-10241. DOI: 10.3390/ijms160510228

[61] Mfouo-Tynga I, Houreld NN, Abrahamse H. Mint: Induced cell death pathway post photodynamic therapy using a metallophthalocyanine photosensitizer in breast cancer cells. Photomedicine and Laser Surgery. 2014;**32**(4):1-7. DOI: 10.1089/pho.2013.3650

[62] Buytaert E, Dewaele M, Agostinis P. Mint: Molecular effectors of multiple cell death pathways initiated by photodynamic therapy. Biochimica et Biophysica Acta. 2007;**1776**:86-107. DOI: 10.1016/j.bbcan.2007.07.001

[63] Mroz P, Yaroslavsky A, Kharkwal GB, Hamblin MR. Mint: Cell death pathways in photodynamic therapy of cancer. Cancer. 2011;**3**:2516-2539. DOI: 10.3390/cancers3022516

[64] Nagata S, Obana A, Gohto Y, Nakajima S. Mint: Necrotic and apoptotic cell death of human malignant melanoma cells following photodynamic therapy using an amphiphilic photosensitizer, ATX-S10 (Na). Lasers in Surgery and Medicine. 2003;**33**:64-70. DOI: 10.1002/lsm.10190

[65] Adigun R, Bhimji SS, Necrosis, Cell (Liquefactive, Coagulative, Caseous, Fat, Fibrinoid, and Gangrenous). In: StatPearls [Internet]. Treasure Island (FL): StatPearls Publishing; 2017 Jun-. Available from: https://www.ncbi.nlm.nih.gov/books/NBK430935/ [Accessed: 2017-12-02]

[66] Castano AP, Mroz P, Hamblin MR. Mint: Photodynamic therapy and anti-tumour immunity. Nature Reviews. Cancer. 2006;**6**:535-545. DOI: 10.1038/nrc1894

[67] Hsieh YJ, Wu CC, Chang CJ, Yu JS. Mint: Subcellular localization of photofrin determines the death phenotype of human epidermoid carcinoma A431 cells triggered by photodynamic therapy: When plasma membranes are the main targets. Journal of Cellular Physiology. 2003;**194**:363-375. DOI: 10.1002/jcp.10273

[68] Liu J, Zheng L, Li Y, Zhang Z, Zhang L, Shen L, Zhang X, Qiao H. Mint: Effect of DTPP-mediated photodynamic therapy on cell morphology, viability, cell cycle, and cytotoxicity in a murine lung adenocarcinoma cell line. Lasers in Medical Science. 2015;**30**(1): 181-191. DOI: 10.1007/s10103-013-1270-0

[69] Levine B, Klionsky DJ. Mint: Development by self-digestion: Molecular mechanisms and biological functions of autophagy. Developmental Cell. 2004;**6**:463-477. DOI: 10.1016/S1534-5807(04)00099-1

[70] Kessel DH, Price M, Reiners JJ Jr. Mint: ATG7 deficiency suppresses apoptosis and cell death induced by lysosomal photodamage. Autophagy. 2012;**8**:1333-1341. DOI: 10.4161/auto.20792

[71] Inguscio V, Panzarini E, Dini L. Mint: Autophagy contributes to the death/survival balance in cancer photodynamic therapy. Cell. 2012;**1**:464-491. DOI: 10.3390/cells1030464

[72] Xue LY, Chiu SM, Azizuddin K, Joseph S, Oleinick NL. Mint: The death of human cancer cells following photodynamic therapy: Apoptosis competence is necessary for Bcl-2 protection but not for induction of autophagy. Photochemistry and Photobiology. 2007;**83**:1016-1023. DOI: 10.1111/j.1751-1097.2007.00159.x

[73] Kessel D, Oleinick NL. Mint: Initiation of autophagy by photodynamic therapy. Methods in Enzymology. 2009;**453**:1-16. DOI: 10.1016/S0076-6879(08)04001-9

[74] Liu H, Lin L, Yang K. Mint: Chemotherapy targeting cancer stem cells. American Journal of Cancer Research. 2015;**5**(3):880-893

[75] Beck B, Blanpain C. Mint: Unravelling cancer stem cell potential. Nature Reviews Cancer. 2013;**13**(10):727-738. DOI: 10.1038/nrc3597

[76] Kreso A, Dick JE. Mint: Evolution of the cancer stem cell model. Cell Stem Cell. 2014; **14**(3):275-291. DOI: 10.1016/j.stem.2014.02.006

[77] Hodgkinson N, Kruger CA, Abrahamse H. Mint: Targeted photodynamic therapy as potential treatment modality for the eradication of colon cancer and colon cancer stem cells. Tumour Biology. 2017;**39**(10):1010428317734691

[78] Lin L, Xiong L, Wen Y, Lei S, Deng X, Liu Z, Chen W, Miao X. Mint: Active targeting of Nano-photosensitizer delivery Systems for Photodynamic Therapy of cancer stem cells. Journal of Biomedical Nanotechnology. 2015;**11**(4):531-554

[79] Kobayashi H, Watanabe R, Choyke PL. Mint: Improving conventional enhanced permeability and retention (EPR) effects; what is the appropriate target? Theranostics. 2013; **4**(1):81-89. DOI: 10.7150/thno.7193

[80] Wang H, Lu Z, Wang L, Guo T, Wu J, Wan J, Zhou L, Li H, Li Z, Jiang D, Song P, Xie H, Zhou L, Xu X, Zheng S. Mint: New generation nanomedicines constructed from self-assembling small molecule prodrugs alleviate cancer drug toxicity. Cancer Research. 2017;**2017**:0984.2017. DOI: 10.1158/0008-5472.CAN-17-0984

[81] Wakaskar RR. Mint: Passive and active targeting in tumor microenvironment. International journal of drug development and research. 2017;**9**:37-41

[82] Sotiropoulou PA, Christodoulou MS, Silvani A, Herold-Mende C, Passarella D. Mint: Chemical approaches to targeting drug resistance in cancer stem cells. Drug Discovery Today. 2014;**19**:1547-1562. DOI: 10.1016/j.drudis.2014.05.002

[83] Chiang CS, Hu SH, Liao BJ, Chang YC, Chen SY. Mint: Enhancement of cancer therapy efficacy by trastuzumab-conjugated and pH-sensitive nanocapsules with the simultaneous encapsulation of hydrophilic and hydrophobic compounds. Nanomedicine. 2014;**10**:99-107. DOI: 10.1016/j.nano.2013.07.009

[84] Suryawanshi YR, Zhang T, Essani K. Mint: Oncolytic viruses: Emerging options for the treatment of breast cancer. Medical Oncology. 2017;**34**(3):43. DOI: 10.1007/s12032-017-0899-0

[85] Yu LY, Tang J, Zhang CM, Zeng WJ, Yan H, Li MP, Chen XP. Mint: New immunotherapy strategies in breast cancer. International Journal of Environmental Research and Public Health. 2017;**14**(1):68. DOI: 10.3390/ijerph14010068

[86] Fougère M, Gaudineau B, Barbier J, Guaddachi F, Feugeas JP, Auboeuf D, Jauliac S. Mint: NFAT3 transcription factor inhibits breast cancer cell motility by targeting the Lipocalin 2 gene. Oncogene. 2010;**29**(15):2292-2301. DOI: 10.1038/onc.2009.499

[87] Gaudineau B, Fougère M, Guaddachi F, Lemoine F, de la Grange P, Jauliac S. Mint: Lipocalin 2 (LCN2), the TNF-like receptor TWEAKR and its ligand TWEAK act downstream of NFAT1 to regulate breast cancer cell invasion. Journal of Cell Science. 2012; **125**(19):4475-4486. DOI: 10.1242/jcs.099879

[88] Duffy MJ. Mint: Biochemical markers in breast cancer: Which ones are clinically useful? Clinical Biochemistry. 2001;**34**(5):347-352. DOI: 10.1016/S0009-9120(00)00201-0

[89] Mohammadzadeh F, Mosayebi G, Montazeri V, Darabi M, Fayezi S, Shaaker M, et al. Mint: Fatty acid composition of tissue cultured breast carcinoma and the effect of Stearoyl-CoA Desaturase 1 inhibition. Journal of Breast Cancer. 2014;**17**(2):136-142. DOI: 10.4048/jbc.2014.17.2.136

[90] Kytölä S, Rummukainen J, Nordgren A, Karhu R, Farnebo F, Isola J, Larsson C. Mint: Chromosomal alterations in 15 breast cancer cell lines by comparative genomic hybridization and spectral karyotyping. Genes, Chromosomes & Cancer. 2000;**28**(3):308-317

7

The Clinical Relevance of Circulating Tumor Cells in Early Breast Cancer

Malgorzata Banys-Paluchowski,
Florian Reinhardt and Tanja Fehm

Abstract

Circulating tumor cells (CTCs) are considered to be evading cancer cells that have been shed or actively invaded from the primary tumor into the blood circulation or lymphatic system and which may finally extravasate to found metastases. CTCs as "liquid biopsy" hold great promise to be a powerful non-invasive real-time measurable biomarker for predicting clinical outcomes and cancer treatment response. Several studies evaluated the role of CTC presence and count in the neoadjuvant and adjuvant setting of early breast cancer (EBC) and revealed their significant prognostic value. In this chapter, we highlight the clinical relevance of CTCs in early breast cancer (EBC) and state the urgency for further research in this field to definitely translate this marker from bench to bedside.

Keywords: early breast cancer, circulating tumor cells, liquid biopsy, survival, clinical relevance

1. Introduction

Circulating tumor cells (CTCs) are deemed to be evading cancer cells that have been shed or actively invaded from the primary tumor into the blood circulation or lymphatic system and which may finally extravasate to found metastases. CTCs as "liquid biopsy" hold great promise to be a powerful non-invasive real-time measurable biomarker for predicting clinical outcome and cancer treatment response [1]. Several studies evaluated the role of CTC presence and count in the neoadjuvant and adjuvant setting of breast cancer (BC) and revealed their significant prognostic value. In this chapter, we highlight the clinical relevance of CTCs in early

BC and state the urgency for further research in this field to definitely translate this marker from bench to bedside.

2. CTCs as a screening tool

Several studies observed the presence of CTCs in patients with no clinically detected metastatic lesion [2, 3]. Illie et al. revealed association of CTC presence with early carcinogenesis and risk of cancer [4]. However, the use of CTC presence as a screening tool to diagnose early breast cancer (EBC) is challenged by the low sensitivity of current CTC detection methods. Current CTC detection platforms such as the FDA-approved CellSearch™ system can only detect CTCs in about 70% of patients with metastatic breast cancer [5]. One of the solutions to improve sensitivity may be the previous performance of leukapheresis. Compared to 20–30% of CTC detection by the CellSearch™ system in early breast cancer, the combination of leukapheresis and the CellSearch™ system has revealed to be able to identify CTCs in 90% of patients with early breast cancer [6]. Respectively, rise of sensitivity due to enrichment techniques may pave the way to use CTCs for early breast cancer screening or diagnosis. An ongoing trial is currently enrolling patients who do not have a prior history of invasive breast carcinoma or clinically apparent metastatic disease to investigate the potential role of CTCs as a screening tool (NCT01322750).

3. CTCs for prediction of prognosis

Cancer cells may leave the primary tumor and enter blood circulation long before the disease becomes clinically detectable and are considered a potential source of metastatic spread. Accordingly, numerous studies reported that early BC patients with detectable CTCs have significantly worse clinical outcomes than CTC-negative patients (**Table 1**). Among these, the largest data set was provided by the German SUCCESS trial (EUDRA-CT No. 2005-000490-21, NCT02181101). Briefly, blood samples from over 2000 average-to-high risk non-metastatic BC patients before chemotherapy and nearly 1500 patients after chemotherapy were examined [8]. Patients with CTCs at baseline had significantly shorter disease-free and overall survival. Further, the trial explored the relationship between CTC counts and prognosis in order to determine the optimal cut-off (i.e., no CTCs vs. ≥ 1; 0–1 vs. ≥ 2; 0–4 vs. ≥ 5 CTCs in 30 ml blood). A statistically significant impact on the clinical outcome was demonstrated for all cut-offs while patients with ≥5 CTCs had the highest relapse risk. Results from the SUCCESS trial are in accordance with smaller studies with longer follow-up [11, 14].

Janni et al. performed a large, multicenter pooled analysis of the available trials and confirmed CTC presence in early BC as an independent predictor of shorter disease-free, overall, breast cancer-specific, and distant disease-free survival [7]. Interestingly, CTC positivity was not associated with survival in low-risk, small node-negative tumors, suggesting that early-stage

Author	Number of patients	Patients	Method	CTC positivity n (%)	Follow up (median, months)	Prognostic significance
Janni pooled analysis [7]*	3173	Stage I–III	CellSearch	641 (20%)	63	DFS, DDFS, BCSS, OS
Rack, SUCCESS trial [8]	2026	Stage I–III, node-positive or high risk node-negative, all pts. received chemotherapy	CellSearch	435 (21%)	36	DFS, DDFS, BCSS, OS
Molloy [9]	733	Stage I–II	qRT-PCR (CK19, p1B, EGP-2, PS2, MmGI)	58 (8%)	91	MFS, BCSS
Ignatiadis [10]	444	Stage I–III, all pts. received adjuvant chemotherapy	RT-PCR (CK19)	181 (41%)	54	DFS, OS
Franken [11]	404	Stage I–III	CellSearch	76 (19%)	48	DDFS, BCSS
Lucci [3]	302	Stage I–III	CellSearch	73 (24%)	35	DFS, OS
Kuniyoshi [12]	167	Stage I–III	RT-PCR (CK19, c-erbB-2)	n.a.	n.a.	None
Hwang [13]	166	Stage I–IIIa	RT-PCR (CK20)	37 (22%)	100	MFS, OS
REMAGUS02 trial [14]	95	Neoadjuvant trial, Stage II–III, ineligible for breast conserving surgery at diagnosis or high-risk	CellSearch	22 (23%)	70	DDFS, OS

n.s.: not significant; BCSS: breast cancer-specific survival; DDFS: distant disease-free survival; DFS: disease-free survival; OS: overall survival; MFS: metastasis-free survival.
*including data from five centers, some previously published as [3, 8, 11, 14].

Table 1. The prognostic relevance of CTC presence in patients with non-metastatic BC.

BC can be treated successfully despite the presence of minimal residual disease in the blood. In high-risk patients, the strong prognostic value of CTCs underlines the necessity to establish new treatment strategies for this particular patient group. Further, CTCs predicted clinical outcomes in women with triple-negative and luminal (i.e., hormone-receptor positive, including luminal B HER2-positive subtype) tumors, but no association was found in case of patients with HER2-positive, hormone receptor-negative disease [7]. This observation is in contrast with the previous study by Ignatiadis et al. who reported that CTCs were highly predictive of clinical outcomes in the triple-negative and HER2-subtype but not in luminal tumors [10, 15]. Similar findings were reported by others [13, 16, 17]. Possibly, the relatively short follow-up may contribute to these partly contradictory results since none of the abovementioned trials reported a follow-up longer than 100 months. Longer follow-up might be necessary to fully understand the relevance of CTCs in patients with luminal tumors who are more at risk for a late relapse compared to women with more aggressive subtypes [18].

4. Therapy monitoring

Gold standard for evaluation of therapy response involves clinical examination, measurement of tumor markers, and radiologic imaging. CTCs provide a blood biomarker for early carcinogenesis, cancer progression, and treatment effectiveness. The identification of circulating tumor cells under therapy correlates with poor prognosis in metastatic breast cancer, but there are few data describing the importance of circulating tumor cells in patients with early breast cancer.

Regarding adjuvant treatment modalities of patients with early breast cancer, the SUCCESS trial and a trial by Xenidis et al. are the only trials in which CTCs were monitored [8, 19]. In the SUCCESS trial, CTCs were analyzed in 1492 patients with early breast cancer before adjuvant chemotherapy and post-chemotherapy using the CellSearch™ system [8]. The 36-month OS was 92.8% for persistently CTC-positive patients and 97.6% for persistently CTC-negative patients. Regarding the DFS, the Kaplan-Meyer estimate was 85.9% for persistently CTC-positive patients and 93.9% for persistently CTC-negative patients. This large prospective trial of patients with early breast cancer suggests the independent prognostic relevance of CTCs both before and after adjuvant chemotherapy. In line, the presence of persistent CTCs 2 years after completion of adjuvant chemotherapy in clinically disease-free patients predicted worse clinical survival [20]. Xenidis et al. analyzed blood samples of 237 patients who were initially positive before start of taxane-based or taxane-free adjuvant chemotherapy [19]. After a median follow-up of 71 months, patients treated with taxane-based regimen had a longer DFS compared to patients receiving taxane-free regimen. Positive effects on median survival in the taxane group were reflected by a shift toward CTC-negative status: 50% of patients in the taxane-treated group turned CTC negative compared to only 33% of patients in the taxane-free arm [19]. In the phase III SUCCESS C trial (NCT00847444), 3547 patients with HER2-negative early breast cancer were randomized to either six cycles of docetaxel and cyclophosphamide (DOC-C) or to epirubicin, 5-fluorouracil, and cyclophosphamide followed by three cycles of docetaxel (FEC-DOC). Data on CTC prevalence after adjuvant chemotherapy between both treatment arms were available for 1766 patients. First results revealed no significant difference of CTC prevalence at the time of last chemotherapy cycle between patients randomized to FEC-DOC or DOC-C (11.5 vs. 13.6%). The comparable prevalence of CTCs may indicate that anthracycline-free chemotherapy is equally effective to anthracycline-containing chemotherapy in HER2-negative, hormone receptor-positive early breast cancer. However, this interpretation needs to be confirmed by data of the final survival analysis [21].

In the neoadjuvant setting, four studies explored the association of CTCs and clinical outcomes. In a small study of Hall et al. focusing on 57 patients with triple negative breast cancer, CTC persistence after neoadjuvant treatment was an independent predictor of worse clinical outcomes [22]. The study showed a significant correlation between CTC presence and shorter relapse-free and overall survival after completion of neoadjuvant therapy. This is in contrast to other studies in which conflicting results were reported in the neoadjuvant setting [14, 23, 24]. These studies also aimed to explore the signatures of CTC dynamics and pathological changes in the primary tumor during neoadjuvant chemotherapy. In several clinical trials pathological complete response is used as an endpoint because of its ability to predict long-term survival.

However, changes in CTC count generally did not correlate with tumor's response to neoadjuvant chemotherapy. In the REMAGUS02 trial, the CTC count of 85 patients was analyzed after neoadjuvant chemotherapy [25]. No correlation between CTC dynamics and pathological response was found after neoadjuvant treatment. Analog results were shown in the Gepar Quattro trial [26]. Riethdorf et al. analyzed blood samples from 213 non-metastasized breast cancer patients before and after preoperative chemotherapy. Interestingly, in 22% of patients, CTCs could be detected by CellSearch™ before neoadjuvant treatment, whereas positivity rates decreased to 11% after chemotherapy. However, neither CTC count before nor after preoperative chemotherapy was predictive to pathological response of the primary tumor.

5. Treatment decisions based on CTCs

Although there are several ongoing trials investigating the role of CTCs as a decision tool in metastatic breast cancer, there are only few studies investigating the clinical utility of isolated tumor cells encountered in the blood stream in early breast cancer. This might be due to technical challenges of CTC research in early breast cancer. Up to date, treatment decisions in early breast cancer are still based on the phenotype of the primary tumor without considering the disease evolution. Nevertheless, features of minimal residual disease may differ from those of the primary tumor. Riethdorf et al. examined the HER2 status of CTCs in HER2-negative primary breast cancer [26]. In 19% of patients with HER2-negative BC, CTCs expressing the HER2 receptor were detected in peripheral blood [26]. Anti-HER2-targeted treatment is not eligible for these patients, which might result in undertherapy and higher risk for relapse. Georgoulias et al. showed an increased DFS and reduced number of relapses among patients with persistent HER2-positive CTCs detected after completion of adjuvant therapy and administration of trastuzumab [27]. In this small Phase II trial (n = 75), additional therapy with trastuzumab resulted in a 75% reduction of patients with detectable CTCs in the trastuzumab arm compared to 17.9% in the control group. Based on these results, this therapeutic approach is currently investigated in the TREAT CTC randomized trial (NCT01548677) [28]. Patients with HER2 negative early breast cancer with persistent CTCs after (neo) adjuvant chemotherapy were randomized concerning additional trastuzumab treatment. HER2 status of CTCs was assessed; nevertheless, treatment decisions were only based on CTC presence. However, the TREAT CTC trial was closed for patient recruitment. To date, there are no published results yet.

Concerning treatment decisions, additional molecular profiling of CTCs may provide important additional information to CTC count. Several studies revealed intra- and intertumoral heterogeneity and demonstrated differences in phenotypes and genotypes between CTCs and primary tumors [29]. Therefore, detection and molecular characterization of CTCs are of great interest for selection of proper medical treatments and prevention of therapeutic resistance. In metastatic breast cancer, clinical significance of CTC subtype for guiding treatment decisions and evaluating therapy response is currently investigated within the German DETECT trials (NCT01619111).

6. Limitations of current methods for CTC detection

In this context, one needs to keep the limitations of current methods for CTC detection in mind. Epithelial cell adhesion molecule (EpCAM)-dependent enrichment techniques are the most widely used with the CellSearch™ system being so far the only FDA-approved system [30]. However, detection of CTCs is limited by the CellSearch™ system to cells with expression of EPCAM and cytokeratin 8/18/19. Respectively, the CellSearch system can certainly miss the detection of subpopulations of CTCs with decreased epithelial marker expression as a result of CTCs that have undergone epithelial-mesenchymal transition (EMT) [31]. It was observed that tumor cells which already initiated EMT are correlated with worse prognosis and therapy resistance [32]. Therefore, many EpCAM-independent methods are currently being developed and tested for CTC characterization. Translation into clinical routine practice of these new methods seems to be currently difficult. Multicenter assessment studies are lacking, and thus their reproducibility, sensitivity and specificity remain to be evaluated.

7. Conclusions

Circulating tumor cells are currently considered one of the most promising biomarkers for prediction of survival and monitoring of therapy in solid malignancies. While their prognostic significance has long been proven in early and metastatic breast cancer, further research is urgently needed to examine the possibility of guiding treatment decisions based on the presence and phenotype/genotype of CTCs (**Table 2**).

Potential	Early BC	Metastatic BC
Prognostication	Yes; CTCs are significantly associated with disease-free and overall survival	Yes (level I evidence); high CTC levels correlate with shorter progression-free and overall survival (cut-off: 5 CTCs/7.5 ml PB)
Therapy monitoring	Unclear; presence of CTCs 2 years after completion of chemotherapy predicts worse survival; contradictory results with regard to association between CTC changes and response to neoadjuvant treatment	Possibly relevant; High CTC levels after start of first-line chemotherapy can adequately predict progression; however, patients do not benefit from a switch to another regimen (clinical trials: SWOG 0500, ongoing: CirCe01)
Treatment selection based on CTCs	Possibly relevant; evidence pending (clinical trials: TREAT CTC, active, closed to patient entry)	Possibly relevant; evidence pending (ongoing clinical trials: STIC CTC METABREAST, DETECT III/IVa/IVb/V)

Modified after Ref. [33].

Table 2. Clinical role of CTCs in early and metastatic breast cancer.

Author details

Malgorzata Banys-Paluchowski[1]*, Florian Reinhardt[2] and Tanja Fehm[2]

*Address all correspondence to: banys.malgorzata@yahoo.com

1 Department of Gynecology and Obstetrics, Marienkrankenhaus Hamburg, Hamburg, Germany

2 Department of Gynecology and Obstetrics, University Hospital Duesseldorf, University of Duesseldorf, Duesseldorf, Germany

References

[1] Banys-Paluchowski M, Krawczyk N, Fehm T. Potential role of circulating tumor cell detection and monitoring in breast cancer: A review of current evidence. Frontiers in Oncology. 2016;**6**:255

[2] Krishnamurthy S et al. Detection of minimal residual disease in blood and bone marrow in early stage breast cancer. Cancer. 2010;**116**(14):3330-3337

[3] Lucci A et al. Circulating tumour cells in non-metastatic breast cancer: A prospective study. The Lancet Oncology. 2012;**13**(7):688-695

[4] Ilie M et al. "Sentinel" circulating tumor cells allow early diagnosis of lung cancer in patients with chronic obstructive pulmonary disease. PLoS One. 2014;**9**(10):e111597

[5] Sarangi S et al. The evolving role of circulating tumor cells in the personalized management of breast cancer: From enumeration to molecular characterization. Current Breast Cancer Reports. 2014;**6**(3):146-153

[6] Fischer JC et al. Diagnostic leukapheresis enables reliable detection of circulating tumor cells of nonmetastatic cancer patients. Proceedings of the National Academy of Sciences of the United States of America. 2013;**110**(41):16580-16585

[7] Janni WJ et al. Pooled analysis of the prognostic relevance of circulating tumor cells in primary breast cancer. Clinical Cancer Research. 2016;**22**(10):2583-2593

[8] Rack B et al. Circulating tumor cells predict survival in early average-to-high risk breast cancer patients. Journal of the National Cancer Institute. 2014;**106**(5):1-11

[9] Molloy TJ et al. The prognostic significance of tumour cell detection in the peripheral blood versus the bone marrow in 733 early-stage breast cancer patients. Breast Cancer Research. 2011;**13**(3):R61

[10] Ignatiadis M et al. Different prognostic value of cytokeratin-19 mRNA positive circulating tumor cells according to estrogen receptor and HER2 status in early-stage breast cancer. Journal of Clinical Oncology. 2007;**25**(33):5194-5202

[11] Franken B et al. Circulating tumor cells, disease recurrence and survival in newly diagnosed breast cancer. Breast Cancer Research. 2012;**14**(5):R133

[12] Kuniyoshi RK et al. Gene profiling and circulating tumor cells as biomarker to prognostic of patients with locoregional breast cancer. Tumour Biology. 2015;**36**:8075-8083

[13] Hwang SB et al. Circulating tumor cells detected by RT-PCR for CK-20 before surgery indicate worse prognostic impact in triple-negative and HER2 subtype breast cancer. Journal of Breast Cancer. 2012;**15**(1):34-42

[14] Bidard FC et al. Time-dependent prognostic impact of circulating tumor cells detection in non-metastatic breast cancer: 70-Month analysis of the REMAGUS02 study. International Journal of Breast Cancer. 2013;**2013**:130470

[15] Ignatiadis M et al. Molecular detection and prognostic value of circulating cytokeratin-19 messenger RNA-positive and HER2 messenger RNA-positive cells in the peripheral blood of women with early-stage breast cancer. Clinical Breast Cancer. 2007;**7**(11):883-889

[16] Karhade M et al. Circulating tumor cells in non-metastatic triple-negative breast cancer. Breast Cancer Research and Treatment. 2014;**147**(2):325-333

[17] Banys-Paluchowski M et al. Prognostic relevance of circulating tumor cells in molecular subtypes of breast cancer. Geburtshilfe und Frauenheilkunde. 2015;**75**(3):232-237

[18] Lim E, Metzger-Filho O, Winer EP. The natural history of hormone receptor-positive breast cancer. Oncology (Williston Park). 2012;**26**(8):688-694 696

[19] Xenidis N et al. Differential effect of adjuvant taxane-based and taxane-free chemotherapy regimens on the CK-19 mRNA-positive circulating tumour cells in patients with early breast cancer. British Journal of Cancer. 2013;**108**(3):549-556

[20] Janni W, Rack B, Fasching P, Haeberle L, Friedl T, Tesch H, et al. Persistence of circulating tumor cells in high risk early breast cancer patients during follow-up care suggests poor prognosis-results from the adjuvant SUCCESS A trial. In: 2015 San Antanio Breast Cancer Symposium, S02-S03, San Antonio; 2015

[21] Schramm A et al. Prevalence of circulating tumor cells after adjuvant chemotherapy with or without Anthracyclines in patients with HER2-negative, hormone receptor-positive early breast Cancer. Clinical Breast Cancer. 2017;**17**(4):279-285

[22] Hall C et al. Circulating tumor cells after neoadjuvant chemotherapy in stage I-III triple-negative breast cancer. Annals of Surgical Oncology. 2015;**22**(Suppl 3):S552-S558

[23] Kasimir-Bauer S et al. Does primary neoadjuvant systemic therapy eradicate minimal residual disease? Analysis of disseminated and circulating tumor cells before and after therapy. Breast Cancer Research. 2016;**18**(1):20

[24] Bidard FC et al. Single circulating tumor cell detection and overall survival in nonmetastatic breast cancer. Annals of Oncology. 2010;**21**(4):729-733

[25] Pierga JY et al. Circulating tumor cell detection predicts early metastatic relapse after neoadjuvant chemotherapy in large operable and locally advanced breast cancer in a phase II randomized trial. Clinical Cancer Research. 2008;**14**(21):7004-7010

[26] Riethdorf S et al. Detection and HER2 expression of circulating tumor cells: Prospective monitoring in breast cancer patients treated in the neoadjuvant GeparQuattro trial. Clinical Cancer Research. 2010;**16**(9):2634-2645

[27] Georgoulias V et al. Trastuzumab decreases the incidence of clinical relapses in patients with early breast cancer presenting chemotherapy-resistant CK-19mRNA-positive circulating tumor cells: Results of a randomized phase II study. Annals of Oncology. 2012;**23**(7): 1744-1750

[28] Ignatiadis M et al. Liquid biopsy-based clinical research in early breast cancer: The EORTC 90091-10093 Treat CTC trial. European Journal of Cancer. 2016;**63**:97-104

[29] Reinhardt F et al. Navigation through inter- and intratumoral heterogeneity of endocrine resistance mechanisms in breast cancer: A potential role for liquid biopsies? Tumour Biology. 2017;**39**(11):1010428317731511

[30] Banys M et al. Circulating tumor cells in breast cancer. Clinica Chimica Acta. 2013;**423**:39-45

[31] Wicha MS, Hayes DF. Circulating tumor cells: Not all detected cells are bad and not all bad cells are detected. Journal of Clinical Oncology. 2011;**29**(12):1508-1511

[32] Tiwari N et al. EMT as the ultimate survival mechanism of cancer cells. Seminars in Cancer Biology. 2012;**22**(3):194-207

[33] Banys-Paluchowski M et al. Circulating tumor cells in breast cancer-current status and perspectives. Critical Reviews in Oncology/Hematology. 2016;**97**:22-29

8

Adjuvant Systemic Treatment in Hormone Receptor Positive, HER2 Negative Breast Cancer

Fatma Sen

Abstract

The introduction of adjuvant systemic therapy led to a significant improvement in post-surgical survival and a reduction in disease relapse. Approximately 75–80% of all breast cancers are hormone-dependent based on the presence of ER and/or PR on tumor cells. Patients with HR+ breast cancer less than 5 mm and treated with only endocrine therapy have usually very good prognosis. They typically are not treated with adjuvant chemotherapy. The patients with stage III HR+ breast cancer still require adjuvant chemotherapy since they carry high risk of recurrence without chemotherapy. Many patients with HR+ HER2 negative breast cancer fall in between these two categories, and they are called as intermediate risk group based on clinicopathological variables, genomic tests or online risk calculators. The minimum duration of adjuvant endocrine treatment is 5 years; however, patients with high risk factors including positive lymph node should be treated with the endocrine therapy up to 10 years either with tamoxifen alone or sequentially with aromatase inhibitors (AI) in postmenopausal women. Adjuvant bisphosphonates reduce bone recurrence and improve survival in postmenopausal women with early stage breast cancer.

Keywords: adjuvant chemotherapy, breast cancer, endocrine therapy, hormone receptor, molecular assays

1. Introduction

Breast cancer is the most common cancer accounting for 25.1% of all cancers in women according to GLOBOCAN and the second most common cancer overall worldwide [1]. Over 1.5 million women are diagnosed with breast cancer every year, and half million women die due to breast cancer in the world each year. Although it is the fifth most common cause of death from cancer in women, during last 3 decades, deaths due to breast cancer have decreased by one-third or more. It is due in part to increased screening, as well as more effective loco-regional and systemic treatment options have been established over last decades.

The risk of relapse varies substantially on the basis of individual disease. Thus, accurate estimates regarding recurrence and survival are critical for selecting patients with breast cancer who will benefit from adjuvant therapy. Decisions about the type of treatment have traditionally been based on the histopathologic parameters including lymph node status, tumor size, histologic grade, histologic subtype, patient age, and estrogen receptor (ER)/progesterone receptor (PR) status. However, these characteristics fail to characterize the biologic heterogeneity of tumors, which has important implications for treatment benefit. The advent of microarray gene expression profiles as well as sequencing of the whole genome has brought several multigene platforms into clinical use. Many of these platforms incorporate traditional markers (e.g., ER, PR, and HER2) as well as additional cancer-associated genes. Approximately 75–80% of all breast cancers are luminal A or luminal B subtypes which are hormone-dependent based on the presence of ER and/or PR on tumor cells [2].

Here, the genetic and online tools which guide the adjuvant systemic treatment, options of endocrine therapy and systemic cytotoxic chemotherapy in patients with early stage HR+, HER2 -negative breast cancer will be discussed.

2. Treatment decision tools

Adjuvant systemic treatments reduce the risk of breast cancer recurrence following the local treatment of primary stage I–III breast cancers. International expert groups recommend determining the histologic grade and ER, PR, Ki-67 and HER2 status in all breast cancer patients, in order to assist prognosis and determine therapeutic options, including hormone therapy, chemotherapy and anti-HER2 therapy.

For patients with HR+ breast cancers receiving hormonal therapy, the risk of distant recurrence is under 20% and therefore, many patients may potentially be spared of chemotherapy. The web-based prognostification and treatment benefit tools and genomic assays have been incorporated into treatment planning for patients with early-stage HR+ breast cancer, which lead to get more information about prognosis and prediction of treatment response. These assays supplement the traditional histopathologic markers and help identify patients at high risk of recurrence. They also provide a more quantitative approach to risk assessment and enable individualization of treatment. This has both quality of life and health care cost implications because patients who will not benefit from a certain treatment can be spared both the toxicity and the expense [3].

One of the available genetic prognostic platforms (MammaPrint®, Oncotype DX®, Prosigna® or EndoPredict®) may be used in node-negative ER+ patients to establish a prognostic category and decide with the patient whether adjuvant treatment may be limited to hormonal therapy.

2.1. Genomic tools: oncotype Dx

Oncotype DX contains five reference genes (ACTB, GAPDH, GUS, RPLPO and TFRC) and 16 cancer-related genes. RNA is extracted from formalin-fixed paraffin-embedded tumor tissue, using quantitative real-time reverse transcriptase polymerase chain reaction (qRT-PCR). The recurrence score (RS) is the result of a mathematical formula of the weighted expression of each gene, ranging from 0 to 100. The cutoff points are divided into three categories: low risk (RS < 18), intermediate risk (RS 18–30), and high risk (RS > 31). The RS has been proved to be a predictor of 10-year distant recurrence for early breast cancer through NSABP B-14 in multivariate analyses including age, tumor size, tumor grade, ER status and HER2 status [4]. Furthermore, patients with low or intermediate RS had large improvements in disease-free survival (DFS) if treated with tamoxifen (TAM), which indicated that RS was helpful in evaluating treatment response to endocrine therapy in early breast cancer. Habel et al. [5] conducted a case–control study among women with ER+, node-negative breast cancer treated with TAM and compared these with untreated patients. The RS was associated with the risk of breast cancer death in both groups (P = 0.003 and P = 0.03). Thus, the RS was strongly related to long-term mortality of breast cancer among ER+ breast cancer patients treated with endocrine therapy.

Paik et al. not only evaluated the relationship between the RS and clinical result of ER+, node-negative early breast cancer but also explored the prognostic ability in late recurrence of breast cancer [4]. The 10-year distant recurrence rate was 6.8% in low-risk group, 14.3% in intermediate-risk group and 30.5% in high-risk group. The RS was shown to be related to distant relapse in patients who did not receive adjuvant chemotherapy, regardless of age and tumor size and performed better than both of them (P < 0.001).

RS can predict chemotherapy sensitivity in patients with ER+, node-negative breast cancer [6]. Paik et al. studied 651 cases of breast cancer who were enrolled in NSABP B-20 and randomly assigned them into a TAM group and a TAM combined with the chemotherapy group [chemotherapy regimen for cyclophosphamide & methotrexate & fluorouracil (CMF) or MF regimen, TAM + CMF/MF group] [4]. The 10-year follow-up results showed that patients with high RS had benefited from cytotoxic chemotherapy, with the 10-year metastasis rate being decreased by 27.6%. In contrast, the 10-year distant metastasis rate was decreased by an average of −1.1% in patients with low RS who received adjuvant chemotherapy. Therefore, patients with ER+ early breast cancer and high RS should benefit from chemotherapy, while patients with low RS cannot. RS can help select patients who experience little benefit of chemotherapy and can avoid the toxic effects of chemotherapy.

In a phase III trial, the Trial Assigning Individualized Options for Treatment (TAILORx), there was a prospective phase to further validate the function of RS in patients with HR+, HER2-negative, node-negative breast cancer. The results from TAILORx indicated that patients with very low RS results (<11) had excellent clinical outcome with a rate of 5-year freedom from distant recurrence with endocrine therapy at 99.3% and a rate of overall survival (OS) of 98.0%, even without chemotherapy [7]. As for its excellent utility in identifying patients with good outcome, Oncotype DX RS became the only gene-expression assay that was recommended at level I evidence in the AJCC Prognostic Stage Group. In patients with HR+, node-negative breast cancer, the RS showed excellent clinical utility to predict clinical outcomes.

In ECOG E2197, the predictive utility of RS on loco-regional recurrence (LRR) was evaluated in 388 patients with N0-N1 involvement and treated with breast conserving surgery, chemo-endocrine therapy and breast irradiation. The 10-year rates of LRR for HR+ tumors were shown to be 3.8, 5.1 and 12.0% for low, intermediate and high risk of RS (P = 0.12) [8].

In NSABP B-28 trial, RS was shown to be a statistically predictor of LRR, with 10-year cumulative incidence of LRR of 3.3, 7.2 and 12.2% in low, intermediate and high RS (P < 0.001) [9]. RS is a strongly predictive factor of LRR for HR+ breast cancer regardless of node status. Another study, PACS 01 trial, with a median of 7.7 years follow-up, showed that RS was a significant predictor of distant recurrence free interval survival, disease-free survival (DFS) and OS (P < 0.001) in HR+, node-positive patients treated with chemotherapy plus endocrine therapy [10].

The Southwest Oncology Group (SWOG)-8814 focused on exploring the benefit of therapy in patients with HR+, node-positive breast cancer. It enrolled postmenopausal women treated with chemotherapy or simple endocrine adjuvant therapy, of which 367 cases (40%) received an RS detection. RS had a definite predictive value (P = 0.016) for adjuvant treatment benefit over 5 years and was poorly predicted for treatment beyond 5 years (P = 0.87). High-risk patients receiving chemotherapy combined with endocrine therapy compared with simple endocrine therapy benefit significantly (P = 0.033). SWOG-8814 trial showed that the RS was also prognostic for TAM-treated patients with positive nodes and predicts significant benefit of chemotherapy [cyclophosphamide & adriamycin & fluorouracil (CAF)] in tumors with a high RS [11].

In a recent prospective phase III trial, West German Study Group Plan B, 348 patients (15.8%) with RS ≤ 11 had excellent 3-year survival even if they omitted chemotherapy. The 3-year DFS in patients with RS ≤ 11 was 98%, in which 41.1% had node-positive and 32.5% were grade 3 disease. These were the first prospective data to report clinical outcome when RS was used to make physical decision in patients with HR+ breast cancer regardless of lymph node invasion [12].

Rx for Positive Node, Endocrine Responsive Breast Cancer (RxPONDER) trial is an ongoing multicenter phase III trial revealed that patients with node positive breast cancer who had low to intermediate RS results could benefit from chemotherapy [13]. The trial also determined whether there is an optimal RS cutoff for these patients above which chemotherapy should be recommended in clinical practice. RxPONDER trial randomized patients with HR+, HER2-negative and 1–3 lymph nodes breast cancer with RS ≤ 25, to improve the risk of stratification in patients with low or intermediate RS.

2.2. MammaPrint

MammaPrint was first developed by the Netherlands Cancer Institute group. van't Veer et al. [14] used a gene-expression panel to detect 78 frozen tumor tissues from patients with pT1-2cN0 invasive breast carcinoma who had received standard treatment. Ribonucleic acid was isolated from fresh frozen tumor tissue to obtain complementary DNA. The gene-expression panel contains 70 genes related to early risk of metastasis, including tumor invasion, metastasis, interstitial invasion, and angiogenesis-related genes.

The MINDACT study was a randomized trial that included 6693 women with histologically proven operable N0/N1 invasive breast cancer without distant metastases [15]. Patients were recruited from 2007 to 2011. Initially, only patients without regional lymph node metastasis were enrolled. The study was amended to include patients with 1–3+ nodes in 2009. MammaPrint assay was used to determine participant's genomic risk and a modified version of Adjuvant! Online (version 8.0 with HER2 status) was used to determine clinical risk [16, 17]. Patients with both low clinical and low genomic risk were not treated with adjuvant chemotherapy; on the other hand, patients with high clinical and high genomic risk received adjuvant chemotherapy. The patients with discordant clinical and genomic risk results (high/low or low/high) were randomized to receive chemotherapy or not to receive chemotherapy. All patients were recommended to receive 7 years of hormonal therapy.

Patients at low clinical risk but high genomic risk who received chemotherapy had a 5-year distant metastasis free survival of 95.8% compared with 95.0% among those who did not receive chemotherapy. The adjusted hazard ratio for distant metastasis or death with chemotherapy versus no chemotherapy in this group was 1.17 (P = 0.66). Thus, a chemotherapy benefit is unlikely in women with tumors at low clinical risk regardless of genomic subtype. If a patient has ER/PgR-positive, HER2-negative, node negative, breast cancer, the MammaPrint (Agendia) assay should not be used in those with low clinical risk per MINDACT categorization to inform decisions on withholding adjuvant systemic chemotherapy because women in the low clinical risk category had excellent outcomes and did not appear to benefit from chemotherapy even with a genomic high-risk cancer.

If a patient has HR+, HER2-negative, node-negative breast cancer, the MammaPrint assay may be used in those with high clinical risk to inform decisions on withholding adjuvant systemic chemotherapy due to its ability to identify a good-prognosis population with potentially limited chemotherapy benefit. Women in the low clinical risk category did not benefit from chemotherapy regardless of genomic MammaPrint risk group. Therefore, the MammaPrint assay does not have clinical utility in such patients.

If a patient has HR+, HER2-negative, node-positive breast cancer, the MammaPrint assay may be used in patients with 1–3 positive nodes and a high clinical risk to inform decisions on withholding adjuvant systemic chemotherapy. However, such patients should be informed that a benefit from chemotherapy cannot be excluded, particularly in patients with greater than one involved lymph node.

The clinician should not use the MammaPrint assay to guide decisions on adjuvant systemic therapy in patients with HR+, HER2-negative, node-positive breast cancer at low clinical risk, nor any patient with HER2-positive or triple-negative breast cancer, because of the lack of definitive data in these populations [18].

2.3. PAM-50: PROSIGNA

The PAM50 Breast Cancer Intrinsic Classifier™ assay (ARUP Laboratories, Salt Lake City, UT) is a standardized test measuring 50 classifier genes and five control genes, amenable to assay by techniques such as quantitative real-time reverse transcriptase PCR [19]. It was originally developed in a microarray-based cohort of node-negative, untreated breast cancer patients. It accurately identifies the major intrinsic biological subtypes of breast cancer commonly known as luminal A, luminal B, HER2 enriched, and basal-like [20] and predicts the risk of recurrence (ROR) at 10 years. Tumors that are named as luminal A in PAM50 intrinsic subtype indicate usually very good prognosis with only adjuvant endocrine therapy, whereas luminal B subtypes have increased risk of recurrence without adjuvant chemotherapy.

Four versions of ROR exist in the research setting: ROR based on subtype information (ROR-S), ROR-S with proliferation (ROR-P), ROR-S with tumor size (ROR-T), and ROR-P with tumor size (ROR-PT) [20]. The minimum ROR score of all Luminal B scores was assigned as the low-risk threshold for each model and the maximum ROR score of all Luminal A scores as the high-risk threshold [20]. Large validation studies (ATAC and ABCSG8) for the PAM50 assay were performed using the standardized version with pre-specified cutoffs based on actual survival outcomes (<10, 10–20, and > 20% risk of distant relapse at 10 years) and not subtype distribution [21].

The Prosigna Breast Cancer Prognostic Gene Signature Assay is an in vitro diagnostic assay, which is performed on the NanoString nCounter® Dx Analysis System using FFPE breast tumor tissue previously diagnosed as invasive breast carcinoma. The Prosigna Score is a numerical value on a 0–100 scale that correlates with the probability of distant recurrence within 10 years. The gene expression profile of a patient's tumor is compared with each of the four PAM50 prototypical molecular profiles to determine the degree of similarity. The results in combination with a proliferation score and tumor size produce an individualized Prosigna Score. This qualitative assay utilizes gene expression data, weighted together with clinical variables to generate a risk category and numerical score, to assess a patient's risk of distant recurrence of disease.

In node-negative patients, the 10-year distant recurrence-free survival (DRFS) rates were > 95% for the low-risk group, 90.4% for the intermediate-risk group, and < 85% for the high-risk group [22, 23]. In node-positive patients, the 10-year DRFS rates were 94.2% for the low-risk group and 75.8% for the high-risk group [22].

The Prosigna Breast Cancer Prognostic Gene Signature Assay is indicated in female breast cancer patients who have undergone surgery in conjunction with locoregional treatment consistent with standard of care, either as:

i. A prognostic indicator for distant recurrence-free survival at 10 years in postmenopausal women with HR+, lymph node-negative, stage I or II breast cancer to be treated with adjuvant endocrine therapy alone, when used in conjunction with other clinicopathological factors.

ii. A prognostic indicator for distant recurrence-free survival at 10 years in postmenopausal women with HR+, lymph node-positive (1–3 positive nodes), stage II breast cancer to be treated with adjuvant endocrine therapy alone, when used in conjunction with other clinicopathological factors.

The assay should not be used for patients with four or more positive nodes.

2.4. EndoPredict

The EndoPredict (EP) assay combines the expression of three proliferative and five ER-signaling/differentiation-associated genes and is normalized by three housekeeping genes [24]. EP may be measured in formalin-fixed, paraffin-embedded tissue sections by quantitative real-time polymerase chain reaction in decentralized laboratories and provides a score that ranges between 0 and 15 after scaling [25].

EPclin was derived from EP by incorporating nodal status and tumor size to create an integrated diagnostic algorithm for clinical decisions [24]. Both EP and EPclin were trained on a cohort of 964 patients with ER+, HER2-negative carcinomas treated with adjuvant endocrine therapy only. Thresholds for EP and EPclin to differentiate between patients at low or high risk corresponding to a 10% probability of distant recurrence at 10 years were set at 5 and 3.3, respectively. Patients with an EP score < 5 (EPclin score < 3.3) were classified as low risk for distance recurrence, whereas patients with an EP score ≥5 (EPclin score ≥3.3) were stratified as high risk. Both EP and EPclin were shown to be prognostic for early and late distant recurrence in the ABCSG-6 and ABCSG-8 trials involving patients with ER+/HER2-negative breast cancer treated with adjuvant endocrine therapy only [26]. EndoPredict provides prognostic information beyond all common clinicopathological parameters and clinical guidelines.

There are several prognostic multigene-based tests for managing breast cancer, but limited data comparing them in the same cohort. The prognostic performance of the EP test was compared with the research-based PAM50 non-standardized qRT-PCR assay in node-positive ER+ and HER2-negative breast cancer patients receiving adjuvant chemotherapy followed by endocrine therapy (ET) in the GEICAM/9906 trial [27]. EP and PAM50 ROR scores [based on subtype (ROR-S) and on subtype and proliferation (ROR-P)] were compared in 536 ER+/HER2−patients. Scores combined with clinical information were evaluated: ROR-T (ROR-S, tumor size), ROR-PT (ROR-P, tumor size), and EPclin (EP, tumor size, nodal status). Patients were assigned to risk categories according to prespecified cutoffs. ROR-S, ROR-P, and EP scores identified a low-risk group with a relative better outcome (10-year distant metastasis-free survival: ROR-S 87%; ROR-P 89%; EP 93%). No significant difference between tests was found. Predictors including clinical information showed superior prognostic performance compared to molecular scores alone (10-year MFS, low-risk group: ROR-T 88%; ROR-PT 92%; EPclin 100%). The EPclin-based risk stratification achieved a significantly improved prediction of MFS compared to ROR-T, but not ROR-PT. All signatures added prognostic information to common clinical parameters.

EPclin provided independent prognostic information beyond ROR-T and ROR-PT. ROR and EP can reliably predict risk of distant metastasis in node-positive ER+/HER2 negative breast cancer patients treated with chemotherapy and ET. Addition of clinical parameters into risk scores improves their prognostic ability.

Recently, in a secondary analysis of a randomized clinical trial, the prognostic value of six multigene signatures was compared in women with early ER+ breast cancer [28]. In this study, 774 postmenopausal women with ER+, HER2-negative disease, 591 had node-negative disease and patients received endocrine therapy for 5 years (the Anastrozole or Tamoxifen Alone or Combined randomized clinical trial comparing 5-year treatment with anastrozole vs. tamoxifen) in addition to the Clinical Treatment Score (nodal status, tumor size, grade, age, and endocrine treatment) for distant recurrence for 0–10 years and 5–10 years after diagnosis [28]. The signatures included the Oncotype Dx recurrence score, ROR, Breast Cancer Index (BCI), EPclin, Clinical Treatment Score, and 4-marker immunohistochemical score. The ROR (HR, 2.56), followed by the BCI (HR, 2.46) and EPclin (HR, 2.14) were shown to be the signatures which have the most prognostic information. Each provided significantly more information than the Clinical Treatment Score (HR, 1.99), the recurrence score (HR, 1.69), and the 4-marker immunohistochemical score (HR, 1.95). Substantially less information was provided by all six molecular tests for the 183 patients with 1–3 positive nodes, but the BCI and EPclin provided more additional prognostic information than the other signatures. For women with node-negative disease, the ROR, BCI, and EPclin were shown to be significantly more prognostic for overall and late distant recurrence. For women with 1–3 positive nodes, limited independent information was available from any test.

2.5. Breast cancer index

The breast cancer index assay previously has been developed and validated. It consists of two independently developed gene expression biomarkers: molecular grade index (MGI) and HOXB13/IL17BR (H/I) [20, 26]. MGI, a 5-gene predictor that recapitulates tumor grade/proliferation, is highly prognostic in ER+ breast cancer patients. H/I, which was developed independent of tumor grade/proliferation, is prognostic for early and late distant recurrences and is predictive of extended adjuvant AI benefit in early stage of ER+ breast cancer patients.

2.6. Online prognostification and prediction tools

The online tools referred to earlier primarily use clinicopathological variables and cancer registry data as the basis of risk prediction. The clinical pathological variables used include age, tumor size and grade, mode of detection, number of lymph nodes involved, ER status, HER2 status, Ki67 status and type of chemotherapy [29].

2.6.1. Adjuvant online

Adjuvant!Online is a free online tool and probably the most widely used tool that estimate risks and benefits of adjuvant endocrine therapy and chemotherapy after breast cancer surgery based on factors, such as the patient's stage, pathologic features, age and comorbidity level. Entering information on age and selected tumor characteristics (tumor size and grade, number of positive axillary nodes, and hormone receptors status) allows for prediction of the 10-year risk of relapse-free and overall survival.

Despite these strengths, Adjuvant! has several limitations. The relapse estimates include local-regional recurrence as well as distant metastases; this is important as the proportions of both may vary greatly depending on stage and tumor phenotype. The baseline risk estimation for Adjuvant! Online was derived from the SEER (surveillance, epidemiology and end results) database [30]. The SEER database program is a collation of nine databases covering one-sixth of the US population. There have been concerns regarding the quality of the data about cause of death [31]. Additionally, the SEER database specifically includes patients between 35 and 69 years and provides limited information on the socio-economic status of people.

Adjuvant! Online tends to overestimate the number of patients at high risk. Cardoso et al. reported that Adjuvant! Online classified 23% of patients as high clinical risk when Oncotype DX classified them as low genomic risk [15].

Olivotto et al. performed a population-based validation study and suggested that Adjuvant! Online would overestimate survival in patients under 35 years of age with lymphovascular invasion. It was also found that Adjuvant! Online tends to overestimate the survival rates of younger women with ER+ breast cancer [16] and that it overestimated the added value of chemotherapy for older patients [32].

The validity of the predictive score is calculated by Adjuvant! Online was deemed weak in the clinician-based validation [33]. Predictions on loco-regional relapse and distant metastases may vary greatly, making it difficult to make clear recommendations for adjuvant treatment [34]. This is reflected in two studies that suggest that when patients are involved in a discussion to decide on adjuvant chemotherapy, they are less likely to choose chemotherapy if using Adjuvant! Online [35].

The database does not include information regarding the benefits of adjuvant trastuzumab, thereby reducing the utility of Adjuvant! Online in clinical decisions about HER2-positive disease treatment [31]. This deficiency of Adjuvant! Online with regard to HER2-positive disease has significant implications for the prediction of metastatic spread. In a recent in vitro study using murine models, the HER2 status of cells predicted the response to progesterone-induced signaling, with HER2-deficient cells being more likely to migrate and HER2-enriched cells tending toward increased proliferation [36]. This recent evidence underlines the importance of HER2 in predicting prognosis and highlights the significance of this inherent shortcoming in online cancer registry-based prognostic tools.

The ethnic variation in the data on which these online tools are based seriously affects the generalizability of these online tools. The SEER database is representative of the usual US population in terms of age, sex and ethnic distribution. However, the ethnic mix of the US population is different from that of England and Wales [37].

2.6.2. Predict

Predict is an another online prognostication and treatment benefit tool based on UK cancer registry data and included information on 5694 women treated in East Anglia from 1999 to 2003 [38]. It is designed to help clinicians and patients make informed decisions about treatment following breast cancer surgery. The model was validated in a second UK cancer registry dataset. It would able to provide not only the accurate prediction of survival but also subsequent calculation of treatment benefit.

Data of an individual patient including patient age, tumor size, tumor grade, number of positive nodes, ER status, HER2 status, KI67 status and mode of detection are submitted to online PREDICT tool. It originally did not include HER2 status and KI67 status, but in 2011,

HER2 status was included (PREDICT version 1.1) and later KI67 was added to model (PREDICT version 1.2) to improve the estimates of breast cancer-specific mortality, especially in HER2-positive patients [29, 39].

While the overall fit of the model has been good in multiple independent case series, PREDICT has been shown to underestimate breast cancer specific mortality in women diagnosed under the age of 40, particularly those with ER+ disease. Another limitation of the model is the use of discrete categories for tumor size and node status which result in "step" changes in risk estimates on moving from one category to the next. For example, a woman with an 18 or 19 mm tumor will be predicted to have the same breast cancer specific mortality if all the other prognostic factors are the same whereas breast cancer-specific morality of women with a 19 or 20 mm tumor will differ. The PREDICT prognostic model was refitted using the original cohort of cases from East Anglia with updated survival time in order to take into account age at diagnosis and to smooth out the survival function for tumor size and node status. The fit of the model has been tested in three independent data sets that had also been used to validate the original version of PREDICT [40].

KI67 positivity for the PREDICT model was defined as greater than 10% of tumor cells staining positive. Survival estimates, with and without adjuvant therapy, are presented in visual and text formats. Treatment benefits for hormone therapy and chemotherapy are calculated by applying relative risk reductions from the Oxford overview to the breast cancer specific mortality. Predicted mortality reductions are available for both second-generation (anthracycline-containing, >4 cycles or equivalent) and third-generation (taxane-containing) chemotherapy regimens. The survival estimates, presented both with and without adjuvant hormone therapy, chemotherapy and trastuzumab, are provided for 5 and 10 years.

The Cambridge Breast Unit uses the absolute 10-year survival benefit from chemotherapy to guide decision-making for adjuvant chemotherapy as follows: <3% no chemotherapy; 3–5% chemotherapy discussed as a possible option; >5% chemotherapy recommended.

Online tools are valuable in guiding adjuvant treatment, especially in resource-constrained countries. However, in the era of personalized therapy, molecular profiling appears to be superior in predicting clinical outcome and guiding therapy.

The AJCC Prognostic Stage Group containing multigene panels has been globally used from January 1, 2018. It suggests that prognostic stage grouping should be used in countries where biomarker tests are routinely performed, indicating that multigene molecular profiling will become part of cancer stage evaluation and will need to be taken into consideration when making clinical decisions [41].

Oncotype DX and MammaPrint have the strongest evidence supporting their clinical utility and decision effectiveness in HR+ breast cancer [42]. The future of multigene panels is promising in personalizing treatment as more studies continue. However, many issues remain to be solved before multigene panels have a wider influence on breast cancer treatment. Importantly new issues, such as how to accurately predicate late recurrence in ER+ cancer and how to provide more access to multigene panels, should be solved in the future.

Newer technologies including next-generation sequencing, liquid biopsy, tumor-infiltrating lymphocytes or PD-1 determination are at this investigational point.

3. Adjuvant chemotherapy

Several pathological factors including histological subtype, ER or PR expression, tumor grade, lymphovascular invasion, tumor stage, and clinical factors such as patient age, preferences and comorbidities should be taken into consideration during adjuvant chemotherapy indication is being decided. The genomic tests and benefit–risk calculators which were developed to be used in determining appropriate candidates for adjuvant chemotherapy in early stage HR+ breast cancer have been discussed in previous section.

Patients with HR+ breast cancer less than 5 mm and treated with only endocrine therapy have usually very good prognosis. Thus, they typically are not treated with adjuvant chemotherapy. However, patients with stage III HR+ breast cancer still require adjuvant chemotherapy since they carry high risk of recurrence without chemotherapy. Many patients with HR+ HER2 negative breast cancer fall in between these two categories, and they are called as intermediate risk group based on clinicopathological variables, genomic tests or online risk calculators.

Clinicians should inform the patients who required adjuvant chemotherapy about the risks and benefits of chemotherapy. Risks include acute or long-term toxicities such as emesis, alopecia, myelosuppression, neuropathy, cardiotoxicity, infertility and leukemias.

Breast cancer is the most frequent malignancy in women of reproductive age. Treatments for breast cancer may eliminate or diminish fertility. Additionally, even in patients who do not require chemotherapy, long duration of adjuvant endocrine therapy often leads natural decline in ovarian reserve during adjuvant treatment.

The chemotherapy-related risk of premature ovarian insufficiency is influenced by age, body mass index, the type and duration of therapy. After six cycles of CMF, the risk of amenorrhea is 33 and 81% in patients <40 and ≥ 40 years of age, respectively. Newer chemotherapy regimens including adriamycin & cyclophosphamide (AC), adriamycin & cyclophosphamide & taxane (ACT), fluorouracil & adriamycin & cyclophosphamide (FAC) and fluorouracil & adriamycin & cyclophosphamide & taxane (FACT) result in lower rates of persisting amenorrhea. The risk of amenorrhea is 10–20 and 13–68% in patients <30 years and in patients >30 years, respectively [43]. Hence, the rate of infertility risk with particular chemotherapy regimen at particular age should be discussed with patients prior to initiation of gonadotoxic therapies. Furthermore, premenopausal women who are willing to be pregnant in the future should be referred to a fertility specialist to be informed about various techniques of fertility preservation.

Although methods of fertility preservation in breast cancer should be a subject of a separate chapter, fertility preservation methods can be summarized as

- established methods: oocyte or embryo cryopreservation

- experimental methods: ovarian suppression with gonadotropin-releasing hormone (GnRH) agonists (GnRHa) and ovarian tissue cryopreservation [44].

3.1. Chemotherapy regimen

Several polychemotherapy regimens are accepted as adjuvant chemotherapy regimen with strong evidence in patients with early stage breast cancer. The preferred regimens vary according to characteristics of disease, patients' comorbidities, patients' preferences, age, prescribing doctor, institution, or country.

Early Breast Cancer Trialists' Collaborative Group (EBCTCG) reports a meta-analysis periodically to review the data on adjuvant treatment of breast cancer. The previous data supported the adjuvant chemotherapy particularly cyclophosphamide, methotrexate and fluorouracil (CMF), anthracyclines and taxane compared with no treatment in adjuvant setting.

Trials with CMF-treated controls revealed that standard 4 AC and standard CMF were equivalent (P = 0·67), but that anthracycline-based regimens with substantially higher cumulative dosage than standard 4 AC [e.g., CAF or cyclophosphamide & epirubicin & fluorouracil (CEF)] were superior to standard CMF (RR 0.78, P = 0.0004) [45]. However, NSABP B-36 randomized phase III trial compared six cycles of FEC-100 with four cycles of standard AC in pts. with T1-3 N0 breast cancer [46]. Primary and secondary endpoint analyses at 8 years did not reveal any significant differences in DFS, OS, recurrence free interval (RFI), or distant RFI, although patients and tumor characteristics were equally distributed between the two groups (<50 years old: 40%, lumpectomy: 68%, and hormone positivity: 65%). Overall, Grade 3 and 4 expected toxicities were more frequent in the FEC arm. Thus, international guidelines excluded six cycles of FEC-100 from adjuvant breast cancer treatment recommendations.

In trials adding four separate cycles of a taxane to a fixed anthracycline-based control regimen, extending treatment duration, breast cancer mortality was reduced (RR 0.86, SE 0.04, two-sided significance P = 0.0005) [45].

In all meta-analyses involving taxane-based or anthracycline-based regimens, proportional risk reductions were little affected by age, nodal status, tumor diameter or differentiation, ER status, or adjuvant tamoxifen. Hence, largely independently of age (up to at least 70 years) or the tumor characteristics currently available to us for the patients selected to be in these trials, some taxane-plus-anthracycline-based or higher-cumulative-dosage anthracycline-based regimens (not requiring stem cells) reduced breast cancer mortality about one-third.

Thus, based on these strong evidences, AC followed by a taxane (either triweekly docetaxel, paclitaxel or two weekly or weekly paclitaxel) is now usually preferred regimen in most cases in whom adjuvant chemotherapy is indicated.

Nonanthracycline-based chemotherapy regimens should be preferred in certain patients with lower risk disease (node-negative), cardiac contraindication, advanced age, previous chest wall irradiation or patients who do not accept the risks of anthracycline-based therapy. In these patients, four cycles of docetaxel and cyclophosphamide (TC) are most preferred regimen.

When adjuvant chemotherapy is indicated in HR+ HER2-negative early breast cancer, taxane is mostly added to anthracycline-based regimen based on scientific data. However, patients who cannot receive taxane due to risks of allergic reactions or peripheral neuropathy, CMF can be administered instead of anthracycline or taxane- based regimens.

Dose-dense chemotherapy plays a controversial role in the adjuvant treatment of breast cancer patients. Whereas meta-analyses persistently describe a significant superiority for dose-dense treatment, the results of large phase III trials remain contradictory [47]. Some of these trials showed important differences between the dose-dense and conventional groups regarding number of cycles, type of drug, and total dose. Other trials are accepted and interpreted as dose-dense but present a mixture of dose-dense and conventional schedules.

Goldvaser et al. performed a systemic review and meta-analysis of clinical trials in which patients with early stage breast cancer were treated with adjuvant dose-dense chemotherapy [48]. Dose-dense treatment significantly improved DFS (HR 0.85, $P < 0.001$) and OS (HR 0.86, $P = 0.008$). A significantly greater relative magnitude of benefit was observed in pre-menopausal women and those with nodal involvement, but there was no influence of hormone receptor status on results. Adjuvant dose-dense regimens improve breast cancer outcomes. It remains uncertain whether the observed benefit reflects the impact of dose density or the inferiority of paclitaxel every 3 weeks as a control group.

Although a direct head-to-head comparison is missing, intense dose-dense epirubicin, paclitaxel, and cyclophosphamide (iddETC) or four cycles each of dose-dense epirubicin/cyclophosphamide followed by paclitaxel are the preferred adjuvant regimens for patients at risk. Patients with four positive lymph nodes should preferentially be treated with iddETC.

However, in EBCTCG meta-analyses, information was lacking about tumor gene expression markers or quantitative immunohistochemistry that might help to predict risk, chemosensitivity, or both.

4. Adjuvant endocrine therapy

Estrogen receptor expression is the main indicator of potential responses to endocrine therapy (ET) which block estrogen-driven tumor growth through a variety of mechanisms. The use of hormonal therapy in breast cancer has improved the overall outcome for patients with early-stage hormone receptor-positive disease. The choice of hormone therapy is related to multiple factors, including menopausal state, patient preference, and potential side effects. Molecular profiling has allowed therapy to be tailored for an individual patient to some extent. However, further molecular studies are needed to individualize the choice and length of adjuvant hormone therapy.

Adjuvant ET currently consists of (i) ovarian suppression, (ii) selective estrogen receptor modulators (SERMs) and down-regulators, and (iii) AIs.

In patients with ER+ tumors, pharmacologic ovary suppression with gonadotropin-releasing hormone agonists in combination with standard adjuvant therapy is generally more effective than adjuvant chemotherapy alone.

Tamoxifen is the best established SERM, has favorable effects on breast cancer control and bone metabolism, but also has adverse effects due to its estrogenic activity in other tissues. For these reasons, other SERMs have been developed.

Fulvestrant is an ER down-regulator with several potential advantages over SERMs, including a 100-fold increase in its affinity for ER compared with tamoxifen and no estrogen-like activity in the uterus.

The inhibition of the aromatase system with third-generation AIs is associated with improved survival in patients with advanced breast cancer compared with SERMs. In postmenopausal patients with ER+ breast cancer adjuvant treatment with AIs should be performed, either as sequential treatment after tamoxifen or as upfront therapy.

According to NCCN guidelines [49], subdivide the adjuvant endocrine therapy recommendations in HR+ breast cancer patients based on the menopausal status of women. Three main subgroups are (i) postmenopausal at initial diagnosis, (ii) premenopausal at initial diagnosis and remain premenopausal after 5 years of adjuvant ET, (iii) premenopausal at initial diagnosis, but become postmenopausal during adjuvant ET.

i. postmenopausal at initial diagnosis:

- an AI as initial adjuvant therapy for 5 years (category 1),
- initially tamoxifen for 2–3 years followed by an AI to complete 5 years of adjuvant ET (category 1),
- initially tamoxifen for 2–3 years followed by 5 years of AI (category 2B),
- tamoxifen for 4.5–6 years followed by 5 years of an AI (category 1) or consideration of tamoxifen for up to 10 years.
- Five years up to 10 years of tamoxifen without AI should only be given to patients who have a contraindication to AI.

ii. premenopausal at initial diagnosis and remain premenopausal after 5 years of adjuvant ET

- tamoxifen with or without ovarian suppression for 5 years (category 1)
- an AI with ovarian suppression for 5 years (category 1)
- tamoxifen continuing up to 10 years

iii. premenopausal at initial diagnosis, but become postmenopausal during adjuvant ET.

Decision of menopausal status is the most important point because amenorrhea does not mean menopause, because ovaries may continue to product estrogens in amenorrheic women. Thus, before starting AI without ovarian suppression, serum LH, FSH and estradiol must be evaluated.

- After or during 5 years of tamoxifen, extend the adjuvant ET with an AI up to 5 years (category 1)
- After 5 years of tamoxifen, consider five additional years of tamoxifen

4.1. Combination of ovarian suppression either exemestane or tamoxifen in premenopausal women

The initial results from the Suppression of Ovarian Function Trial (SOFT) indicate that tamoxifen is a suitable therapy for premenopausal women with low risk clinical-pathologic features. For women at sufficient risk to receive chemotherapy who have premenopausal E2 levels within 8 months of completion, the addition of ovarian suppression to tamoxifen for 5 years resulted in some reduction of recurrence. The use of ovarian suppression combined with an AI exemestane for 5 years resulted in further reduction of recurrence [50, 51].

The joint analysis of SOFT and Tamoxifen and Exemestane Trial (TEXT) found the combination of ovarian suppression and exemestane significantly reduced recurrence, compared with ovarian suppression plus tamoxifen. Premenopausal women with ER+ve HER2-negative breast cancer with high-risk features can derive a meaningful improvement in 5-year invasive breast cancer-free interval with exemestane plus ovarian suppression, as an alternative to tamoxifen. Very young women under age 35 with ER+ve breast cancer have higher risks of recurrence, and the use of ovarian suppression with oral endocrine therapy should be considered.

4.2. Extended adjuvant endocrine therapy beyond 5 years

Adjuvant endocrine therapy for 5 years is the standard adjuvant treatment for ER+ breast cancer while the benefits of extended adjuvant endocrine therapy (EAET) beyond 5 years are still controversial. In a recent meta-analysis, 5 years of adjuvant endocrine therapy only was compared with EAET [52]. Eleven controlled trials including 29,000 women were analyzed. There was no advantage of EAET in OS from all causes mortality ($P = 0.67$). On the other hand, compared with standard therapy, the pooled effects showed that EAET was associated with improvement in breast cancer-specific survival ($OR = 0.87$; $P = 0.004$), DFS ($OR = 0.87$; $P = 0.002$), disease recurrence ($OR = 0.76$; $P = 0.001$), and contralateral breast recurrence ($OR = 0.74$; $P = 0.008$). Improvement in DFS or disease recurrence was not shown in studies that compared 5 years of tamoxifen versus tamoxifen beyond 5 years. Subgroup analysis showed that EAET conferred more benefit for patients with positive lymph nodes. Rates of positive lymph nodes, the study size, and the median duration of follow-up were identified as variables that explained most of the demonstrated data heterogeneity. EAET should be considered as a preferred strategy for high-risk hormone-positive early breast cancer patients with positive lymph nodes; however, the benefit on OS could not be demonstrated.

Extended adjuvant endocrine therapy results in increased toxicity based on the type of extended endocrine agents. Risk of bone fractures is reported to be higher with AI, whereas the risk of endometrial cancer and venous thromboembolism are more frequently than with TAM. No difference was shown between AI (mono- or sequenced therapy) and TAM for cardiovascular events, whereas sequenced therapy compared with AI had lower risk of cardiovascular events (moderate level of evidence).

4.3. Concurrent or sequential ovarian function suppression

Breast cancer treatment guidelines recommend that higher risk premenopausal patients should receive ovarian function suppression as part of adjuvant endocrine therapy. However, if chemotherapy is also given, until recently, it was uncertain whether concurrent or sequential sequential ovarian function suppression (OFS) initiation has any detrimental effect on prognosis or menstruation resumption.

Recently, in a phase 3, open-label, parallel, randomized controlled trial, 216 premenopausal patients younger than 45 years with invasive ER+ breast cancer were randomized at a 1:1 ratio to receive (neo)adjuvant chemotherapy combined with sequential or simultaneous GnRHa treatment between July 2009 to May 2013 [53]. All patients were advised to receive GnRHa for at least 2 years. The rates of early menopause were 22.8% (21/92) in the sequential group and 23.1% (18/78) in the simultaneous group (simultaneous vs. sequential: OR 1.01; P = 0.969; age-adjusted OR 1.13; P = 0.737). The median menstruation resumption period was 12.0 months and 10.3 months for the sequential and simultaneous groups, respectively (HR 0.83; P = 0.274; age-adjusted HR 0.90; P = 0.567). During a median follow-up time of 56.9 months (IQR 49.5–72.4 months), there were no significant differences in disease-free survival (P = 0.290) or in overall survival (P = 0.514) between the two groups.

In **an exploratory analysis of phase III TEXT and SOFT trials,** 1872 patients who received adjuvant chemotherapy for HR+, HER2-negative breast cancer and upon randomization to an OFS-containing adjuvant endocrine therapy, initiated GnRHa triptorelin were analyzed [54]. Breast cancer-free interval (BCFI) was compared between patients who received OFS concurrently with chemotherapy in TEXT (n = 1242) versus sequentially post-chemotherapy in SOFT (n = 630). Because timing of trial enrollment relative to adjuvant chemotherapy differed, landmark analysis was implemented to re-define BCFI beginning 1 year after final dose of chemotherapy (median, 15.5 months in TEXT and 8.1 months from enrollment to landmark in SOFT). The median duration of adjuvant chemotherapy was 18 weeks in both groups. Patients who were premenopausal post-chemotherapy in SOFT were younger on average. After post-landmark median follow-up of about 5 years, post-landmark BCFI was found to be statistically similar between concurrent use of triptorelin with chemotherapy and sequential use of triptorelin after chemotherapy, either in the overall population (HR = 1.11; P = 0.72; 4-year BCFI 89% in both groups), or in the subgroup of 692 women < 40 years at diagnosis (HR = 1.13) who are less likely to develop chemotherapy-induced amenorrhea.

Because the sequential use of GnRHa and chemotherapy showed similar ovarian preservation and survival outcomes when compared with simultaneous use ER+ premenopausal patients, addition of GnRHa to oncologic treatment can probably be delayed until menstruation resumption after chemotherapy. However, based on comparative-effectiveness modeling of TEXT and SOFT after about 5 years median follow-up, concurrent administration of OFS with chemotherapy is neither detrimental nor beneficial effect on the efficacy of adjuvant therapy which includes chemotherapy, with limited statistical power especially for the subgroup < 40 years.

5. Adjuvant bisphosphonates

Cancer Care Ontario and ASCO convened a Working Group and Expert Panel to develop evidence-based recommendations by a systematic review of the literature [55]. The women with natural menopause or the women who were postmenopausal induced by ovarian suppression or ablation were included. Adjuvant bisphosphonates were reported to reduce bone recurrence and improve survival in postmenopausal women with early stage breast cancer. Absolute benefit was found to be greater in patients who are at higher risk of recurrence, and almost all trials were conducted in patients who also received systemic therapy. The data are extremely limited for bisphosphonates other than zoledronic acid or clodronate due to most studies performed with these two bisphosphonates. ASCO clinical guidelines recommends that, if available, zoledronic acid (4 mg intravenously every 6 months) or clodronate (1600 mg/d orally) be considered as an adjuvant therapy for postmenopausal patients with breast cancer who are deemed candidates for adjuvant systemic therapy. However, further research comparing different bone-modifying agents, doses, dosing intervals, and durations is required. Risk factors for osteonecrosis of the jaw and renal impairment should be assessed, and any pending dental or oral health problems should be dealt with prior to starting treatment. While adjuvant denosumab reduces fractures and it looks promising in adjuvant setting, long-term survival data are still insufficient to make any recommendation. The use of these agents to reduce fragility fractures in patients with low bone mineral density is beyond the scope of the guideline.

6. Promising targeted agents

Ongoing studies are evaluating the role of additional targeted therapies, such as CDK4/6 inhibitors including ribociclib, palbociclib, to further improve outcome for patients with early-stage HR+ breast cancer.

Conflict of interest

I confirm there are no conflicts of interest.

Author details

Fatma Sen

Address all correspondence to: fatmasen840@gmail.com

Avrasya Hospital, Medical Oncology Unit, Zeytinburnu, Istanbul, Turkey

References

[1] Ghoncheh M, Pournamdar Z, Salehiniya H. Incidence and mortality and epidemiology of breast cancer in the world. Asian Pacific Journal of Cancer Prevention. 2016;**17**(S3):43-46. DOI: 10.7314/APJCP.2016.17.S3.43

[2] Cancer Genome Atlas Network. Comprehensive molecular portraits of human breast tumours. Nature 2012;**490**(7418):61-70. DOI: 10.1038/nature11412

[3] Hayes DF. Do we need prognostic factors in nodal-negative breast cancer? Arbiter: European Journal of Cancer. 2000;**36**(3):302-306

[4] Paik S, Shak S, Tang G, Kim C, Baker J, Cronin M, Baehner FL, Walker MG, Watson D, Park T, Hiller W, Fisher ER, Wickerham DL, Bryant J, Wolmark N. A multigene assay to predict recurrence of tamoxifen-treated, node-negative breast cancer. The New England Journal of Medicine. 2004;**351**(27):2817-2826. DOI: 10.1056/NEJMoa041588

[5] Habel LA, Shak S, Jacobs MK, Capra A, Alexander C, Pho M, Baker J, Walker M, Watson D, Hackett J, Blick NT, Greenberg D, Fehrenbacher L, Langholz B, Quesenberry CP. A population-based study of tumor gene expression and risk of breast cancer death among lymph node-negative patients. Breast Cancer Research. 2006;**8**(3):R25. DOI: 10.1186/bcr1412

[6] Xin L, Liu YH, Martin TA, Jiang WG. The era of multigene panels comes? The clinical utility of oncotype DX and MammaPrint. World Journal of Oncology. 2017;**8**(2):34-40. DOI: 10.14740/wjon1019w

[7] Sparano JA, Gray RJ, Makower DF, Pritchard KI, Albain KS, Hayes DF, Geyer Jr CE, Dees EC, Perez EA, Olson Jr JA, Zujewski J, Lively T, Badve SS, Saphner TJ, Wagner LI, Whelan TJ, Ellis MJ, Paik S, Wood WC, Ravdin P, Keane MM, Gomez Moreno HL, Reddy PS, Goggins TF, Mayer IA, Brufsky AM, Toppmeyer DL, Kaklamani VG, Atkins JN, Berenberg JL, Sledge GW. Prospective validation of a 21-gene expression assay in breast cancer. The New England Journal of Medicine. 2015;**373**(21):2005-2014. DOI: 10.1056/NEJMoa1510764

[8] Solin LJ, Gray R, Goldstein LJ, Recht A, Baehner FL, Shak S, Badve S, Perez EA, Shulman LN, Martino S, Davidson NE, Sledge Jr GW, Sparano JA. Prognostic value of biologic subtype and the 21-gene recurrence score relative to local recurrence after breast conservation treatment with radiation for early stage breast carcinoma: Results from the Eastern Cooperative Oncology Group E2197 study. Breast Cancer Research and Treatment. 2012; **134**(2):683-692. DOI: 10.1007/s10549-012-2072-y

[9] Solin LJ, Gray R, Goldstein LJ, Recht A, Baehner FL, Shak S, Badve S, et al. Prognostic value of biologic subtype and the 21-gene recurrence score relative to local recurrence after breast conservation treatment with radiation for early stage breast carcinoma: Results from the eastern cooperative oncology group E2197 study. Breast Cancer Research and Treatment. 2012;**134**(2):683-692. DOI: 10.1007/s10549-012-2072-y

[10] Penault-Llorca FMFT, Asselain B, et al. Prediction of recurrence with the Onco type DX recurrence score in node-positive, HR+, breast cancer patients treated with adjuvant chemotherapy: Results from PACS01 trial. Journal of Clinical Oncology. 2014;**32**(suppl)

[11] Albain KS, Barlow WE, Shak S, Hortobagyi GN, Livingston RB, Yeh IT, Ravdin P, Bugarini R, Baehner FL, Davidson NE, Sledge GW, Winer EP, Hudis C, Ingle JN, Perez EA, Pritchard KI, Shepherd L, Gralow JR, Yoshizawa C, Allred DC, Osborne CK, Hayes DF, Breast Cancer Intergroup of North America. Prognostic and predictive value of the 21-gene recurrence score assay in postmenopausal women with node-positive, oestrogen-receptor-positive breast cancer on chemotherapy: A retrospective analysis of a randomised trial. The Lancet Oncology. 2010;**11**(1):55-65. DOI: 10.1016/S1470-2045(09)70314-6

[12] Gluz O, Nitz UA, Christgen M, Kates RE, Shak S, Clemens M, Kraemer S, Aktas B, Kuemmel S, Reimer T, Kusche M, Heyl V, Lorenz-Salehi F, Just M, Hofmann D, Degenhardt T, Liedtke C, Svedman C, Wuerstlein R, Kreipe HH, Harbeck N. West German Study Group phase III PlanB trial: First prospective outcome data for the 21-gene recurrence score assay and concordance of prognostic markers by central and local pathology assessment. Journal of Clinical Oncology. 2016;**34**(20):2341-2349. DOI: 10.1200/JCO.2015.63.5383

[13] Jasem J, Fisher CM, Amini A, Shagisultanova E, Rabinovitch R, Borges VF, Elias A, Kabos P. The 21-gene recurrence score assay for node-positive, early-stage breast cancer and impact of RxPONDER trial on chemotherapy decision-making: Have clinicians already decided? Journal of the National Comprehensive Cancer Network. 2017;**15**(4):494-503. DOI: 10.6004/jnccn.2017.0049

[14] van't Veer LJ, Dai H, van de Vijver MJ, He YD, Hart AA, Mao M, Peterse HL, van der Kooy K, Marton MJ, Witteveen AT, Schreiber GJ, Kerkhoven RM, Roberts C, Linsley PS, Bernards R, Friend SH. Gene expression profiling predicts clinical outcome of breast cancer. Nature. 2002;**415**(6871):530-536. DOI: 10.1038/415530a

[15] Cardoso F, van't Veer LJ, Bogaerts J, Slaets L, Viale G, Delaloge S, Pierga JY, Brain E, Causeret S, DeLorenzi M, Glas AM, Golfinopoulos V, Goulioti T, Knox S, Matos E, Meulemans B, Neijenhuis PA, Nitz U, Passalacqua R, Ravdin P, Rubio IT, Saghatchian M, Smilde TJ, Sotiriou C, Stork L, Straehle C, Thomas G, Thompson AM, van der Hoeven JM, Vuylsteke P, Bernards R, Tryfonidis K, Rutgers E, Piccart M, MINDACT Investigators. 70-Gene signature as an aid to treatment decisions in early-stage breast cancer. The New England Journal of Medicine 2016;**375**(8):717-729. DOI: 10.1056/NEJMoa1602253

[16] Olivotto IA, Bajdik CD, Ravdin PM, Speers CH, Coldman AJ, Norris BD, Davis GJ, Chia SK, Gelmon KA. Population-based validation of the prognostic model ADJUVANT! For early breast cancer. Journal of Clinical Oncology. 2005;**23**(12):2716-2725. DOI: 10.1200/JCO.2005.06.178

[17] Harris L, Fritsche H, Mennel R, Norton L, Ravdin P, Taube S, Somerfield MR, Hayes DF, Bast Jr RC, American Society of Clinical Oncology. American Society of Clinical Oncology

2007 update of recommendations for the use of tumor markers in breast cancer. Journal of Clinical Oncology 2007;**25**(33):5287-5312. DOI: 10.1200/JCO.2007.14.2364

[18] Krop I, Ismaila N, Andre F, Bast RC, Barlow W, Collyar DE, Hammond ME, Kuderer NM, Liu MC, Mennel RG, Van Poznak C, Wolff AC, Stearns V. Use of biomarkers to guide decisions on adjuvant systemic therapy for women with early-stage invasive breast cancer: American Society of Clinical Oncology clinical practice guideline focused update. Journal of Clinical Oncology. 2017;**35**(24):2838-2847. DOI: 10.1200/JCO.2017.74.0472

[19] Parker JS, Mullins M, Cheang MC, Leung S, Voduc D, Vickery T, Davies S, Fauron C, He X, Hu Z, Quackenbush JF, Stijleman IJ, Palazzo J, Marron JS, Nobel AB, Mardis E, Nielsen TO, Ellis MJ, Perou CM, Bernard PS. Supervised risk predictor of breast cancer based on intrinsic subtypes. Journal of Clinical Oncology. 2009;**27**:1160-1167. DOI: 10.1200/JCO.2008.18.1370

[20] Nielsen TO, Parker JS, Leung S, Voduc D, Ebbert M, Vickery T, Davies SR, Snider J, Stijleman IJ, Reed J, Cheang MC, Mardis ER, Perou CM, Bernard PS, Ellis MJ. A comparison of PAM50 intrinsic subtyping with immunohistochemistry and clinical prognostic factors in tamoxifen-treated estrogen receptor-positive breast cancer. Clinical Cancer Research. 2010;**16**:5222-5232. DOI: 10.1158/1078-0432.CCR-10-1282

[21] Dowsett M, Sestak I, Lopez-Knowles E, Sidhu K, Dunbier AK, Cowens JW, Ferree S, Storhoff J, Schaper C, Cuzick J. Comparison of PAM50 risk of recurrence score with oncotype DX and IHC4 for predicting risk of distant recurrence after endocrine therapy. Journal of Clinical Oncology. 2013;**31**(22):2783-2790. DOI: 10.1200/JCO.2012.46.1558

[22] Prosigna [Package Insert]. Seattle, WA: NanoString Technologies, Inc.; 2013

[23] Gnant M, Filipits M, Greil R, Stoeger H, Rudas M, Bago-Horvath Z, Mlineritsch B, Kwasny W, Knauer M, Singer C, Jakesz R, Dubsky P, Fitzal F, Bartsch R, Steger G, Balic M, Ressler S, Cowens JW, Storhoff J, Ferree S, Schaper C, Liu S, Fesl C, Nielsen TO, Austrian Breast and Colorectal Cancer Study Group, Austrian Breast and Colorectal Cancer Study Group. Predicting distant recurrence in receptor-positive breast cancer patients with limited clinicopathological risk: using the PAM50 Risk of Recurrence score in 1478 postmenopausal patients of the ABCSG-8 trial treated with adjuvant endocrine therapy alone. Annals of Oncology. 2014;**25**(2):339-345. DOI: 10.1093/annonc/mdt494

[24] Filipits M, Rudas M, Jakesz R, Dubsky P, Fitzal F, Singer CF, Dietze O, Greil R, Jelen A, Sevelda P, Freibauer C, Müller V, Jänicke F, Schmidt M, Kölbl H, Rody A, Kaufmann M, Schroth W, Brauch H, Schwab M, Fritz P, Weber KE, Feder IS, Hennig G, Kronenwett R, Gehrmann M, Gnant M, Investigators EP. A new molecular predictor of distant recurrence in ER+, HER2-negative breast cancer adds independent information to conventional clinical risk factors. Clinical Cancer Research. 2011;**17**(18):6012-6020. DOI: 10.1158/1078-0432.CCR-11-0926

[25] Denkert C, Kronenwett R, Schlake W, Bohmann K, Penzel R, Weber KE, Höfler H, Lehmann U, Schirmacher P, Specht K, Rudas M, Kreipe HH, Schraml P, Schlake G, Bago-Horvath Z, Tiecke F, Varga Z, Moch H, Schmidt M, Prinzler J, Kerjaschki D, Sinn BV, Müller BM, Filipits M, Petry C, Dietel M. Decentral gene expression analysis for ER+/

HER2-breast cancer: Results of a proficiency testing program for the EndoPredict assay. Virchows Archiv. 2012;**460**(3):251-259. DOI: 10.1007/s00428-012-1204-4

[26] Dubsky P, Brase JC, Jakesz R, Rudas M, Singer CF, Greil R, Dietze O, Luisser I, Klug E, Sedivy R, Bachner M, Mayr D, Schmidt M, Gehrmann MC, Petry C, Weber KE, Fisch K, Kronenwett R, Gnant M, Filipits M, Austrian Breast and Colorectal Cancer Study Group (ABCSG). The EndoPredict score provides prognostic information on late distant metastases in ER+/HER2-breast cancer patients. British Journal of Cancer 2013;**109**(12):2959-2964. DOI: 10.1038/bjc.2013.671

[27] Martin M, Brase JC, Ruiz A, Prat A, Kronenwett R, Calvo L, Petry C, Bernard PS, Ruiz-Borrego M, Weber KE, Rodriguez CA, Alvarez IM, Segui MA, Perou CM, Casas M, Carrasco E, Caballero R, Rodriguez-Lescure A. Prognostic ability of EndoPredict compared to research-based versions of the PAM50 risk of recurrence (ROR) scores in node-positive, estrogen receptor-positive, and HER2-negative breast cancer. A GEICAM/9906 sub-study. Breast Cancer Research and Treatment. 2016;**156**(1):81-89. DOI: 10.1007/s10549-016-3725-z

[28] Sestak I, Buus R, Cuzick J, Dubsky P, Kronenwett R, Denkert C, Ferree S, Sgroi D, Schnabel C, Baehner FL, Mallon E, Dowsett M. Comparison of the Performance of 6 Prognostic Signatures for Estrogen Receptor-Positive Breast Cancer: A Secondary Analysis of a Randomized Clinical Trial. JAMA Oncol. AMA Oncol. 2018 Apr 1;**4**(4):545-553. DOI: 10.1001/jamaoncol.2017.5524

[29] Wishart GC, Bajdik CD, Dicks E, Provenzano E, Schmidt MK, Sherman M, Greenberg DC, Green AR, Gelmon KA, Kosma VM, Olson JE, Beckmann MW, Winqvist R, Cross SS, Severi G, Huntsman D, Pylkäs K, Ellis I, Nielsen TO, Giles G, Blomqvist C, Fasching PA, Couch FJ, Rakha E, Foulkes WD, Blows FM, Bégin LR, van't Veer LJ, Southey M, Nevanlinna H, Mannermaa A, Cox A, Cheang M, Baglietto L, Caldas C, Garcia-Closas M, Pharoah PD. PREDICT plus: Development and validation of a prognostic model for early breast cancer that includes HER2. British Journal of Cancer. 2012;**107**(5):800-807. DOI: 10.1038/bjc.2012.338

[30] Ravdin PM. A computer program to assist in making breast cancer adjuvant therapy decisions. Seminars in Oncology. 1996;**23**(1 Suppl 2):43-50

[31] Warren JL, Klabunde CN, Schrag D, et al. Overview of the SEER-Medicare data: Content, research applications, and generalizability to the United States elderly population. Medical Care. 2002;**40**(8 Suppl):IV-3-18

[32] de Glas NA, van de Water W, Engelhardt EG, Bastiaannet E, de Craen AJ, Kroep JR, Putter H, Stiggelbout AM, Weijl NI, van de Velde CJ, Portielje JE, Liefers GJ. Validity of adjuvant! Online program in older patients with breast cancer: A population-based study. The Lancet Oncology. 2014;**15**(7):722-729. DOI: 10.1016/S1470-2045(14)70200-1

[33] Loprinzi CL, Thome SD. Understanding the utility of adjuvant systemic therapy for primary breast cancer. Journal of Clinical Oncology. 2001;**19**(4):972-979. DOI: 10.1200/JCO.2001.19.4.972

[34] Shachar SS, Muss HB. Internet tools to enhance breast cancer care. NPJ Breast Cancer. 2016;**2**:16011. DOI: 10.1038/npjbcancer.2016.11

[35] Peele PB, Siminoff LA, Xu Y, Ravdin PM. Decreased use of adjuvant breast cancer therapy in a randomized controlled trial of a decision aid with individualized risk information. Medical Decision Making. 2005;**25**(3):301-307. DOI: 10.1177/0272989X05276851

[36] Hosseini H, Obradović MM, Hoffmann M, Harper K, Sosa MS, Werner-Klein M, Nanduri LK, Werno C, Ehrl C, Maneck M, Patwary N, Haunschild G, Gužvić M, Reimelt C, Grauvogl M, Eichner N, Weber F, Hartkopf AD, Taran FA, Brucker SY, Fehm T, Rack B, Buchholz S, Spang R, Meister G, Aguirre-Ghiso JA, Klein CA. Early dissemination seeds metastasis in breast cancer. Nature. 2016. DOI: 10.1038/nature20785

[37] Wazir U, Mokbel K, Carmichael A, Mokbel K. Are online prediction tools a valid alternative to genomic profiling in the context of systemic treatment of ER+ breast cancer? Cellular & Molecular Biology Letters. 2017;**22**:20. DOI: 10.1186/s11658-017-0049-x. eCollection 2017

[38] Wishart GC, Azzato EM, Greenberg DC, Rashbass J, Kearins O, Lawrence G, Caldas C, Pharoah PD. PREDICT: A new UK prognostic model that predicts survival following surgery for invasive breast cancer. Breast Cancer Research. 2010;**12**(1):R1. DOI: 10.1186/bcr2464. Epub 2010 Jan 6. Erratum in: Breast Cancer Research. 2010;**12**(2):401

[39] Wishart GC, Rakha E, Green A, Ellis I, Ali HR, Provenzano E, Blows FM, Caldas C, Pharoah PD. Inclusion of KI67 significantly improves performance of the PREDICT prognostication and prediction model for early breast cancer. BMC Cancer. 2014;**14**:908. DOI: 10.1186/1471-2407-14-908

[40] Candido Dos Reis FJ, Wishart GC, Dicks EM, Greenberg D, Rashbass J, Schmidt MK, van den Broek AJ, Ellis IO, Green A, Rakha E, Maishman T, Eccles DM, Pharoah PDP. An updated PREDICT breast cancer prognostication and treatment benefit prediction model with independent validation. Breast Cancer Research. 2017;**19**(1):58. DOI: 10.1186/s13058-017-0852-3

[41] Amin MB, Edge S, Greene FL. AJCC Cancer Staging Manual. 8th ed. New York: Springer; 2016

[42] Markopoulos C, van de Velde C, Zarca D, Ozmen V, Masetti R. Clinical evidence supporting genomic tests in early breast cancer: Do all genomic tests provide the same information? European Journal of Surgical Oncology. 2017;**43**(5):909-920

[43] Schüring AN, Fehm T, Behringer K, Goeckenjan M, Wimberger P, Henes M, Henes J, Fey MF, von Wolff M. Practical recommendations for fertility preservation in women by the FertiPROTEKT network. Part I: Indications for fertility preservation. Archives of Gynecology and Obstetrics. 2018;**297**(1):241-255. DOI: 10.1007/s00404-017-4594-3

[44] Constance ES, Moravek MB, Jeruss JS. Strategies to maintain fertility in young breast cancer patients. Cancer Treatment and Research 2018;**173**:1-13. DOI: 10.1007/978-3-319-70197-4_1

[45] Early Breast Cancer Trialists' Collaborative Group (EBCTCG), Peto R, Davies C, Godwin J, Gray R, Pan HC, Clarke M, Cutter D, Darby S, McGale P, Taylor C, Wang YC, Bergh J, Di

Leo A, Albain K, Swain S, Piccart M, Pritchard K. Comparisons between different polychemotherapy regimens for early breast cancer: Meta-analyses of long-term outcome among 100,000 women in 123 randomised trials. Lancet 2012;**379**(9814):432-444. DOI: 10.1016/S0140-6736(11)61625-5

[46] Samuel JA, Wilson JW, Bandos H, et al. [S3-02] NSABP B-36: A randomized phase III trial comparing six cycles of 5-fluorouracil (5-FU), epirubicin, and cyclophosphamide (FEC) to four cycles of adriamycin and cyclophosphamide (AC) in patients (pts) with node-negative breast cancer. 2014 San Antonio Breast Cancer Symposium. Abstract S3-02. Presented Dec 11, 2014

[47] Möbus V. Adjuvant dose-dense chemotherapy in breast cancer: Standard of Care in High-Risk Patients. Breast Care (Basel). 2016;**11**(1):8-12. DOI: 10.1159/000444004

[48] Goldvaser H, Majeed H, Ribnikar D, Šeruga B, Ocaña A, Cescon DW, Amir E. Influence of control group therapy on the benefit from dose-dense chemotherapy in early breast cancer: A systemic review and meta-analysis. Breast Cancer Research and Treatment. 2018 Feb 8. DOI: 10.1007/s10549-018-4710-5

[49] Nccn Clinical Practice Guidelines in Oncology. Breast Cancer Version 4.2017. Feb 8, 2018

[50] Francis PA. Adjuvant endocrine therapy for premenopausal women: Type and duration. Breast. 2017;**34**(Suppl 1):S108-S111. DOI: 10.1016/j.breast.2017.06.040

[51] Pagani O, Regan MM, Francis PA, TEXT and SOFT Investigators, International Breast Cancer Study Group. Exemestane with ovarian suppression in premenopausal breast cancer. The New England Journal of Medicine. 2014;**371**(14):1358-1359. DOI: 10.1056/NEJMc1409366

[52] Ibrahim EM, Al-Hajeili MR, Bayer AM, Abulkhair OA, Refae AA. Extended adjuvant endocrine therapy in early breast cancer: A meta-analysis of published randomized trials. Medical Oncology. 2017;**34**(7):131. DOI: 10.1007/s12032-017-0986-2

[53] Zhang Y, Ji Y, Li J, Lei L, Wu S, Zuo W, Jia X, Wang Y, Mo M, Zhang N, Shen Z, Wu J, Shao Z, Liu G. Sequential versus simultaneous use of chemotherapy and gonadotropin-releasing hormoneagonist (GnRHa) among estrogen receptor (ER)-positive premenopausal breast cancer patients: effects on ovarian function, disease-free survival, and overall survival. Breast Cancer Research and Treatment. Jan 13, 2018. DOI: 10.1007/s10549-018-4660-y

[54] Regan MM, Walley BA, Francis PA, Fleming GF, Láng I, Gómez HL, Colleoni M, Tondini C, Pinotti G, Salim M, Spazzapan S, Parmar V, Ruhstaller T, Abdi EA, Gelber RD, Coates AS, Goldhirsch A, Pagani O. Concurrent and sequential initiation of ovarian function suppression with chemotherapy in premenopausal women with endocrine-responsive early breast cancer: an exploratory analysis of TEXT and SOFT. Ann Oncol. 2017 Sep 1;**28**(9): 2225-2232. DOI: 10.1093/annonc/mdx285

[55] Dhesy-Thind S, Fletcher GG, Blanchette PS, Clemons MJ, Dillmon MS, Frank ES, Gandhi S, Gupta R, Mates M, Moy B, Vandenberg T, Van Poznak CH. Use of adjuvant bisphosphonates and other bone-modifying agents in breast cancer: A Cancer Care Ontario and American Society of Clinical Oncology Clinical Practice Guideline. Journal of Clinical Oncology. 2017; **35**(18):2062-2081. DOI: 10.1200/JCO.2016.70.7257

9

Caring of Breast Cancer Patient

Anggorowati Anggorowati

Abstract

Breast cancer is one of the biggest causes of mortality in some countries. Various conditions contribute to the incidence of breast cancer in either unmarried or married women. Caring in women with breast cancer is the key to successful treatment of breast cancer. The conditions patient when is diagnosed breast cancer, undergoing therapy, and after treatment are different, so caring on breast cancer can be divided into caring at the time of diagnosis, caring during therapy, and caring in follow-up therapy. The results obtained from caring of breast cancer increase survival of breast cancer patients.

Keywords: caring in diagnosis, caring in therapy, caring in follow-up therapy, survival cancer, breast cancer

1. Introduction

Women have risk developing breast cancer in non-breastfeeding women or infertile conditions. The risk of breast cancer was higher among women who currently or recently used contemporary hormonal contraceptives than among who had never used hormonal contraceptives [1].

At the time when women began to feel the complaint with her breasts, few women hasten to check themselves completely. The condition of the emergence of symptoms is the right time for handling so that the rate of recovery is high. Some women are open to complain and hasten for therapy. Stigma is present in women when breast cancer is present in them. This is a management bottleneck in the days before being diagnosed with breast cancer. Attendance of others such as family and healthcare workers who pay attention, fast management, and plenary caring are needed during this period.

Most women diagnosed with breast cancer are already in a late condition where the breasts have given an unpleasant condition, foul smell, and excessive fluid. The existence of women in the family as wives, mothers, and caregivers of families becomes disrupted, and some women undergo self-care.

Caring in women with breast cancer requires a variety of understanding of the development, roles and functions of women with breast cancer, and psycho-spiritual and psychosocial needs. The context of understanding conditions under conditions of diagnosis, therapy, and follow-up after therapy is a caring breast cancer approach.

2. Caring for patient in breast cancer diagnosis

The diagnosis of breast cancer is identified in someone who has breast cancer risk. Most women included in the risk group pay more attention to any changes in their breasts. The following groups are at risk of developing breast cancer [2]:

a. Personal history of breast cancer. Women who had breast cancer in the past have a higher risk of developing breast cancer again. Breast cancer can develop in the same breast as the first cancer or in the other breast.

b. Family history of breast and other cancers. The greatest risk in family history of breast cancer is from mother, sister, or daughter who had breast cancer, especially if they were diagnosed before menopause.

c. Certain genetic conditions. The following rare inherited genetic conditions are linked with a higher risk for breast cancer:

   1. Li-Fraumeni syndrome increases the risk of developing certain types of cancer, including breast cancer, osteosarcoma, soft tissue sarcoma, and leukemia. Most people with Li-Fraumeni syndrome have inherited a mutation in the TP53 gene, which is normally a tumor suppressor gene.

   2. Ataxia telangiectasia (AT) is caused by a mutation of the ATM gene. This gene is responsible for repairing damaged DNA. Certain families with a high rate of breast cancer have mutations of this gene.

   3. Cowden syndrome is caused by a mutation in the PTEN gene, which is normally a tumor suppressor gene. People with this condition are more likely to develop breast cancer, gastrointestinal cancers, and thyroid cancer.

   4. Peutz-Jeghers syndrome may be related to a mutation of the STK11 (also known as LKB1) gene. This gene appears to normally function as a tumor suppressor gene. Peutz-Jeghers syndrome increases the risk of developing gastrointestinal, breast, ovarian, and testicular cancers.

d. Dense breast. Dense breasts have more connective tissue, glands, and milk ducts than fatty tissue. Breast density is an inherited trait. Some studies show that women with dense breast tissue in 75% or more of their breasts are 4–6 times more likely to develop breast cancer than women with little or no dense breast tissue. Breast density can only be seen on a mammogram, but dense breasts also make a mammogram harder to read. On a mammogram, fatty tissue looks dark, while dense tissue looks white, like tumors, so it can hide a tumor.

e. Reproductive history. Estrogen is the main hormone associated with breast cancer. Estrogen affects the growth of breast cells. Experts believe that it plays an important role in the growth of breast cancer cells as well. The type of exposure and how long cells are exposed to estrogen affect the chances that breast cancer will develop. Menopause at a younger age decreases the length of time the breast tissue is exposed to estrogen and other hormones. Women who experience early menarche, late menopause, and late pregnancy at risk of breast cancer. Early menopause is linked with a lower risk of breast cancer. Pregnancy interrupts the exposure of breast cells to circulating estrogen. It also lowers the total number of menstrual cycles a woman has in her lifetime. Women who have their first full-term pregnancy after the age of 30 have a slightly higher risk of breast cancer than women who have at least one full-term pregnancy at an earlier age.

f. Exposure to ionizing radiation. Woman who have received radiation therapy to the chest, neck, and armpit area have a higher risk of developing breast cancer.

g. Hormone replacement therapy. Woman who is taking hormone replacement therapy for a long time increases the risk of breast cancer.

h. Oral contraception. Oral contraceptives that contain both estrogen and progesterone can slightly increase the risk for breast cancer, especially among women who have used oral contraceptives for 10 or more years. The higher risk disappears after the woman stops taking oral contraceptives. However, current and recent (less than 10 years since last use) users have a slightly greater risk than women who have never used oral contraceptives.

i. Atypical hyperplasia. Atypical hyperplasia is a noncancerous (benign) condition where there are a greater number of abnormal (atypical) cells in the breast tissue. Atypical hyperplasia increases a woman's risk of developing breast cancer.

j. Alcohol. Drinking alcohol increases a woman's risk for breast cancer. Even low levels of alcohol consumption (just over 1 drink per day) can increase a woman's risk. The risk increases with the amount of alcohol consumed. One possible reason for the link between alcohol and breast cancer is that alcohol is thought to cause higher levels of estrogen. Alcohol may also lower levels of some essential nutrients that protect against cell damage, such as folate (a type of vitamin B), vitamin A, and vitamin C.

k. Being obese. Obesity increases the risk for breast cancer in postmenopausal women. Studies show that women who have never taken hormone replacement therapy and who have a body mass index (BMI) of 31.1 or higher have a 2.5 times greater risk of developing breast cancer than those with a BMI of 22.6 or lower. Ovarian hormones, estrogens in particular, play an important role in breast cancer. Many of the risk factors for breast cancer are believed to result from the overall dose of estrogen the breast tissue receives over time. The ovaries make most of the body's estrogen, but after menopause fat tissue produces a small amount of estrogen. Having more fat tissue can increase estrogen levels and so increase the chance that breast cancer will develop.

l. Physical inactivity. Physical inactivity increases the risk of breast cancer in both premenopausal and postmenopausal women.

m. High socioeconomic status. Breast cancer risk is slightly higher for women with higher incomes. This may be because of lifestyle factors that are linked to breast cancer, such as having children later in life or having fewer children.

n. Tall adult height. Women who have a slightly higher risk of developing breast cancer after menopause. It is thought that energy intake and diet early in life, which affect adult height, are the factors that increase the risk, rather than just being tall.

During breast cancer diagnosis, patients follow a series of tests. Examinations performed on breast cancer patients include [3]:

1. Physical exam. A physical exam allows your doctor to look for any signs of breast cancer.
2. Clinical breast exam.
3. Diagnostic mammography. Diagnostic mammography is an x-ray that uses small doses of radiation to make an image of the breast. It is used to follow up on abnormal results of a screening mammography or a clinical breast exam. Mammography can also be used to find an abnormal area during a biopsy.
4. Biopsy. A biopsy is the only definite way to diagnose breast cancer. During a biopsy, the doctor removes tissues or cells from the body so they can be tested in a lab. A report from the pathologist will confirm whether or not cancer cells are found in the sample.
5. Hormone receptor status testing. Estrogen and progesterone are hormones that can stimulate the growth of breast cancer cells. Hormone receptor status testing looks for estrogen receptors (ERs) and progesterone receptors (PRs) in the breast cancer cells.
6. HER2 status testing. HER2 status testing is done to find out if breast cancer cells are making more HER2 protein than normal (called overexpression).
7. Tumor marker test. Tumor markers are substances found in the blood, tissues, or fluids removed from the body.
8. X-ray. An X-ray uses small doses of radiation to make an image of parts of the body on film. It is used to find out if breast cancer has spread to the lungs.
9. Bone scan. Bone scan is used to find out if breast cancer has spread to the bones (called bone metastasis).

Most of the patients and their families face some degree of depression, anxiety, and fear when cancer becomes a part of their lives. Breast cancer patients may experience anxiety at different situations as while undergoing a screening test, waiting for the results, receiving a diagnosis, undergoing treatment, or anticipating a recurrence of their cancer. The anxiety associated with cancer may increase feelings of pain, interfere their ability to sleep, cause nausea and vomiting, and interfere with their quality of life. And the severe anxiety may even shorten the patient's life [4].

Interviewing some breast cancer patients reported that their anxiety is characterized by a number of typical symptoms and signs such as shivering or tremor. They find that their feelings of anxiety increase or decrease at different times. They may become more anxious as cancer spreads or treatment becomes more intense. The level of anxiety experienced by one person may differ from the level of anxiety experienced by another. Anxiety in breast cancer patients is associated with death anxiety, fear of death as a result of their symptoms [4].

Caseness in depression significantly increased in the first year of breast cancer diagnosis from baseline (18.5%) to 4 months (21.5%) but decreased to 15.3% at 12 months [5, 6]. This is in accordance with other studies that majority of women newly diagnosed with early breast cancer reported clinical or severe depressive symptoms. The patients presented a controlled emotional coping style. Anger suppression might play a unique role in depressive symptoms among women newly diagnosed with breast cancer [7]. Anxiety is a more significant psychological state that contributed to the feeling of distress in breast cancer than depression [8]. So on the stage diagnosis, the health team should be concern about management of anxiety.

Education in depressed breast cancer patients is adjusted for depression and patient characteristics. Psychoeducation in groups is an intervention given to overcome depression [9]. The role and function of the patient in the family, the pattern of family-patient interaction, the cultural structure in the community, and the religious value of the patient affect the acceptance of breast cancer patients. The severity of depression cannot be separated from the type of cancer suffered. Patients with no history of cancer in the family experienced more severe depression than had a family history of cancer [10]. The severity of the patient's breast cancer level is related to the depressed level of the patient.

The most common types of breast cancer diagnoses are inflammatory breast cancer, Paget disease of the nipple, and triple-negative breast cancer [11–14]. Explanations of each type of breast cancer are as follows:

2.1. Inflammatory breast cancer

Inflammatory breast cancer develops when cancer cells block the lymph vessel; the breast becomes red and swollen. Inflammatory breast cancer develops more often in younger women and women of African ancestry. Inflammatory breast cancer is rare and aggressive, which means that it grows and spreads quickly. In most cases, inflammatory breast cancer has already spread to the lymph nodes or other organs when it is diagnosed. The most common symptom of inflammatory breast cancer is a change to the color of the skin on at least one-third of the breast. The skin becomes very red or purplish in color. Other symptoms of inflammatory breast cancer include:

1. A swollen breast
2. Dimpled or pitted kin that looks like an orange peel (called peau d'orange)

3. Thickened skin or breast tissue
4. A breast that feels warm to the touch
5. An increase in the size of the breast
6. Changes to the nipple such as a nipple that suddenly starts to point inward (called an inverted nipple)
7. Tenderness or pain in the breast
8. Itching or burning
9. A lump in the armpit (called the axilla) or near the collarbone

The symptoms of inflammatory breast cancer are very similar to the symptoms of infection in the breast tissue (mastitis), which is more common in breastfeeding women.

2.2. Paget disease of the breast

Paget disease of the breast is a rare type of breast cancer. It develops as a rash or other skin changes on the nipple, usually on only one breast. This is more common in women over the age of 50. Most women with Paget disease also have invasive ductal carcinoma or ductal carcinoma in situ (DCIS). The cancer can then spread to the dark-colored skin around the nipple (called the areola).

Paget disease of the breast usually causes changes to the nipple, including:

1. Crusting, scaling, or flaking
2. Redness of the nipple and areola
3. Burning or itching
4. Bleeding or discharge
5. The nipple turning inward, or becoming inverted
6. The nipple becoming flat a lump in the breast, often near or under the nipple

2.3. Triple-negative breast cancer

Many breast cancer cells have receptors for estrogen or progesterone. They may also have receptors for a protein called HER2 (also called ERBB2). Triple-negative breast cancer means that the cancer cells do not have any of these receptors. Because it does not have any of these receptors, triple-negative breast cancer is considered a separate type of breast cancer with its own treatment options. Most triple-negative breast cancers are invasive ductal carcinoma. Ductal carcinoma in situ (DCIS) may also be triple negative.

Basal-like breast cancer is similar to triple-negative breast cancer because the cancer cells often do not have receptors for estrogen, progesterone, and HER2. But basal-like breast cancer cells have changes in the proteins that triple-negative breast cancers usually do not have. Most basal-like breast cancers are invasive ductal carcinomas.

It is important to note that not all triple-negative breast cancers are basal-like and not all basal-like breast cancers are triple negative. They are two similar, but distinct, subtypes of breast cancer. Scientists have not yet developed one internationally accepted definition of a basal-like breast cancer. But they know that it is different from other types of breast cancer.

Women under the age of 40 and women of African or Asian ancestry have a higher risk of developing triple-negative breast cancer. Basal-like breast cancers are more likely to be found in younger women and in women of African ancestry.

Many triple-negative and basal-like breast cancers may be called interval cancers because they can develop between regularly scheduled screening mammography.

Most triple-negative and basal-like breast cancers are high-grade, or aggressive, tumors. This means that they tend to grow and spread quickly. Many are diagnosed at a later stage when the cancer has already spread (metastasized) to lymph nodes or other organs. These tumors tend to spread to the brain or lungs more often than breast cancers that are not triple negative. Most triple-negative breast cancers have a less favorable prognosis than other types of breast cancer.

Basal-like breast cancers spread differently than other types of breast cancer. They usually spread to the bloodstream, brain, and lungs. They do not spread to the lymph nodes or the bones as often as other types of breast cancer.

When the patient is diagnosed with breast cancer, a feeling of sadness and fear arises, sad because she did not think she will be diagnosed with breast cancer and will lose her breast due to surgery and patient's fear of illness and death [15].

Role changes begin to occur in women undergoing diagnosis. The role of mother who takes care of her children is time-consuming. Some patients still have children less than 2 years old, so there is a feeling of guilt for not being able to persecute. The role of wife in serving the husband is disturbed because of his physical condition. Women can still meet the sexual needs of couples but the frequency is reduced. This role change affects self-acceptance as a woman. The reaction of a patient diagnosed with breast cancer is to accept, deny, blame yourself, and withdraw [16].

Feeling sad about the diagnosis of cancer that the patient takes requires resistance from yourself so as not to get sucked in sorrow. Patients should have the power to deal with perceived problems. The speed of cancer treatment is proportional to the rate of cancer development itself; the sooner the patient decides to overcome her cancer, the closer she gets in handling it. Psychological support is needed for patients to gain confidence in themselves; the patient believes that the cancer she faces can heal. Family and people closest to her are part of a meaningful social support for patients. Various forms of psychological support, among others, are always present to accompany patients at the time of cancer management. Methods of psychological support, among others, are crisis interventions, psychological counseling, self-support groups, relaxation, and suggestive psychotherapy [17]. The presence of people who are meaningful for the life of the patient will give its own strength, increasing the efficacy

Care	Activities
Make time for self	Try to stay involved in activities and enjoy
	Ask family and friends to help
Care for the body	Eat healthy meals and snacks
	Try to get enough rest
	Continue having checkups
	Avoid using alcohol and cigarette
	Exercise for 15–30 min each day
Deal with uncertainty	Put some plans on hold
	Focus on things you can control
	Have more knowledge about what is happening
Talk to family and friends	Talking how you feel if feeling angry
	Try not to hold in all feelings
Organize your time	Prioritize your weekly tasks and activities
	Use personal planner
	Ask for help from family, friends, or support services
	Concentrate on one task a time
	Avoid multiple trips

Table 1. Activities to take care of themselves for breast cancer patients.

of patients to undergo therapy. Patients will follow various follow-up measures of various cancer intervention options. The nearest mentoring gives meaning to the patient so that the patient has hope for the success of the follow-up to be followed.

Patient should care for themselves to overcome breast cancer problems. **Table 1** shows some of the activities that breast cancer patients do to take care of themselves [18].

Caring shown in these conditions, such as empathy with women, do not blame that women who suffer from breast cancer because of the risks that exist in her. The presence of the nearest person as the person who gives attention to the woman reinforces her.

3. Caring for breast cancer patients during treatment

Breast cancer patients are given treatment, i.e., surgery, radiation, and chemotherapy depending on the stage of breast cancer. Each of these treatments has side effects. Effects after chemotherapy are neutropenia, anemia, nausea, vomiting, and neuropathy [19]. Interventions to increase food intake in breast cancer patient during treatment are cook extra food, make meals a time when patient can sit together and talk, and take extra care when preparing food. These differences include physical changes such as alopecia, depression, decreased body image, emotional changes, and impaired role function and social function [19].

Breast cancer patients who have chemotherapy will experience high distress 55.3%. Symptoms of stress include physical signs, such as trouble sleeping, constant headache, high blood pressure, and other heart problems. Emotional signs may include feeling tired, unwell, and overly sensitive. Activities to reduce stress are exercise regularly, meditate to practice deep breathing, listen to music or read, talk to someone, ask others to help, try to rest and get enough sleep, eat nourishing food to give energy and keep well, and take time to care for self.

Some breast cancer treatments have side effects that affect the heart; the most common side effects are heart dysfunction, chest pain, and irregular heartbeat [20]. Heart dysfunction can occur during cancer treatment or any time up to 2 years after treatment is finished. The symptoms of heart dysfunction are difficulty keeping up level activity, a bloated feeling around the abdomen, feeling less hungry, swelling of ankles and feet, feeling dizzy when changing position, and shortness of breath, at rest or when active.

Patients need basic information about chemotherapy, side effects, and problem-solving skills during therapy. Fulfillment of chemotherapy information prevents depression and anxiety in breast cancer patients [21]. Patients undergoing radiotherapy experience various problems such as skin changes, burning scars, and edema. Patients who dissected experienced losing her breasts affected her body image. Changes in patients with radiotherapy and surgery lead to changes in self-image that affect the psychological health of the patient. After breast surgery studies show that mastectomy as surgical treatment for breast cancer may negatively affect a woman's body image and her self-image [22].

Breast cancer patients maintain a healthy life with various activities. **Table 2** describes healthy activity for the heart of breast cancer patient.

In fact, patients who receive both often have less severe symptoms, have better quality of life, and report they are more satisfied with treatment [23]. So, they needed symptom management, supportive care, or palliative care. Palliative care is given at every step of treatment process. In this part, the patients accept support from caregivers, family, and friends [24]. The other person such as volunteer, clergy, social group providing support for the patient's emotional and social needs, spiritual needs or concern and practical needs.

Healthy living	Activities
Be active	Try to stay active during cancer treatment; exercise or do physical activity each day
	Increasing physical activity after treatment can help: strengthen muscles, improve fitness level, lower blood pressure, and give more energy
Eat well	Eat a variety of foods from the four food groups each day
	Read food label to choose healthier foods
	Limit food and drinks that are high in calories, fat, sugar, and sodium
	Drink little or no alcohol
Do not smoke	Limited smoking or stop smoking

Table 2. Healthy living for breast cancer patients during treatment.

Palliative care starts at diagnosis and continues throughout all stages of the disease. The best palliative care occurs when patients and their families work together with the healthcare team [25].

Caring for this period can occur when there is good communication between patient, family, and health teams. Caring can be achieved if the patient can show some communication skills. For patient, tips to help promote good communication patient with healthcare team are:

a. Ask the doctor to explain the diagnosis, treatment plan, and prognosis.

b. Ask healthcare team to explain if you do not understand an explanation, description, or unfamiliar medical word.

c. Tell the doctors and nurses about any pain, discomfort, or other side effects.

d. Keep track of symptoms and side effects. Write down what they are, how often they occur, and how severe they are.

e. Do not be afraid to ask questions.

For the treatment of breast cancer, the physical symptoms of breast cancer patients affect the needs and fulfillment of the physical, psychological, social, and spiritual aspects [16]. The success of AI therapy depends on patients' ability to adhere to treatment recommendations [26].

The breast cancer patients need friends, which receive the shortcomings, and more attention. During therapy patients should have realistic expectations and interpersonal relationships, remain active in activities, support family and community, and improve their spirituality. The patient's condition enhances the survival abilities of patients undergoing therapy.

4. Caring for following treatment for breast cancer patients

Breast cancer patients who have recovered still have risk to relapse again. Study in the UK showed that after 5 years of adjuvant endocrine therapy, breast cancer recurrences continued to occur steadily throughout from 5 to 20 years [27]. After undergoing therapy, breast cancer patients follow a series of follow-ups. Some follow-ups are doctor visit, mammogram screening, pelvic exams, and bone density test. Completed of follow up assesment breast cancer patients on **Table 3**.

After breast surgery, physical changes can make some women less comfortable with their bodies. There may be a loss of sensation in the affected breast. Other treatments for breast cancer, such as chemotherapy, can change your hormone levels and affect sexual interest and/or response. Partner may worry about how to express love physically and emotionally after treatment, especially after surgery. But breast cancer can be a growth experience for couples—especially when partners take part in decision-making and go along to treatments [29, 30].

From the review of research, Sisler showed that after breast cancer treatment, the survivorship care involves four main tasks: surveillance and screening, management of long-term effect, health promotion, and care condition. Surveillance for recurrence involves only annual

Maneuver	Recommendation
Do	
Primary care visit with history and physical examination	Every 3–6 months for years 1–3 after treatment, every 6–12 months for years 4 and 5, and then annually
	History to focus on symptoms of distant (bone, lung, liver, brain) and local recurrence
	Examination focuses on surgical scar, breasts, chestwall, regional nodes, arms for lymphedema, and common sites of distant spread
	Annual gynecologic examination for patients taking tamoxifen
Breast self-examination	Monthly breast self-examination is recommended in this higher-risk group
Mammography	Annually, starting 1 year after initial mammogram but at least 6 months after radiation therapy is complete, can be performed every 6 months in select cases, no routine imaging of a reconstructed breast is needed
Screen for other cancers	As for average-risk individuals, unless family suggests otherwise
Do not do	
Breast magnetic resonance imaging	Not recommended
Other tests:	Not recommended
Complete blood counts	
Liver function tests	
Routine imaging of the chest, abdomen, or bone	
Tumor markers	
Cardiac imaging	Not recommended after completion of anthracycline (epirubicin, doxorubicin) or trastuzumab therapy unless there are symptoms

Source: Sisler et al. [28].

Table 3. Surveillance and screening for asymptomatic breast cancer survivors.

mammography, and screening for other cancers should be done according to population guidelines Management of the long-term effects of cancer and its treatment addresses common issues of pain, fatigue, lymphedema, distress, and medication side effect. Health promotion emphasizes the benefits of active lifestyle change in cancer survivors, with an emphasis on physical activity [28]. Completed task after treatment breast cancer is shown in **Tables 3–5**.

Caring in breast cancer patients after treatment can be given by group like in Canada there is CanIMPACT (Canadian Team to Improve Community-Based Cancer Care along the Continuum) [31]. Similar teams from either the health team or from community groups are needed by breast cancer patients to survive.

Breast cancer patients are likely to heal. Once cured, there are those who can survive, but there is a relapse. Every woman is at risk of breast cancer. Prevention is done by breastfeeding before the age of 35 years [32].

Category	Recommendations
Cardiovascular health	Monitor lipid level and provide cardiovascular monitoring as indicated
	Educate patient about healthy lifestyle modification (balanced diet, exercise, smoking cessation), potential cardiac risk factors, and when to report relevant symptoms (shortness of breath or fatigue) to healthcare providers
Cognitive dysfunction	Ask about cognitive difficulties
	Assess reversible contributing factors of cognitive impairment and optimally treat when possible
	Refer for neurocognitive assessment and rehabilitation if there are signs of cognitive impairment
	Suggest self-management and coping strategies for cognitive dysfunction (relaxation, stress management, routine exercise)
Distress, depression, and anxiety	Assess for distress, depression, and anxiety
	Assess further if the patient is at higher risk of depression
	Offer counseling and pharmacotherapy or refer to mental health resource as indicated
Fatigue	Assess for fatigue, use severity rating scale, and treat causative factor
	Offer treatment or referral for factors affecting fatigue (mood disorder, sleep disturbance, pain, etc.)
	Encourage regular physical activity, refer for cognitive behavior therapy (CBT) if indicated
	When fatigue is present, provide education and general strategies to manage fatigue and evaluate
	Do not recommend methylphenidate or modafinil to manage fatigue, given insufficient evidence
	Preliminary evidence suggest that yoga is likely to improve fatigue
Referral for genetic counseling	Consider referral for genetic counseling if: • Breast cancer was diagnosed before age 50 years (especially <35 years) • Ovarian cancer at any age (epithelial) • Bilateral breast cancer in the same woman • Both breast and ovarian cancers in the same women or some family • Multiple breast cancers on the same side of the family (paternal or maternal) • Male breast cancer • Ashkenazi Jewish ethnicity
Osteoporosis	Dual-energy X-ray absorptiometry (DEXA) scan at baseline and then every 2 years if the patient is taking aromatase inhibitors or gonadotrophin-releasing hormone (GnRH) agonists
Pain and chemotherapy-induced peripheral neuropathy (CIPN)	Assess for pain and contributing factors with pain scale and history
	Offer interventions such as acetaminophen, nonsteroidal anti-inflammatory drugs (NSAIDs), physical activity, or acupuncture for pain
	Suggest physical activity for neuropathic pain
	Refer to appropriate specialist once the cause of pain has been determined (e.g., lymphedema specialist)
	Consider transcutaneous electrical nerve stimulation (TENS) for CIPN in survivors with contraindications to medication or for whom medication is ineffective
	Consider acupuncture as an adjunct option to treat patients with medication-resistant CIPN
Sexual health	Assess for signs and symptoms of sexual or intimacy problems
	Assess for reversible contributing factors to sexual problems and treat when appropriate
	Offer nonhormonal, water-based lubricants for vaginal dryness
	Refer for psychoeducational therapy and sexual or marital counseling when appropriate

Category	Recommendations
Premature menopause, menopausal symptoms	Offer selective norepinephrine reuptake inhibitors (SNRIs), selective serotonin reuptake inhibitors (SSRIs), or gabapentin and lifestyle modifications to help vasomotor symptoms of premature menopause
	Consider CBT or routine exercise for treatment
	Consider tailored patient education interventions and consultations when appropriate to decrease menopausal symptoms
Lymphedema	Counsel weight loss for overweight or obese patients to prevent or reduce lymphedema risk
	Educate survivors about lymphedema sign and symptoms and assess for lymphedema
	Refer if symptoms are suggestive of lymphedema
Infertility	Refer survivors of childbearing age experiencing infertility to reproductive endocrinology and infertility specialist promptly
Body image concerns	Assess for body image concerns
	Refer to psychosocial resources as indicated

Source: Sisler et al. [28].

Table 4. Assessment and management of long-term effects of breast cancer and its treatments.

Category	Recommendation
Weight management	Counsel patients to achieve and maintain a healthy weight
	Counsel patients who are overweight or obese to change dietary habits and increase physical activity to promote and maintain weight loss
Physical activity	Counsel patients to avoid inactivity and return to daily activities as soon as possible after diagnosis
	Aim for at least 150 min of moderate or 75 min of vigorous physical activity weekly
	Include strength training exercise at least 2 days/week
Nutrition	Counsel patients to have a dietary pattern high in vegetables, fruits, whole grains, and legumes; low in saturated fats; limited in processed and red meats
	Limit alcohol
	Counselor supplements only if deficiencies are demonstrated
Smoking cessation	Counsel patients to avoid smoking; offer or refer for cessation counseling and resources

Source: Sisler et al. [28].

Table 5. Health promotion for breast cancer survivors.

5. Conclusion

Breast cancer occurs in most women who get married late or are not breastfeeding. Acceptance of breast cancer diagnosis affects a person's ability to survive. Caring given since the diagnosis of breast cancer provides the strength for patients to survive.

Breast cancer patients need caring of their own body to keep their health. Patients undergoing therapy require the presence of family and friends to provide care for them. After successfully undergoing therapy, breast cancer patients should always live healthily and always do a series of checks regularly in order to prevent the risk of recurring illness.

Author details

Anggorowati Anggorowati

Address all correspondence to: anggorowati@fk.undip.ac.id

Nursing Department, Medical Faculty, Diponegoro University, Semarang, Indonesia

References

[1] Morch et al. Contemporary hormonal contraception and the risk of breast cancer. The New England Journal of Medicine. 2017;**377**:2228-2239

[2] Canadian Cancer Society. Risk of Breast Cancer. 2017. http://www.cancer.ca/en/cancer-information/cancer-type/breast/risk/?region=on

[3] Canadian Cancer Society. Diagnosis of Breast Cancer. 2017. http://www.cancer.ca/en/cancer-information/cancer-type/breast/diagnosis/?region=on

[4] Baqutayan SMS. The effect of anxiety on breast cancer patients. Indian Journal of Psychological Medicine. 2012;**34**(2):119-123

[5] Burgess C, Cornelius V, Love S, Graham J, Richards M, Ramirez A. Depression and anxiety in women with early breast cancer: five year observational cohort study. BMJ. 2005;**330**(7493):702. DOI: 10.1136/bmj.38343.670868.D3 [PMC free article]

[6] Saboonchi F, Petersson LM, Wennman-Larsen A, Alexanderson K, Brännström R, Vaez M. Changes in caseness of anxiety and depression in breast cancer patients during the first year following surgery: Patterns of transiency and severity of the distress response. European Journal of Oncology Nursing. 2014;**18**(6):598-604. DOI: 10.1016/j.ejon.2014.06.007

[7] Li L, Yang Y, He J, Yi J, Wang Y, Zhang J, et al. Emotional suppression and depressive symptoms in women newly diagnosed with early breast cancer. BMC Women's Health. 2015;**15**:91

[8] Guang Ng C, Mohamed S, Kaur K, Sulaiman AH, Zainal NZ, Taib NS, et al. Perceived distress and its association with depression and anxiety in breast cancer patients. Plos One. March 15, 2017. DOI: 10.1371/journal.pone.0172975

[9] Ram S, Narayanasamy R, Barua A. Effectiveness of group psycho-education on well-being and depression among breast cancer survivor of Malaka, Malaysia. Indian Journal of Palliative Care. 2013;**19**(1):34-39

[10] Dastan NB, Buzlu S. Depression and anxiety levels in early stage Turkish breast cancer patients and related factors. Asian Pacific Journal of Cancer Prevention. 2011;**12**(1):137-141

[11] American Cancer Society. Types of Breast Cancer. 2017. https://www.cancer.org/cancer/breast-cancer/understanding-a-breast-cancer-diagnosis/types-of-breast-cancer.html

[12] Canadian Cancer Society. Types of Breast Cancer. 2017. http://www.cbcf.org/central/aboutbreastcancermain/diagnosis/pages/breastcancertypes.aspx

[13] National Breast Cancer Foundation. Types of Brest Cancer. 2017. http://www.national-breastcancer.org/types-of-breast-cancer

[14] Breast Cancer Network Australia. Types of Breast Cancer. 2017. https://www.bcna.org.au/understanding-breast-cancer/types-of-breast-cancer

[15] Muhbes FJ. Fear of patient with breast cancer. American Journal of Scientific and Industrial Research. 2010;**1**(1):47-50

[16] Gandes A. A phenomenological study: Fulfillment of psychosocial needs of patients with breast cancer undergoing chemotherapy [thesis]. Diponegoro University; 2017

[17] Cieslak K. Professional psychological support and psychotherapy methods for oncology patients. Basic concepts and issues. Reports of Practical Oncology and Radiotherapy. 2013 May;**18**(3):121-126

[18] Goldman et al. Caring for Someone with Cancer. Sydney: Cancer Council Australia; 2011

[19] Barbour SY. Caring for the treatment-experienced breast cancer patient: The pharmacist's role. American Journal of Health-System Pharmacy. May 2008;**65**(10 Supplement 3): S16-S22. DOI: 10.2146/ajhp080090

[20] Belford L. Caring for your Heart during Breast Cancer Treatment. Toronto: University Health Network; 2016

[21] Komatsu H, Hayashi N, Suzuki K, Yagasaki K, Iioka Y, Neumann J, Ueno NT. Guided Self-Help for Prevention of Depression and Anxiety in Women with Breast Cancer. ISRN Nursing; Vol. 2012. 2012. pp. 9. Artical ID: 716367. http://doi.org/10.5402/2012/716367

[22] Kocan S, Gursoy A. Boy image of women with breast cancer after mastectomy: A qualitative research. Journal of Breast Health. 2016 Oct;**12**(4):145-150

[23] Shapiro SL, Lopez AM, Schwartz GE, Bootzin R, Figueredo AJ, Braden CJ, et al. Quality of life and breast cancer: Relationship to psychosocial variables. Journal of Clinical Psychology. 2001;**57**(4):501-519

[24] Heisey R, Carroll JC. Identification and management of women with a family history of breast cancer. Practical guide for clinicians. Canadian Family Physician. 2016;**62**:799-803 (Eng), e572-7 (Fr)

[25] Cancer Net Editorial Board. Caring for the symptoms of cancer and its treatment. https://www.cancer.net/navigating-cancer-care/how-cancer-treated/palliative-care/caring-symptoms-cancer-and-its-treatment, 10/2016

[26] Crew KD, Greenlee H, Capodice J, Raptis G, Brafman L, Fuentes D, et al. Prevalence of joint symptoms in postmenopausal women taking aromatase inhibitors for early-stage breast cancer. Journal of Clinical Oncology. 2007 Sep 1;**25**(25):3877-3883

[27] Pan H et al. 20-year risks of breast-cancer recurrence after stopping endocrine therapy at 5 years. New England Journal of Medicine. 2017;**377**:1836-1846. DOI: 10.1056?NEJMoa1701830

[28] Sisler J, Chaput G, Sussman J, Ozokwelu E. Follow-up after treatment for breast cancer: Practical guide to survivorship care for family physicians. Canadian Family Physician. 2016;**2016**(62):805-811

[29] Rojas MP, Telaro E, Russo A, Moschetti I, Coe L, Fossati R, et al. Follow-up strategies for women treated for early breast cancer. Cochrane Database of Systematic Reviews. 2005;**1**:CD001768

[30] Harris SR, Schmitz KH, Campbell KL, McNeely ML. Clinical practice guidelines for breast cancer rehabilitation: Syntheses of guideline recommendations and qualitative appraisals. Cancer. 2012;**23**:12-24

[31] Grunfiled E. It takes a team. CanIMPACT. Canadian team to improve community-based cancer care along the continuum. Canadian Family Physician. October 2016;**62**(10):781-782

[32] Anggorowati, Susilowati D, Zubaidah. Hormonal images nursing mothers breast cancer risk in Semarang. Bangladesh Journal of Medical Science. 2017;**3**:413-417

10

Endocrine and Cell Surface Receptor Signaling in Breast Carcinogenesis

Ibrahim O. Alanazi and Zahid Khan

Abstract

Breast cancer is the most commonly diagnosed cancer and the leading cause of cancer-related death in female. To better understand the growth and progression as well as therapeutic management, breast cancers are grouped based on histopathological and molecular classification. A number of factors have been implicated in the development of breast cancer. Various cell surface as well as hormone receptor signaling play crucial role in breast cancer initiation and progression. This chapter briefly discusses few of the important receptor signaling pathways and the various strategies in practice as well as at different stages of development to target these pathways.

Keywords: breast cancer, estrogen receptor, HER1, HER2, tyrosine kinase inhibitors, WNT signaling, therapeutic monoclonal antibodies

1. Introduction

Cancer is considered to be the leading cause of death in developed countries and the second in developing countries. The burden of cancer is growing in economically developing countries due to population aging and adaption of cancer-associated lifestyle including smoking and Western diet. In 2008, it has been estimated that around 12.7 million cancer cases and 7.6 million cancer deaths have happened. Of these about 56% of the cases and 64% of the deaths have been recorded in the economically developing countries [1].

Breast cancer in female is the most common diagnosed cancers and the leading cause of cancer-related death in developed and developing countries. It accounted for 1.38 million new cancer cases (23%) and 458,400 (14%) of the total cancer deaths in 2008 worldwide. Of these, about 50% of the cases of breast cancer and 60% of breast cancer deaths takes place in developing countries including Western and Northern Europe, North America, Australia and New Zealand [2]. In the United States, in 2008, the American Cancer Society (ACS) estimates that almost 182,500 women were diagnosed with breast cancer and during the year about 40,500 women lost their life due to breast cancer.

The breast is made up of different types of tissues including fatty, lymphatic and connective tissue. A female breast is organized into 15–20 sections called lobes. Each of these lobes contains many smaller glandular structures called lobules which responsible for milk production. The lobes and lobules are connected through a network of tubes called ducts through which milk flows and reaches the nipple [3].

Majority of breast cancers arise from the cells in the duct or from milk-producing cells in the lobules. Increase in the incidence of breast cancer observed in epidemiological studies is as a result of breast cancer risk factors. About 20–30% of diagnosed cancer cases may be associated with these factors and their activity that lead to deregulation of the normal cellular processes into neoplastic transformation of breast cells [4]. However, about 75–80% of women with breast cancer have no identifiable risk factor [4]. Therefore, different system or model is required to be utilized to examine this cancer.

2. Risk factors of breast cancer

Being a women and getting older are the main influence to have breast cancer. It has been reported that women with age 30has a lower chance (about 1 in 1500) of developing breast cancer compared to women with age 40 (about 1 in 173) [5]. Thus, being 40 years of age or above poses significant risk for developing breast malignancy. There are several other factors that play crucial role in developing breast cancer, such as history of cancer in first-degree relatives, history of mammary gland diseases, early menarche, late menopause, Caucasian race, and late childbearing after 35 years of age. Causes of breast cancer development have also been linked to lifestyle-related factors including alcohol consumption, not being physically active, being overweight or obese and using hormone replacement therapy. Risk of having breast cancer may result from combination for these factors as reviewed by Singletary [6] as can be seen in **Table 1**.

Breast cancer classification systems have been utilized in order to organize the heterogeneity of this disease. Over many decades, these systems have been developed in order to assist in prognosis and treatment. The breast cancer classification models evolved due to advances in cancer research and understanding of the molecular heterogeneity of breast cancers. These classifications are based on histological and molecular variations in breast cancer subtypes [7]. Such classifications assist in understanding the growth and progression of breast cancer as well as in their therapeutic management.

Risk factor	Category at risk	Comparison category	Relative risk
Alcohol intake	2 drinks per day	Non-drinker	1.2
Body mass index	80th percentile, age 55 or greater	20th percentile	1.2
Hormone replacement therapy with estrogen and progesterone23	Current user for at least 5 years	Never used	1.3
Radiation exposure	Repeated fluoroscopy	No exposure	1.6
	Radiation therapy for Hodgkin's disease	No exposure	5.2
Early menarche	Younger than 12 years	Older than 15 years	1.3
Late menopause	Older than 55 years	Younger than 45	1.2–1.5
Age at first childbirth	Nulliparous or first child after 30	First child before 20	1.7–1.9
Current age	65 or older	Less than 65	5.8
Past history of breast cancer	Invasive breast carcinoma	No history of invasive breast carcinoma	6.8
Other histologic findings	Lobular carcinoma in situ	No abnormality detected	16.4
	Ductal carcinoma in situ	No abnormality detected	17.3
Breast biopsy	Hyperplasia without atypia*	No hyperplasia	1.9
	Hyperplasia with atypia	No hyperplasia	5.3
	Hyperplasia with atypia and positive family history	No hyperplasia, negative family history	11
Cytology (fine-needle aspiration, nipple aspiration fluid)	Proliferation without atypia*	No abnormality detected	2.5
	Proliferation with atypia	No abnormality detected	4.9–5
	Proliferation with atypia and positive family history	No abnormality detected	18.1
Family history	1st-degree relative 50 years or older with postmenopausal breast cancer	No 1st- or 2nd-degree relative with breast cancer	1.8
	1st-degree relative with premenopausal breast cancer	No 1st- or 2nd-degree relative with breast cancer	3.3
	2nd-degree relative with breast cancer	No 1st- or 2nd-degree relative with breast cancer	1.5
	Two 1st-degree relatives with breast cancer	No 1st- or 2nd-degree relative with breast cancer	3.6
Germline mutation	Heterozygous for BRCA1, age < 40	Not heterozygous for BRCA1, age < 40	200
	Heterozygous for BRCA1, age 60–69	Not heterozygous for BRAC1, age 60–69	15

*There is controversy over whether pathologic hyperplasia detected in breast biopsy samples is directly equivalent to cytologic hyperplasia detected in samples obtained through FNA or nipple aspiration.

Table 1. Risk factors for breast cancer.

3. Classification of breast cancer

3.1. Histopathological classification

Breast cancer can be broadly classified based on the location and aggressiveness of the disease. Two main classes of breast cancer are in situ carcinoma and invasive (infiltrating) carcinoma. Breast carcinoma in situ can be divided into two types. Ductal carcinoma in situ (DCIS) originates from the cells lining the ducts that transport milk to the nipple while lobular carcinoma in situ (LCIS) occurs in the cells of lobules, the milk-producing glands at the end of breast ducts [3, 7]. Both DCIS and LCIS are premalignant lesions that do not invade deeper or spread through the body. Women with these lesions have higher likelihood of getting cured but also have increased risk of developing invasive breast cancer in the future. DCIS is significantly more common accounting for 80–90%, while LCIS accounts for 10–20% of breast cancer cases [3]. DCIS has been traditionally sub-classified to five well-recognized subtypes as Solid, Papillary, Micropapillary, Cribriform and Comedo based on the architectural features of the tumor [8]. Invasive carcinomas, similar to in situ carcinomas are differentiated into histological subtypes. These subtypes include infiltrating

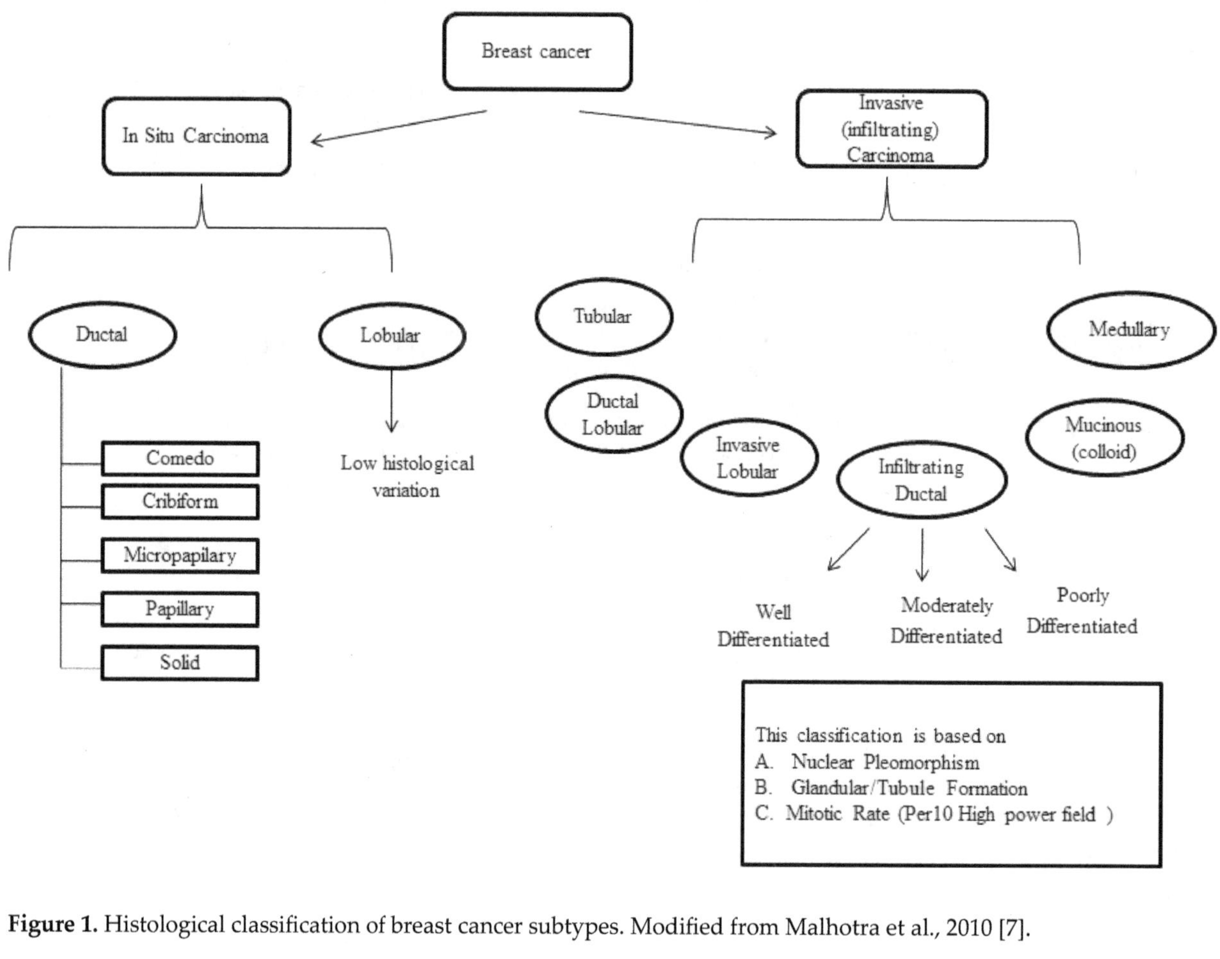

Figure 1. Histological classification of breast cancer subtypes. Modified from Malhotra et al., 2010 [7].

ductal (IDC), invasive lobular (ILC), mucinous (colloid), medullary, tubular and papillary carcinomas (**Figure 1**) [7]. IDC is considered as the most common histological subtype of breast cancer, and it accounts for 70–80% of all invasive lesions [9], while ILC is the second most prevalent and accounts for roughly 10% of all breast cancers. These subtypes differ from each other based on clinicopathologic aspects, natural history, epidemiology and molecular alterations [10].

3.2. Molecular classification

Breast cancer is a heterogeneous disease with diverse histological and molecular variations determining the biological behavior and therapeutic response. The occurrence as well as death due to breast cancer is on the rise globally despite advances in the development of diagnostic techniques and medications. There are many factors including age, family history, receptor status and others that have been investigated to assess patients' risk and treatment selection. It has been proven that receptor status is the most valuable in determining prognosis and responsiveness to therapy [11, 12]. Based on the receptor status, breast cancers are divided into three main groups. The first group includes estrogen receptor (ER) or progesterone receptor (PR) positive, while the second group comprises tumors that tested positive for human epidermal growth factor receptor 2 (HER2) with or without ER and PR positivity. Finally, triple-negative breast cancer (TNBC) is defined by the absence of ER/PR expression and HER2 amplification [11]. Targeted therapy is available for breast cancer patients that express ER, PR or HER2 receptors; however, no standard treatment options are in practice for TNBC patients. Traditional chemotherapeutic regimens are utilized for this type of patients [13].

A number of techniques including immunohistochemistry (IHC), DNA microarray technology, fluorescent in situ hybridization (FISH) are utilized to reveal molecular differences within the same or different histopathological specimens [14–16]. Using IHC and DNA microarrays lead to the identification of five discrete subtypes of breast cancer. These subtypes include luminal A (ER^+ and/or PR^+ and $HER2^-$), luminal B (ER^+ and/or PR^+ and $HER2^+$), HER2 overexpressing (ER^- and PR^-, $HER2^+$), basal-like ($ER^-/PR^-/HER2^-$, cytokeratin $5^+/6^+$ and/or epidermal growth factor receptor $(EGFR)^+$) and normal breast-like. These different breast cancer subtypes are diverse in prognosis and therapeutic management [11]. Microarray classification of breast cancer is represented in **Table 2**. This classification is based on two types of epithelial cells including luminal and basal cells (and/or myoepithelial) in human mammary gland. These cells can be identified using IHC technique as luminal cells express ER and PR receptors and keratins $8^+/18^+$, whereas basal cells are keratins $5^+/6^+$ and 17^+ [17, 18].On the other hand, TNBC can be identified by ER^-, PR^- and $HER2^-$ using IHC range between 0 and 1 or by FISH negative if 2+ on IHC [15].

Various receptors including estrogen receptor (ER) and other growth factor receptor signaling pathways play an important role in breast cancer initiation and progression. Targeting these receptors by specific inhibitors may lead to the inhibition of tumor growth [20].

Subtypes	ER, PgR, Her 2 Status	Other IHC features	Cell of origin	Other characteristics
Luminal A	ER + or PgR + or both, Her 2-	Keratin 8/18 + ve	Luminal epithelial cell	Younger age Best prognosis Low rates of recurrence Higher survival rate
Luminal B	ER + or PgR + or both, Her 2+	Keratin 8/18 + ve	Luminal epithelial cell	Higher tumor grade Poorer prognosis
Basal-like	ER-, PgR-, Her2−/+	Keratin 5/6/17 + ve EGFR + ve	Basal/myoepithelial cell/ Bipotent progenitor	15% Younger age Associated with hereditary BRCA 1 Poorer prognosis compared to other types Spread to axillary nodes, less common to bones
Her 2+	ER-, PgR-, Her2+	–	Late luminal progenitor	20–25% Poorer grade Lymph nodes positive Early distant metastases Poor prognosis Frequent relapse
Normal breast-like	Tumors that do not fill into any of these categories	–	Luminal epithelial cell	6–10% of all breast cancers Small tumors Good prognosis More common in postmenopausal Associated with fibroadenomas
Claudin low	ER-, PR-, Her2-	Mesenchymal markers	Stem cell	5–10% of all tumors Typically triple negative Low expression of cell-cell junction proteins (like E-Cadherin) Lymphocytic infiltrates

IHC, immunohistochemistry; ER, estrogen receptor; PgR, progesterone receptor, +, positive, − negative.

Table 2. Microarray classification of breast cancer [19].

4. Breast cancer receptors (ER, PR and HER2) and their involvement in cancer progression

4.1. Estrogen receptor (ER)

Despite the fact that a large number of potentially valuable factors have been identified, only three receptors, the estrogen receptor-alpha (ERα), the progesterone receptor (PgR), and the HER2 are utilized in clinical practice, and their assessment is obligatory [21]. Approximately 70% of all breast cancers, which belong to the molecular subtypes luminal A or luminal B, express ERα. There is strong evidence demonstrating that estrogen plays an important role in the progression and development of breast cancers, although the causes behind these malignancies still remains uncertain [22]. ER alpha positive breast cancers depend on estrogen signaling for proliferation. Binding of estrogen to ERs leads to dimerization of the receptor which then translocates to the nucleus and binds estrogen response elements in the DNA sequence. This leads to cell proliferation as a result of stimulation of target genes [23]. ERα mediates a number of molecular signaling such as mitogen-activated protein kinase (MAPK) and phosphoinositide 3-kinase (PI3K) pathways which are involved in cell growth and proliferation [24] as can be seen in **Figure 2**.

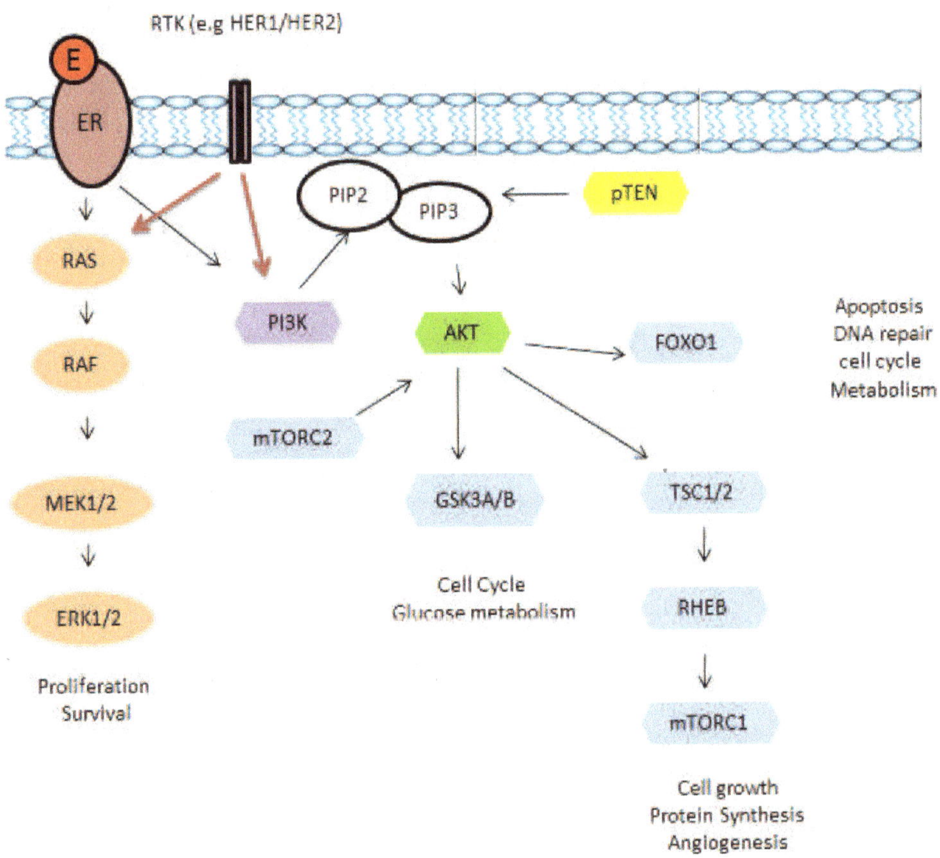

Figure 2. The PI3K/AKT/mTOR and the RAS/RAF/MEK/MAPK pathways. Modified from Toss and Cristofanilli [25].

ERα-positive breast cancer depends on these signaling for proliferation. Therefore, the most effective approach to terminate or slow the growth of this type of cancer is by blocking estrogen action in the tumor using hormone therapies. For the past few decades, one of the most widely used drug for the treatment of breast cancer is tamoxifen, which is a selective ER modulator and acts as anantagonizer for ERα function. It has been utilized as a long-term adjuvant therapy and as preventative agent in a lot of women at increased risk for the disease. Also, fulvestrant, which acts as an anti-estrogen, downregulates ERα and has been approved for clinical use [22].

Another class of breast cancer treatment drugs that have evolved are called aromatase inhibitors (AIs). These inhibitors include anastrozole, letrozole and exemestane as detailed in **Table 3**. AIs are able to inhibit the aromatase enzyme (a cytochrome P450 heme-containing protein), which is required for estrogen synthesis [26] During menopause, the level of estrogen decreases due to cessation of estrogen production by the ovaries. Hence, locally synthesized estrogen via breast adipose tissue plays crucial role in the survival and growth of ERα-positive breast tumors [27].Unfortunately, majority of patients treated with endocrine therapy develop resistance. This leads to the progression of disease and fatality. Several signal transduction pathways such as MAPK and PI3K are involved in tamoxifen resistance. These pathways are activated by growth factors including human epidermal growth factor receptor 2 (HER2). It has been noticed that MCF-7/HER2–18 tamoxifen-resistant model system that overexpress HER2 shows increased growth when cells are treated with tamoxifen. Several studies indicate that there exists a molecular cross-talk between the ER and HER2 pathways [28, 29]. Also, the mechanisms associated with AIs resistance share similarities with tamoxifen resistance, particularly in the upregulation of growth factor pathway such as HER2 and its dimerization partner epidermal growth factor receptor (EGFR/HER1) [30].

Retinoblastoma (RB) is the tumor suppressor protein that plays an important role in regulating the progression of cell cycle. This occurs by the RB inhibitory action on E2Fs which are a family of transcription factors that are crucial for the expression of S-phase genes. It has been noticed that deregulation in the RB pathway occurs in various cancers including breast cancer 2. About 50% of breast cancers overexpress cyclin D1 that lead to an aberrant phosphorylation of RB facilitating cell cycle progression [31]. Adjuvant tamoxifen-treated ER positive breast cancer patients having functional RB pathway have fewer breast cancer recurrences, while those with RB non-functional tumors have no benefit of tamoxifen. Therefore, knowing the RB status in breast cancer can be utilized as predictive factor to identify patients who will benefit from tamoxifen therapy [32]. Further, it has been observed that histone demethylase retinoblastoma-binding protein 2 (RBP2) has a potential to develop endocrine therapy resistance in breast cancer. Choi et al. demonstrated that tamoxifen resistance in vitro and in vivo occurs as a result of RBP2 overexpression, while knocking down RBP2 imparted tamoxifen sensitivity. The cooperation between RBP2 and ER coactivators and corepressors regulates a number of tamoxifen resistance-associated genes. Moreover, RBP2 increased IGF1R-HER2 cross-talk that lead to PI3K-AKT activation through demethylase activity-independent HER2 protein stabilization. Therefore, RBP2-mediated tamoxifen resistance might be overcome using combinational treatment with PI3K inhibitor and tamoxifen. ER-IGF1R-HER2 signaling cascade can be activated in various ways by RBP2 to induce tamoxifen resistance, thus making RBP2

Drug	Target	Indications/trials
Tamoxifen	ER	Treatment of metastatic estrogen receptor positive breast cancer. Adjuvant treatment of node-positive breast cancer in postmenopausal women following total mastectomy or segmental mastectomy. Adjuvant treatment of axillary node-negative breast cancer in women following total mastectomy or segmental mastectomy.
Fulvestrant	ER	Hormone receptor (HR)-positive, human epidermal growth factor receptor 2 (HER2)-negative advanced breast cancer in postmenopausal women who have not been previously treated with endocrine therapy. HR-positive advanced breast cancer in postmenopausal women whose disease has progressed after endocrine therapy HR-positive, HER2-negative advanced breast cancer or breast cancer that has spread to other parts of the body (metastatic), in combination with palbociclib or abemaciclib in women whose disease has progressed after endocrine therapy.
Anastrozole	Aromatase enzyme	Adjuvant treatment (treatment following surgery with or without radiation) of postmenopausal women with hormone receptor positive early breast cancer approved for the initial treatment of postmenopausal women with hormone receptor positive or hormone receptor-unknown locally advanced or metastatic breast cancer and for the treatment of postmenopausal women with advanced breast cancer that has progressed following treatment with tamoxifen.
Letrozole	Aromatase enzyme	Adjuvant treatment of postmenopausal women with estrogen receptor positive early breast cancer.
Exemestane	Aromatase enzyme	Adjuvant treatment of postmenopausal women with estrogen receptor positive early breast cancer who have received 2–3 years of tamoxifen and are switched to exemestane for completion of a total of five consecutive years of adjuvant hormonal therapy.
Trastuzumab	HER2	Treatment of patients with HER2-overexpressing breast cancer.
Pertuzumab	HER2	Used in combination with trastuzumab and chemotherapy as adjuvant treatment of patients with HER2-positive early breast cancer at high risk of recurrence.
T-DM1	HER2	Used for the treatment of patients with metastatic HER2-positive breast cancer.
Cetuximab	HER1	Pre-clinical and clinical studies especially in combination therapy to treat triple-negative breast cancer.
Panitumumab	HER1	Phase II study of Panitumumab, Nab-paclitaxel, and Carboplatin for patients with primary inflammatory breast cancer (IBC) without HER2 overexpression.
Erlotinib	HER1	Phase I study of Erlotinib and Metformin in triple-negative breast cancer. Pre-clinical studies in triple-negative breast cancer.
Lapatinib	HER2/HER1	Treatment of postmenopausal women with hormone receptor positive metastatic breast cancer that overexpresses the HER2 receptor and for whom hormonal therapy is indicated.
Neratinib	HER2/HER1	Adjuvant treatment of adult patients with early stage HER2-overexpressed/amplified breast cancer, to follow adjuvant trastuzumab-based therapy.

Drug	Target	Indications/trials
RO4929097	γ-secretase inhibitor (NOTCH Pathway)	Pre-clinical and early clinical trial.
MRK-003	γ-secretase inhibitor (NOTCH Pathway)	Pre-clinical studies in animal models
MK-0752	γ-secretase inhibitor (NOTCH Pathway)	A pilot study in combination with tamoxifen or letrozole in patients with early stage breast cancer prior to surgery.
PF-03084014	γ-secretase inhibitor (NOTCH Pathway)	Pre-clinical studies and phase 2 trial in patients with advanced triple-negative breast cancer with or without genomic alterations in notch receptors
Salinomycin	LRP6 (Wnt/β-catenin pathway)	Pre-clinical studies in animal models.
OMP-18R5	FZD7 (Wnt/β-catenin pathway)	A phase 1b dose escalation in combination with paclitaxel in patients with locally recurrent or metastatic breast cancer.
OMP-54F28	FZD8 (Wnt/β-catenin pathway)	Phase I study in patients with advanced solid tumors.
OTSA101	FZD10 (Wnt/β-catenin pathway)	Yttrium 90-radiolabeled OTSA101 in phase I trial in patients with relapsed or refractory non-resectable synovial sarcomas

Table 3. Approved and investigational drugs targeting estrogen receptor and other signaling pathway components.

as a potential therapeutic target for ER-driven cancer [33]. Despite these findings the mechanisms of endocrine therapy resistance are poorly understood making it a major challenge in the clinical management of this disease.

4.2. Progesterone receptor (PR)

Human breast cancers rely on estrogen and/or progesterone hormones for growth, and this effect is mediated through ERs and PRs. ER or PR positive tumors represent up to two thirds of invasive breast cancers in women whose age are less than 50 years, while about 80% of tumors in women with age above 50 years are ER positive [34]. ERα regulates the expression of PR. Therefore, the detection of PR normally indicates that the estrogen-ERα pathway is intact and functional. Once PR is expressed, the hormone progesterone activates PR leading to the upregulation of several crucial cellular function such as proliferation contributing to breast cancer growth [21]. One of the most important parameter in breast cancer management is determining the response of tumor to hormone therapy as not all patients benefit from these therapies. Patients with breast cancer overexpressing ERs and PRs are more likely to respond to hormone therapy, while tumors negative for these receptors are unlikely to get benefit from them and respond better to chemotherapy [35]. Hormone therapy provides better quality of living and improves survival. Higher expression level of PR is associated with better hormone therapy response, increased survival rate and longer time for treatment failure. It has been noticed that PR$^+$ is correlated with higher hormone therapy response rate independent of ER despite the fact that the expression levels of ER and PR are correlated. Tumors with ER^+/PR^+ have higher response rate compared to ER^+/PR^-tumors. Thus, the status of PR provides essential information about how tumors will respond to hormone therapies [35].

4.3. Human epidermal growth factor receptor 2 (HER2)

Transmembrane receptor tyrosine kinases family (RTKs) consists of HER1 (epidermal growth factor receptor [EGFR]), HER2, HER3 and HER4. These receptors are involved in regulating a range of cellular processes that controls cell growth, differentiation, survival and migration. HER2 gene overexpression has been reported in 20–30% of patients with breast cancer [16, 36]. HER receptors are located at the plasma membrane and get activated by ligand binding to the extracellular domain. This binding induces the formation of homodimers or heterodimers [36]. While HER2 does not have a known ligand, HER3 is kinase-inactive and thus both these receptors signal by heterodimerization. Dimerization of these receptors leads to the phosphorylation of tyrosine residues within the receptor intracellular tyrosine kinase domain (cytoplasmic domain). These residues work as docking sites for adaptor proteins containing Src homology 2 and phosphotyrosine binding domains (PTB). These proteins activate a large number of signal transduction molecules such as stress-activated protein kinase and signal transducer and activator of transcription (STATs) and protein kinase B (PKB or AKT) and subsequent stimulation of downstream signaling pathways including STAT, PI3K and MAPK pathways. These signaling pathways are able to activate a wide range of cellular responses such as survival, proliferation, cell motility and differentiation [16]. Overexpression of HER2 and HER1 is responsible for poor clinical prognosis including unfavorable response to endocrine therapy in breast cancer patients.

4.4. HER1 and HER2 as therapeutic targets

There are two types of therapeutic strategies that have been utilized against breast cancers overexpressing HER1 and HER2 receptors. The first includes monoclonal antibodies (MAbs) that bind to the extracellular domain of the receptor interfering with the binding of endogenous ligands that activates these receptors. In the second strategy, small molecule inhibitors (tyrosine kinase inhibitors [TKIs]) bind to the tyrosine kinase domain and inhibit its kinase activity and subsequent downstream signaling (**Figure 3** and **Table 3**) [16].

Anti-HER2 antibodies have been successfully utilized in the treatment of various cancers overexpressing HER2 including breast cancer. These antibodies target the extracellular domain of HER2 and prevent receptor activation. Several monoclonal antibodies have been used including trastuzumab and Pertuzumab. They bind to extracellular domain of HER2 in order to suppress its activity by preventing receptor dimerization and subsequent phosphorylation of the tyrosine kinase domain. As a result, the initiation of downstream signaling pathways gets precluded [37].In addition, a number of TKIs such as gefitinib, lapatinib and neratinib that are approved for treatment of breast cancers binds to HER1 and HER2 tyrosine kinase domains and inhibits their downstream signaling pathways [38]. A major clinical challenge in the treatment of HER2-positive breast cancer is due to resistance to the HER2-targeted antibody trastuzumab. Aghazadeh and Yazdanparast indicated that the over-activation of signal

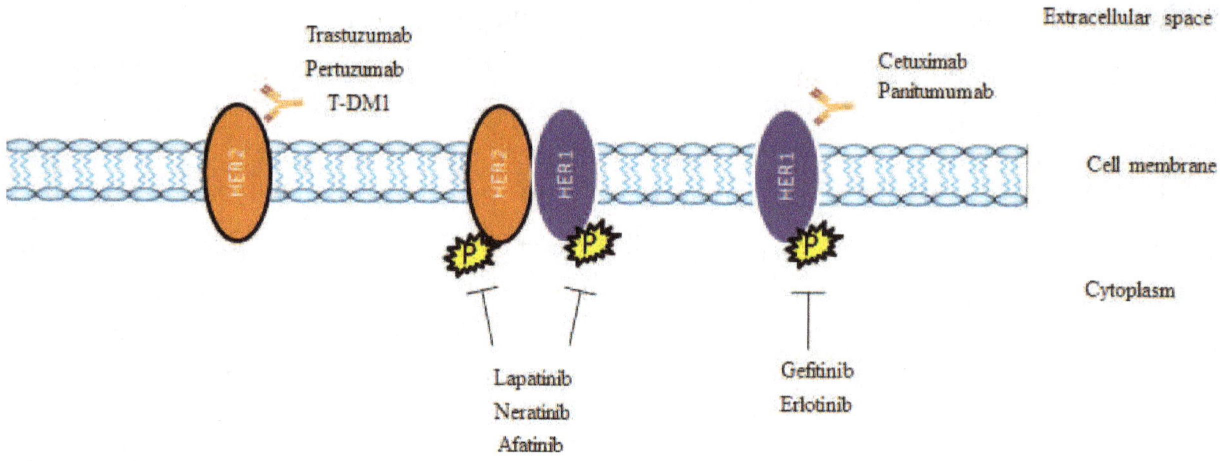

Figure 3. TKIs and MAbs target HERs for the treatment of breast, lung and several other types of cancer. Modified from Alanazi and Khan [16].

transducer and activator of transcription protein 3 (STAT3) has been associated with trastuzumab resistance. This suggests that STAT3 acts as a prognostic indicator of trastuzumab resistance in primary HER2-positive breast cancer [39]. More than 50% of breast cancer patients with aggressive and chemotherapeutic resistant condition have been detected with the phosphorylation of STAT3. Abnormal STAT3 activation due to alterations in HER2, HER1, BRCA1, and ER leads to deregulation of cell proliferation, migration, survival and angiogenesis. Several up-regulated genes including hypoxia inducible factor 1 alpha (HIF-1α) as a result of unexpected STAT3 activation have been implicated in trastuzumab resistance. During their study, Aghazadeh and Yazdanparast found that HIF-1α is an essential signaling element required to downregulate phosphatase and tensin homolog (PTEN) via Hes Family BHLH Transcription Factor 1 (HES-1) repressor during the induction of trastuzumab resistance [39]. Similarly, Sonnenblick et al. provide convincing evidence for a link between phosphorylation of STAT3 and trastuzumab resistance in HER2 positive primary breast cancers. Patients with activated STAT3 may suggest novel approaches to block the STAT3 pathway in combination with trastuzumab treatment particularly in PTEN-deleted breast cancer [40]. Additionally, it has been observed that inhibition of IL6-STAT3 pathway in PTEN-deleted HER2 positive breast cancer leads to decrease in the population of cancer stem cells and inhibits the development of distance metastasis using IL6R antibody alone or in combination with trastuzumab [41].

5. Other receptors involved in breast cancer

5.1. NOTCH signaling pathway

Notch signaling pathway within the breast cancer field attracted a huge number of research scientists over the past decade. It has been observed that Notch signaling is aberrantly activated in breast cancer and affects a number of cellular processes such as apoptosis, proliferation and cancer stem cell activity. The Notch signaling pathway consists of four receptors (Notch1, Notch2, Notch3 and Notch4) and five Delta/Serrate/LAG-2 (DSL) ligands Jagged1,

Jagged2, Delta-like1 (Dll1, Dll3 and Dll4). The activation of Notch signaling pathway occurs by the interaction of DSL ligands with Notch receptors on adjacent cells. This interaction induces a proteolytic cleavage of the Notch protein at the S2 cleavage site mediated by two enzymes, Disintegrin and metalloproteinase domain-containing protein 10 (ADAM10) and Disintegrin and metalloproteinase domain-containing protein 17 (ADAM17). After this cleavage, the remaining part of the Notch protein will be cleaved by the γ-secretase enzyme complex and releases the Notch intracellular domain (NICD). Finally, NICD translocates to the nucleus and forms a complex with DNA-binding protein recombination signal binding protein for immunoglobulin Kappa J region (RBPj) and a member of the mastermind-like (MAML) family transcriptional coactivators (**Figure 4**). This complex activates various target genes of Notch pathway that are associated with tumorigenesis [42], cell growth, differentiation, and cell survival [43].

A number of studies indicate that aberrant activation of Notch signaling has been observed in breast cancer. The high expression of Notch signaling pathway components including Dll1, Dll3 and Dll4, Jagged1–2 and Notch receptors has been observed in invasive breast cancer. This expression is associated with poor prognosis in breast cancer patients [43, 44]. Due to the important role of Notch signaling pathway in breast cancer, it becomes a very attractive therapeutic target. At present, several classes of Notch inhibitors have been developed and are under various clinical trials including γ-secretase inhibitor (GSI), monoclonal antibodies against Notch receptors or ligands and small interfering RNA (siRNA).GSI effectively represses cancer stem cells (CSCs) in *in vitro* studies and triggers apoptosis via inhibiting proteasome activity and enhancing endoplasmic reticulum (ER) stress in tumor cells [45]. Several GSIs have completed pre-clinical and early clinical trials including RO4929097 which significantly sensitizes putative breast cancer stem cells to ionizing radiation and may be effective in treating inflammatory breast cancer (IBC), MRK-003 in combination with trastuzumab induced tumor regression and prevented tumor recurrence post-trastuzumab

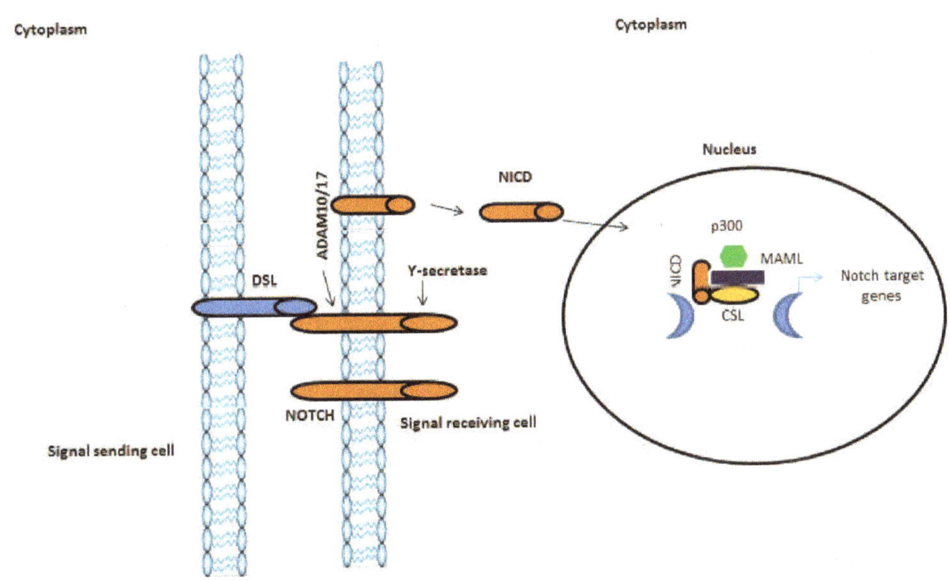

Figure 4. Basics of notch signaling pathway. Modified from Acar et al. [42].

treatment in HER2 positive breast xenografts and partially reverses trastuzumab resistance *in vivo*, MK-0752 reduced breast cancer stem cell subpopulation *in vitro* and in human tissues and PF-03084014 exhibited antitumor and antimetastatic activity in breast xenograft models (**Table 3**) [45].

5.2. The Wnt/β-catenin pathway

The Wnt/β-catenin pathway plays an important role in both normal development and tumorigenesis. The initiation of Wnt/β-catenin pathway occurs via conserved growth factors of the wingless and integration site growth factor (Wnt) family. Nineteen different Wnt genes which share a high level of sequence homology encode Wnts. Binding of Wnts to cell surface receptors lead to the activation of Wnt pathway by triggering signaling cascades that are very crucial in many cellular functions including survival, cell proliferation, specification of cell fate, migration and polarity and self-renewal property of stem cells [46]. Canonical Wnt pathway is also known as β-catenin-dependent Wnt pathway. In the absence of this signaling, β-catenin is maintained at a low level via *ubiquitin/proteasome-mediated degradation*. This can be regulated through protein destruction complex consisting of adenomatous polyposis coli (APC), axin and glycogen synthase kinase-3β (GSK-3β). Binding of Wnt ligand to a seven-pass transmembrane Frizzled (FZD) receptor in combination with its co-receptor, low-density lipoprotein receptor-related protein 6 (LRP6) or its close relative LRP5leads to the activation of Wnt signaling pathway.. The formation of Wnt/FZD/LRP6 complex with the recruitment of the scaffolding protein Disheveled (Dvl) leads to LRP6 phosphorylation and recruitment of the Axin complex to the receptors. As a result, Axin-mediated β-catenin phosphorylation gets inhibited and β-catenin will be stabilized in the cytoplasm. Accumulated β-catenin translocates to the nucleus to form complexes with T cell factor/lymphoid enhancer factor (TCF/LEF) family of proteins and activates target gene expression of Wnt signaling pathway (**Figure 5**) [47].

It has been noticed that aberrant activation of canonical Wnt pathway, which supports the formation and the maintenance of cancer stem cells (CSCs), maintains the pluripotency of the stem cells instead of allowing them to differentiate leading to neoplastic proliferation. Dysregulation in any components of this pathway accelerates tumor growth [46].

Triple-negative breast cancers (TNBC) is considered to be the most difficult subtype to treat due to the lack of effective targeted therapy. It has been observed that Wnt/β-catenin signaling is activated in TNBC patients with the upregulation of its components. The overactivation of this signaling with the upregulation of Wnt receptor expression in TNBC and basal-like breast cancer (BLBC) advocates this signaling pathway might be utilized as therapeutic target for TNBC/BLBC. For instance, salinomycin has been identified as an inhibitor of LRP6 expression and Wnt/β-catenin signaling and also as a selective killer of breast cancer stem cells. Another example is mesoderm development (Mesd), which has been identified as a specialized chaperone for LRP5/6 and acts as an LRP6 antagonist. Several other Wnt pathway inhibitors are in clinical trials such as OMP-18R5, OMP-54F28 and OTSA101 targeting FZD7, FZD8 and FZD10, respectively, as summarized in **Table 3**. Drugs targeting β-catenin

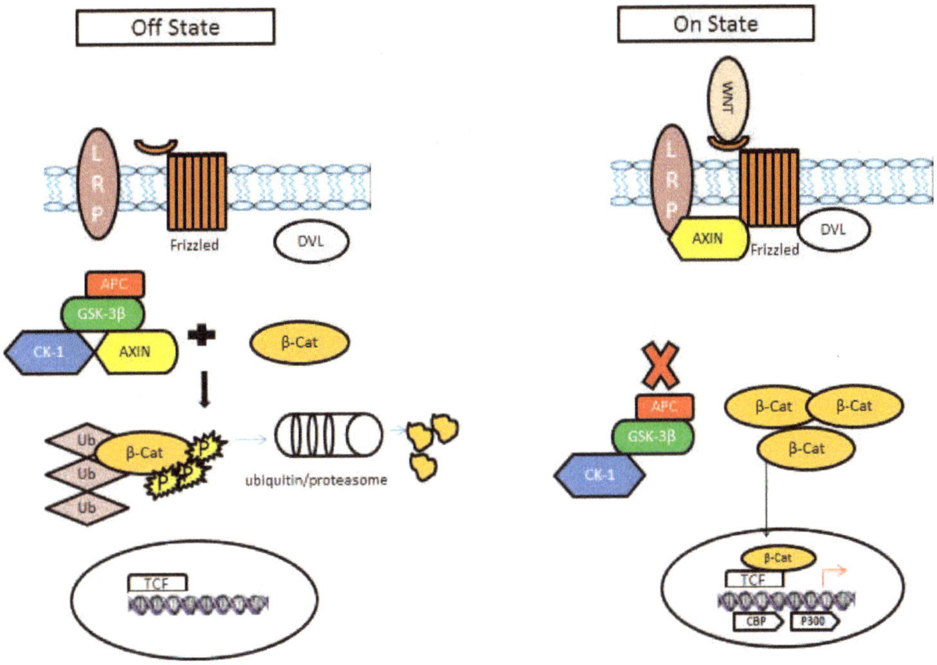

Figure 5. Schematic representation of canonical Wnt signaling pathway. Modified from Kazi et al. [46].

are also being tested [48]. Thus, effective treatment of TNBC by targeting Wnt signaling pathway is highly anticipated and would prove immensely beneficial in conquering this deadly disease.

Acknowledgements

We thank King Abdulaziz City for Science and Technology for their support in this work.

Conflict of interest

The authors declare no conflict of interest.

Abbreviation

APC	adenomatous polyposis coli
ACS	American Cancer Society
AIs	aromatase inhibitors
GSK-3β	axin and glycogen synthase kinase-3β

BLBC	basal-kike breast cancer
CSCs	cancer stem cells
DSL	Delta/Serrate/LAG-2
Dll1	delta-like1
Dvl	Disheveled
DCIS	ductal carcinoma in situ
ER	endoplasmic reticulum
HER2	epidermal growth factor receptor 2
ER	estrogen receptor
FZD	frizzled
IHC	immunohistochemistry
IBC	inflammatory breast cancer
LRP6	lipoprotein receptor-related protein 6
MAML	member of the mastermind-like
ADAM10	metalloproteinase domain-containing protein 10
MAPK	mitogen-activated protein kinase
MAbs	monoclonal antibodies
NICD	notch intracellular domain
PI3K	phosphoinositide 3-kinase
PR	progesterone receptor
PKB Or AKT	protein kinase B
RBPj	recombination signal binding protein for immunoglobulin kappa J region
STATS	signal transducer and activator of transcription
siRNA	small interfering RNA
TKIs	tyrosine kinase inhibitors
TCF/LEF	T cell factor/lymphoid enhancer factor
RTKs	transmembrane receptor tyrosine kinases family
TNBC	triple-negative breast cancer
GSI	γ-secretase inhibitor

Author details

Ibrahim O. Alanazi[1]* and Zahid Khan[2]

*Address all correspondence to: ialenazi@kacst.edu.sa

1 National Center for Biotechnology, King Abdulaziz City for Science and Technology (KACST), Saudi Arabia

2 Genome Research Chair, Department of Biochemistry, College of Science, King Saud University, Riyadh, Kingdom of Saudi Arabia

References

[1] Jemal A et al. Global cancer statistics. CA: A Cancer Journal for Clinicians. 2011;**61**(2):69-90

[2] Jemal A et al. Global patterns of cancer incidence and mortality rates and trends. Cancer Epidemiology, Biomarkers & Prevention. 2010;**19**(8):1893-1907

[3] Sarkar S, Mandal M. Breast cancer: Classification based on molecular etiology influencing prognosis and prediction. Gunduz PM. editor, In: Breast Cancer - Focusing Tumor Microenvironment, Stem cells and Metastasis, 2011. https://www.intechopen.com/books/breast-cancer-focusing-tumor-microenvironment-stem-cells-and-metastasis/breast-cancer-classification-based-on-molecular-etiology-influencing-prognosis-and-prediction

[4] Kaminska M et al. Breast cancer risk factors. Prz Menopauzalny. 2015;**14**(3):196-202

[5] Anders CK et al. Breast cancer before age 40 years. Seminars in Oncology. 2009;**36**(3): 237-249

[6] Singletary SE. Rating the risk factors for breast cancer. Annals of Surgery. 2003;**237**(4): 474-482

[7] Malhotra GK et al. Histological, molecular and functional subtypes of breast cancers. Cancer Biology & Therapy. 2010;**10**(10):955-960

[8] Recommendations for the reporting of breast carcinoma. Association of Directors of Anatomic and Surgical Pathology. American Journal of Clinical Pathology. 1995;**104**(6): 614-619

[9] Lester SC et al. Protocol for the examination of specimens from patients with invasive carcinoma of the breast. Archives of Pathology & Laboratory Medicine. 2009;**133**(10): 1515-1538

[10] Barroso-Sousa R, Metzger-Filho O. Differences between invasive lobular and invasive ductal carcinoma of the breast: Results and therapeutic implications. Therapeutic Advances in Medical Oncology. 2016;**8**(4):261-266

[11] Kumar P, Aggarwal R. An overview of triple-negative breast cancer. Archives of Gynecology and Obstetrics. 2016;**293**(2):247-269

[12] Barnard ME, Boeke CE, Tamimi RM. Established breast cancer risk factors and risk of intrinsic tumor subtypes. Biochimica et Biophysica Acta. 2015;**1856**(1):73-85

[13] Hon JDC et al. Breast cancer molecular subtypes: From TNBC to QNBC. American Journal of Cancer Research. 2016;**6**(9):1864-1872

[14] Nielsen TO et al. Immunohistochemical and clinical characterization of the basal-like subtype of invasive breast carcinoma. Clinical Cancer Research. 2004;**10**(16):5367-5374

[15] Sotiriou C, Pusztai L. Gene-expression signatures in breast cancer. The New England Journal of Medicine. 2009;**360**(8):790-800

[16] Alanazi IO, Khan Z. Understanding EGFR signaling in breast cancer and breast cancer stem cells: Overexpression and therapeutic implications. Asian Pacific Journal of Cancer Prevention. 2016;**17**(2):445-453

[17] Rakha EA et al. Morphological and immunophenotypic analysis of breast carcinomas with basal and myoepithelial differentiation. The Journal of Pathology. 2006;**208**(4):495-506

[18] van de Rijn M et al. Expression of cytokeratins 17 and 5 identifies a group of breast carcinomas with poor clinical outcome. The American Journal of Pathology. 2002;**161**(6):1991-1996

[19] Krishnamurthy S et al. Triple negative breast cancer - our experience and review. Indian Journal of Surgical Oncology. 2012;**3**(1):12-16

[20] Osborne CK et al. Crosstalk between estrogen receptor and growth factor receptor pathways as a cause for endocrine therapy resistance in breast cancer. Clinical Cancer Research. 2005;**11**(2 Pt 2):865s-870s

[21] Allred DC. Issues and updates: Evaluating estrogen receptor-alpha, progesterone receptor, and HER2 in breast cancer. Modern Pathology. 2010;**23**(Suppl 2):S52-S59

[22] Hayes EL, Lewis-Wambi JS. Mechanisms of endocrine resistance in breast cancer: An overview of the proposed roles of noncoding RNA. Breast Cancer Research : BCR. 2015;**17**:40

[23] Hall JM, Couse JF, Korach KS. The multifaceted mechanisms of estradiol and estrogen receptor signaling. The Journal of Biological Chemistry. 2001;**276**(40):36869-36872

[24] Levin ER. Integration of the extranuclear and nuclear actions of estrogen. Molecular Endocrinology (Baltimore, Md.). 2005;**19**(8): pp. 1951-1959

[25] Toss A, Cristofanilli M. Molecular characterization and targeted therapeutic approaches in breast cancer. Breast Cancer Research. 2015;**17**:60

[26] Simpson ER et al. Aromatase cytochrome P450, the enzyme responsible for estrogen biosynthesis. Endocrine Reviews. 1994;**15**(3):342-355

[27] Simpson ER. Sources of estrogen and their importance. The Journal of Steroid Biochemistry and Molecular Biology. 2003;**86**(3-5):225-230

[28] Shou J et al. Mechanisms of tamoxifen resistance: Increased estrogen receptor-HER2/neu cross-talk in ER/HER2-positive breast cancer. Journal of the National Cancer Institute. 2004;**96**(12):926-935

[29] Schettini F et al. Hormone receptor/human epidermal growth factor receptor 2-positive breast cancer: Where we are now and where we are going. Cancer Treatment Reviews. 2016;**46**:20-26

[30] Gilani RA et al. The importance of HER2 signaling in the tumor-initiating cell population in aromatase inhibitor-resistant breast cancer. Breast Cancer Research and Treatment. 2012;**135**(3):681-692

[31] Bosco EE, Knudsen ES. RB in breast cancer: At the crossroads of tumorigenesis and treatment. Cell Cycle. 2007;**6**(6):667-671

[32] Lehn S et al. A non-functional retinoblastoma tumor suppressor (RB) pathway in premenopausal breast cancer is associated with resistance to tamoxifen. Cell Cycle. 2011;**10**(6):956-962

[33] Choi HJ et al. Role of RBP2-induced ER and IGF1R-ErbB signaling in Tamoxifen resistance in breast cancer. Journal of the National Cancer Institute. 2018;**110**(4). DOI: 10.1093/jnci/djx207

[34] Anderson WF et al. Estrogen receptor breast cancer phenotypes in the surveillance, epidemiology, and end results database. Breast Cancer Research and Treatment. 2002;**76**(1):27-36

[35] Sari E, Yalcin S. Clinical aspects of estrogen and progesterone receptors and ERBB2 testing. Aydiner A, İğci A, Soran A, Editors. In: Breast Disease: Diagnosis and Pathology. Cham: Springer International Publishing; 2016. p. 161-185

[36] Spector NL, Blackwell KL. Understanding the mechanisms behind Trastuzumab therapy for human epidermal growth factor receptor 2–positive breast cancer. Journal of Clinical Oncology. 2009;**27**(34):5838-5847

[37] Iqbal N, Iqbal N. Human epidermal growth factor receptor 2 (HER2) in cancers: Overexpression and therapeutic implications. Mol Biol Int. 2014;**2014**:852748

[38] Segovia-Mendoza M et al. Efficacy and mechanism of action of the tyrosine kinase inhibitors gefitinib, lapatinib and neratinib in the treatment of HER2-positive breast cancer: Preclinical and clinical evidence. American Journal of Cancer Research. 2015;**5**(9):2531-2561

[39] Aghazadeh S, Yazdanparast R. Activation of STAT3/HIF-1alpha/Hes-1 axis promotes trastuzumab resistance in HER2-overexpressing breast cancer cells via down-regulation of PTEN. Biochimica et Biophysica Acta. 2017;**1861**(8):1970-1980

[40] Sonnenblick A et al. Constitutive phosphorylated STAT3-associated gene signature is predictive for trastuzumab resistance in primary HER2-positive breast cancer. BMC Medicine. 2015;**13**:177

[41] Korkaya H et al. Activation of an IL6 Inflammatory Loop Mediates Trastuzumab Resistance in HER2+ breast cancer by expanding the cancer stem cell population. Molecular Cell. 2012;**47**(4):570-584

[42] Acar A et al. A role for notch signalling in breast cancer and endocrine resistance. Stem Cells International. 2016;**2016**:2498764

[43] Reedijk M et al. High-level coexpression of JAG1 and NOTCH1 is observed in human breast cancer and is associated with poor overall survival. Cancer Research. 2005;**65**(18):8530-8537

[44] Mittal S et al. Cooperation of notch and Ras/MAPK signaling pathways in human breast carcinogenesis. Molecular Cancer. 2009;**8**(1):128

[45] Yuan X et al. Notch signaling: An emerging therapeutic target for cancer treatment. Cancer Letters. 2015;**369**(1):20-27

[46] Kazi M et al. The potential of Wnt signaling pathway in cancer: A focus on breast cancer. Cancer Translational Medicine. 2016;**2**(2):55-60

[47] MacDonald BT, Tamai K, He X. Wnt/β-catenin signaling: Components, mechanisms, and diseases. Developmental Cell. 2009;**17**(1):9-26

[48] King TD, Suto MJ, Li Y. The wnt/β-catenin signaling pathway: A potential therapeutic target in the treatment of triple negative breast cancer. Journal of Cellular Biochemistry. 2012;**113**(1):13-18

11

Breast Cancer and Flavonoids as Treatment Strategy

Pinar Obakan-Yerlikaya, Elif Damla Arisan,

Ajda Coker-Gurkan and Narcin Palavan-Unsal

Abstract

Breast cancer is the most prevalent cancer type among women. Despite recent progress in early detection and therapeutic strategies, the rate of mortality is increasing. Anti-estrogens or aromatase inhibitors are preferred to treat the women diagnosed with estrogen-receptor (ER) positive tumors. However, breast tumors usually show intra-tumoral heterogeneity with ER-positive and -negative cells. The advanced breast cancer cells lose the estrogen responsiveness and become aggressive by developing new strategies for rapid proliferation such as mutations in cell cycle machinery. New promising drugs are still being investigating against these types of tumors especially to overcome acquired resistance against chemotherapeutic drugs; however, a successful treatment for metastatic tumors is still unclear. Flavonoids, with various pharmacological activities, are plant or fungus secondary metabolites present in human diet. In plants, beside their role in pigmentation, they may also act as messengers, regulators and cell cycle inhibitors. Therefore, they are being tested in ovarian, cervical as well as breast cancer. Due to the positive correlation between flavonoids-rich diet and lower risk of cancer, flavonoids are referred as chemopreventive agents. The current chapter emphasizes the therapeutic potential of flavonoids and their synthetic analogues as anti-cancer agents in breast cancer providing new insights into the molecular mechanisms.

Keywords: breast cancer, chemoprevention, flavonoids

1. Introduction

The use of natural and dietary agents for cancer chemoprevention and therapy received attention for their health benefits. As consumption of fruits or vegetables has been associated with a reduced risk of human cancers especially breast cancer [1], dietary flavonoids, found particularly in these alimentary groups with more than 5000 polyphenolic compounds, have been identified as potential cancer-preventive components [2, 3]. Polyphenols can be divided into ten different classes based on their chemical structure [4]. Flavonoids, phenolic acids, stilbenes, and lignans are the most abundant polyphenols in plants. Polyphenols, mainly flavonoids, possess a number of functions including pollination, pollen tube growth, resorption of minerals, and tolerance to abiotic stress [5]. Flavonoids represented greater attention with the decreased incidence of cancer and cardiovascular diseases in Mediterranean population, which was associated with vegetables, fruits, and red wine consumption. Therefore, they have been under investigation for their therapeutic significance in the protection of human health for decades. Flavonoids are one of the common components in the human diet and generally are present as O-glycosides with sugars bound at C3 position [6].

Breast cancer is the leading cause of cancer death among women worldwide. Despite the presence of new promising advances in therapeutics, the breast cancer mortality rate is still increasing. Recent reports suggest that breast cancer prognosis is lower in countries consuming a healthy, plant-based diet [7]. The possible cause to this scenario has been suggested as flavonoids in fruits and vegetables. Epidemiologic investigations showed that flavonoids exhibit important effects on cancer chemoprevention and chemotherapy. They have been shown to interact with different genes and enzymes including those playing role in antiproliferation, cell cycle arrest, apoptosis, angiogenesis, and multidrug resistance. Therefore, this chapter focuses on the chemopreventive and chemotherapeutical roles of flavonoids in the treatment of breast cancer [6].

2. Structure, classification and metabolism in humans

The chemical structure of flavonoids is based on a C15 skeleton with a chromane ring bearing a second aromatic ring B in position 2, 3, or 4 (**Figure 1**).

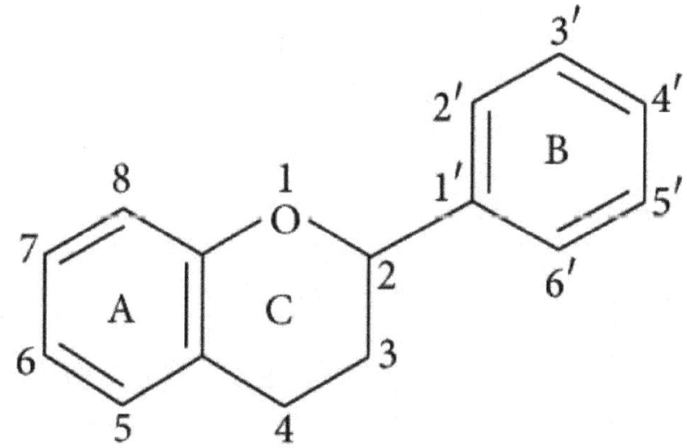

Figure 1. Basic flavonoid structure [8].

Flavonoids are subdivided into different groups based on the nature of C3 element: flavones, flavonols, flavanones, flavanols, anthocyanins, and isoflavones (**Figure 2**).

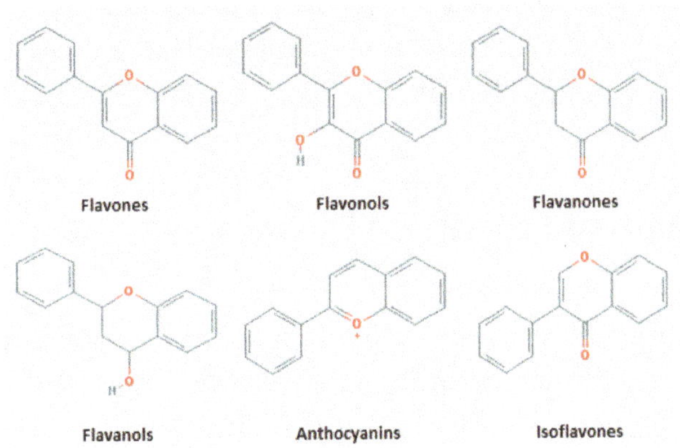

Figure 2. Subclasses of flavonoids (PubChem).

Flavonoids participate light-dependent phase of photosynthesis [9], and they catalyze electron transport. They have been shown to be synthesized from phenylalanine and tyrosine, the aromatic amino acids, with acetates [10]. First, aromatic amino acids are converted to cinnamic acid and parahydroxycinnamic acid, respectively, by phenylalanine and tyrosine ammonia lyase enzymes [11]. Then, parahydroxycinnamic acid accumulates with acetate units to give rise to cinnamoyl, which is the derivative of caffeic acid and chlorogenic acid. Cinnamoyl, then, is converted to ortho-hydroxyacetophenone with a benzaldehyde derivative generating flavonones. If ortho-hydroxyacetophenone condenses with a benzoic acid derivative, flavones are formed. Anthocyanins are naturally occurring glycosides of flavylium (2-phenyl-1-benzopyrylium) ions substituted by hydroxyl and methoxyl groups. Biotransformation of flavonoids occurs in the gut and various secondary metabolites are produced as well such as phenolic acids, lignins, lignans, and stilbenes [11].

Flavonoids, mainly flavanols and quercetin glucosides, are absorbed from the small intestine, while quercetin, quercetin galactoside, and many others are not [12]. Those absorbed by the intestine have been shown to be transported through membrane and use both ATP-dependent pumps and ATP-independent transporters [13]. Following absorption, they are metabolized *via* microbial catabolism and conjugated in the liver and enterocytes [14]. Depending on the subclass, only 5–10% of the amount consumed was shown to be absorbed in the intestine; the rest excreted through the colon where they are further metabolized. The absorbed part in the duodenum is found as methylated, sulfate-conjugated, glucuronide-conjugated, or glycine-conjugated forms [15]. Firstly, in 1992, Hertog et al. measured the content of flavonoids in different fruits, vegetables, and wine. Their findings indicated that mostly quercetin, kaempferol, myricetin, apigenin, and luteolin are found as flavonoid subclasses in the diet. They also suggested that the mean daily intake of flavonoids was higher than the antioxidants β-carotene, vitamin E, and vitamin C [16]. However, the measurement of daily flavonoid intake is difficult to estimate since a standardized method is lacking [17]. Flavonoids, except catechins, exist in nature as glycosides. Following flavonoid intake, the glucosides are cleaved and glucuronated. Glucuronides can be metabolized, released, or stored as aglycones by glucuronidases in a tissue-specific manner [18]. Although the glycosylation of flavonoids has been suggested important for their absorption, the non-glycosylated form of catechin intake has been shown relatively efficient [19]. Flavonoids, especially flavanols, flavonols, and anthocyanins, are relatively abundant in human diet and are shown to play role in cancer, cardiovascular, and neurodegenerative disease disorder prevention [20].

3. Flavonoid-rich food and medicinal plants

The plant extracts have been used as folk remedies against various health problems, including metabolic diseases, cancer, and neurodegenerative disorders. According to in vitro and in vivo studies, a number of plant species have antiproliferative and antitumoral role in breast cancer pathogenesis. In addition, plants which have higher amount of flavonoids are accepted as chemopreventive agents. According to the United States Department of Agriculture (USDA) database, the six subclasses of flavonoids are listed for 506 food items. According to the database, flavonols (quercetin, kaempferol, myricetin, isorhamnetin), flavones (luteolin, apigenin), flavanones (hesperetin, naringenin, eriodictyol), flavan-3-ols ((+)-catechin, (+)-gallocatechin (GC), (−)-epicatechin (EC), (−)-epigallocatechin (EGC), (−)-epicatechin 3-gallate, (−)-epigallocatechin 3-gallate, theaflavin, theaflavin 3-gallate, theaflavin 3′-gallate, theaflavin 3,3′ digallate, thearubigins), anthocyanidins (cyanidin, delphinidin, malvidin, pelargonidin, peonidin, petunidin), and isoflavones (genistein, daidzein, glycitein) are listed.

Generally, these dietary compounds are known with their antioxidant, anti-inflammatory, and anticarcinogenic effects. According to the Seven Countries Study report, the average consumption of quercetin, kaempferol, myricetin, luteolin, and apigenin in composite food samples have ranged from 6 mg/day in Finland to 64 mg/day in Japan, with intermediate intakes in the United States (13 mg/day), Italy (27 mg/day), and the Netherlands (33 mg/day). In a similar study report, average flavonoid intake in Hungarian population was lower compared to Dutch, Danish, and Finnish citizens. The intake of five flavonoids in 17 different diets was estimated. When diet types were compared to each other according to flavonoid consumption ratio, it was shown that South African diet is the lowest flavonoid consumed diet type as 1–9 mg/day consumption. In contrary, Scandinavian diet in correlation with population-based study outcomes was the higher flavonoid intake diet type (75–81 mg/day).

In addition dietary origin of the flavonoids varied between countries. While tea is the main dietary source of flavanoids in Japan by 95% and the Netherlands by 64%, alcoholic beverages such as famous resveratrol based popularity of red wine and beer in Italy by 46%. The vegetables and fruits are the most common dietary sources of Scandinavian countries such as Finland by 100%. Similar ratio was also observed in the United States by 80%. In Australia, tea is the major source of flavonoid, and flavan-3-ols are 75% of whole intake. Therefore, it is important to evaluate the chemopreventive and chemotherapeutic potential of flavonoids in breast cancer disease.

In this section, it is aimed to discuss potential molecular mechanism of above-listed flavanoids in breast cancer studies.

3.1. Flavanols

3.1.1. *Quercetin*

Quercetin is a natural dietary flavonoid which exerts antioxidant, anti-inflammatory and anticancer properties. Quercetin is found in barks of many plants, fruits, and vegetables. It is one of the well-established grape polyphenols like other members, resveratrol, naringenin, and catechin, can exert antitumoral, antioxidant, anti-angiogenic properties and modify selectively estrogen-receptor (ER). According to a recent study, it is found that quercetin at IC50 value (37 μM) modulated Twist and p38 MAPK signaling, which lead to apoptosis in MCF-7 and MDA-MB-231 breast cancer cells [21]. In addition it is well documented that quercetin exerts its therapeutic effect through modulating different cellular targets. According to the previous study, it was shown that quercetin induced p21 CDK inhibitor with a concomitant decrease of phosphorylation of retinoblastoma (Rb), which inhibits the G1/S cell cycle progression by trapping E2F1. A low dose of quercetin induced mild DNA damage and Chk2 activation, which is the main regulator of p21 expression by quercetin. In addition, quercetin downregulated the cyclin B1 and CDK1, essential components of G2/M cell cycle progression. Inhibition of the recruitment of key transcription factor NF-Y to cyclin B1 gene promoter by quercetin led to transcriptional inhibition SKBR3, MDA-MB-453, and MDA-MB-231 cells [22, 23].

Similar to previous findings, MCF-7 breast cancer cells were exposed to the increasing concentrations of quercetin; consequently, cell viability ratios were decreased, and apoptosis was triggered. Following exposure of cells to moderate cytotoxic dose of quercetin for 48 h, cells undergo apoptosis due to activation of caspases. In addition, quercetin mediates the disruption of Bcl-2/Bax ratio in MCF-7 cells [24].

3.1.2. *Kaempferol*

A dietary flavonoid, kaempferol (3,5,7-trihydroxy-2-(4-hydroxyphenyl)-4H-1-benzopyran-4-one), is found in edible plants such as kale, beans, endive, tea, broccoli, cabbage, tomato, and grapes, is commonly used in traditional medicine (e.g., *Ginkgo biloba*, *Tilia* spp., *Equisetum* spp., *Moringa oleifera*, *Sophora japonica*, and propolis) has been reported as antimicrobial, anticancer, antioxidant, neuroprotective, cardioprotective, and antiallergic activity [25]. Kaempferol leads to anti-angiogenic effect via reducing vascular endothelial growth factor (VEGF) expression in ovarian cancer cells [26]. Moreover, it enhanced the effect of cisplatin in ovarian cancer and induced cell cycle arrest and apoptosis by modulating Bcl-2-Bax expression. In vitro studies about kaempferol on breast cancer cases, time-dependent exposure of cells to flavonoid (50 μM) induced G2/M arrest *via* inhibiting CDK1; cyclin A, and cyclin B and induced apoptosis by p53 phosphorylation in MDA-MB-453 breast cancer cell [27]. Although kaempferol treatment significantly induced cell viability loss in MCF-7 cells, no significant effect has been reported in MDA-MB-231 breast cancer cells or HC-11 mammary epithelial cells. Kaempferol-induced ERK activated apoptotic cell death and reactive oxygen species (ROS) generation and N-acetyl cysteine (NAC) co-treatment prevented kaempferol-mediated poly (ADP-ribose) polymerase (PARP) cleavage in MCF-7 breast cancer cells [28]. Kaempferol could be extracted from *Murraya koenigii* leaf, which was reported to induce caspase-3-dependent apoptotic cell death and inhibited endogenous 26S proteasomal enzyme activity in MDA-MB-231 breast cancer cells. Moreover, dose-dependent kaempferol treatment reduced the tumor growth through inhibiting the expression of angiogenic and antiapoptotic genes in breast cancer xenografts [29]. In vivo breast cancer xenograft mice models, kaempferol-mediated anticancer effect reported *via* downregulation of IRS-1, pAkt, pMEK1/2, and ERK gene expression and decreased the tumor growth and volume. In addition, kaempferol treatment prevents breast cancer invasion and metastasis in MDA-MB-231 breast cancer cells due to reduction in MMP-2 and MMP-9 expressions, suppression of transcription factor activator protein-1 (AP-1) and MAPK signaling [30]. Lymphangiogenesis, a new lymphatic vessels formation process, is a major step in spreading of tumor cells. Lymphangiogenesis inhibitors might be focused as an important drug target strategy in breast cancer cells. A VEGFR2/3 kinase inhibitor, kaempferol, inhibited mammalian lymphangiogenesis in metastatic breast cancer xenograft models [31].

3.1.3. Myricetin

The use of plant derivatives, which exert biological functions, has gained importance in recent years. Myricetin (3,5,7,3′,4′,5′-hexahydroxyflavone cannabiscetin) is a natural flavonol, which has a unique hydrophobic chemical structure found in different varieties of fruits, vegetables, tea, berries, etc. [32]. The dietary intake of myricetin from our foods is about 0.98–1.1 mg per day, which is quite higher than some other flavonols [33]. Recent studies showed that myricetin is an antioxidant and it possesses cytoprotective, anticarcinogenic, antiviral, and antimicrobial effects [34].

3.1.4. Isorhamnetin

Isorhamnetin is one of the important flavanols found in *G. biloba* leaf extracts. Isorhamnetin is also found in parsley, and thereby it is a common dietary flavonoid as the metabolite of quercetin. Generally, it is well known as antagonist of peroxisome proliferator-activated receptor γ (PPARγ), which inhibits adipocyte differentiation induced by the PPARγ agonist rosiglitazone [35]. Isorhamnetin is a naturally occurring compound in fruits and vegetables; recent study showed that isorhamnetin could significantly inhibit the invasion of MDA-MB-231 cells by downregulating matrix metalloproteinases (MMP-2 and MMP-9) through inhibiting p38 MAPK and STAT3 [36]. Similar results were also obtained in another study, which showed that isorhamnetin inhibited cell proliferation and led to apoptosis. In addition, isorhamnetin was found effective on Akt/mTOR/MAPKs signaling axis. It was established that isorhamnetin-induced autophagy can be reversed by the co-treatment of 3-methyl-adenine in lung cancer cells. The results indicated that isorhamnetin exerts antitumor effect in breast cancer through targeting multiple molecular targets [37].

3.1.5. Silymarin

In recent years, chemopreventive potential of fruits, vegetables, and medicinal herbs such as tea due to ingredients rich in phytochemicals that act as an antioxidant become an important agent. One of the polyphenolic flavonoids silymarin that is isolated from milk thistle (*Silybum marianum* (L.) *Gaertn*) has been shown for its antioxidant action against liver toxicity [38]. Recently, studies reported the anticarcinogenic effect of silymarin in several mouse skin tumorigenic samples and cervical, prostate, liver, and breast cancers. The molecular machinery of silymarin was more frequently shown in the treatment of human umbilical vein endothelial cells (HUVECs), and downregulation of survivin, Akt, and nuclear factor (NF)-κB was observed [39]. Beside cell growth and proliferation inhibition, silymarin was demonstrated as an inhibitor of MMPs and *in vitro* angiogenesis. Silymarin induced liver cancer prevention due to membrane stabilizing antioxidant effect through acting on tumor necrosis factor alpha (TNF-α) expression in hepatocellular carcinoma cells [40]. Moreover, VEGF secretion suppression instead of normal epithelial cells, in prostate and breast cancer epithelial cells, has also been reported in Ref. [41]. In MCF-7 breast cancer cells, silymarin treatment inhibited cell growth *via* upregulating ERB. However, ER alpha (ERα) downregulation is reported to be an important key player in drug-induced autophagy and apoptosis in MCF-7 breast cancer cells *via* Akt/mTOR/ERK signaling pathway [42].

3.2. Flavanes

3.2.1. Luteolin

Luteolin (3′,4′,5,7-tetrahydroxyflavone) which belongs to flavonoids is a heat-stable and non-toxic compound. It is found in vegetables and fruits such as celery, parsley, broccoli, onion leaves, carrots, peppers, cabbages, apple skins, and mignonette and chrysanthemum flowers. As well as other flavanoids, cardiovascular protection, immune system stimulation, antioxidant, anti-inflammatory, and anticarcinogenesis capacities of luteolin have been shown in previous studies [43]. Luteolin exerts its molecular effect *via* inducing different signaling routes in dose-dependent manner. According to previous studies, it is well documented that lutein is both pro- and antioxidant compound. The pro-oxidant activity of flavonoids may be related to their ability to undergo autoxidation catalyzed by transition metals to produce superoxide anions [44]. Due to structural differences including bioactive phenolic ring, prooxidant status of luteolin may increase the cytotoxicity in cells. Luteolin is important in ER-expressing cells. It was shown that luteolin at low concentrations is an antiestrogenic agent and reduces cell proliferation. In addition, luteolin may inhibit aromatase whose function is to catalyze the production of estrogens [44]. A recent study indicated that luteolin downregulates ER and thus caused the degeneration of ER protein. Because the etiology of breast cancer is strongly correlated with nuclear hormone receptor activity, the consumption of luteolin in diet may reduce risk through regulation of estrogen-induced cellular effects. In vitro and in vivo studies showed that luteolin prevented estrogen-induced cell proliferation. It was shown that luteolin impaired estrogen signaling pathway (ESP) in MCF-7 cells by microarray analysis [45]. Luteolin altered cell cycle regulation signaling targets, including CCNA2, PLK1, PCNA, and CDKN1A. This result was considered as the final consequence of ESP modulation, which suppresses cell proliferation in breast cancer cells. A previous study showed that luteolin (5 μM) could be utilized as a chemosensitizing mechanism to target the expression level of cyclin E2 and to overcome tamoxifen resistance in breast cancer patients. In vivo studies also showed that luteolin may exert its effect *via* modulating miRNA expressions such as miR-34a and miR-181a which bidirectionally reduced notch and suppressed invasion mechanism [46].

3.2.2. Apigenin

Apigenin is known as the phytoestrogen, used in postmenapausal symptom treatment, and presented in various plant species. Although it is a nontoxic and non-mutagenic plant derivative, it exerts antitumoral activity in different types of cancers and induces oxidative stress in breast cancer cells [47]. However, there are contradictory reports showing that apigenin might stimulate cell proliferation in ERα-positive MCF-7 and T47D cells, but not effective in ERα-negative MDA-MB-435 breast cancer cells [48]. The molecular mechanism of apigenin-induced apoptotic cell death was caspase-dependent, mitochondria [49] and NF-κB, STAT signaling-mediated [50]. Moreover, apigenin inhibited cell growth, metastasis, and invasion in breast cancer cells *via* acting on PI3K/Akt signaling and beta 4 integrin in MDA-MB-231 breast cancer cells [51].

3.3. Flavanones

It was shown that flavanone-rich diet mediated 0.1–100 μM physiologically achievable concentration in the plasma. One of the mostly known flavanones is naringenin, which is especially abundant in the Mediterranean diet, rich for consumption of grapes, tomato, and citrus. Naringenin was shown with anticancerous effect in various cancer cells. According to in vitro studies, it was shown that naringenin modulated NF-κB to induce apoptosis in the cells. Naringenin was effective in MCF-7 ERα+/ERβ + cell line, but not in ER-independent SKBR-3 (ERα−/ERβ−) cell line [52–55]. *Thymus vulgaris* ethanol extraction originated in naringenin induced cell cycle arrest at S and G2/M phases, which led to apoptotic induction in HTB26 and HTB132 breast cancer cells [52]. The apoptotic efficiency of naringenin was found due to alteration of different cell cycles and apoptosis-related genes such as cyclin-dependent kinases and Bcl-2 family members. Naringenin may activate T cells to induce antitumoral activity in mice and lead to increased interferon (IFN)-γ and interleukin (IL)-2 expressing T cell population [54, 56]. Naringenin promotes the therapeutic effect of tamoxifen in breast cancer cells [57, 58]. Thus, naringenin might promote the potential therapy outcomes and good prognosis in breast cancer cases.

Similar to naringenin, eriodictyol has promising therapeutic effects in cancer cells. Eriodictyol, a flavanone, activated Nrf2 and induced phase II proteins to exert its antioxidant effects [59, 60]. However, there are less studies to evaluate the molecular mechanism of eriodictyol compared to naringenin.

Hesperetin is also a promising flavanone and induced cell cycle arrest at G1 phase. According to the previous study, hesperetin regulated CDK4 and p21 (Cip1) in MCF-7 cells and led to block of cell cycle. Hesperetin is also known with its apoptotic effect in breast cancer cells without effecting normal mammary epithelial cells. It was shown that hesperetin induced apoptosis in dose- and time-dependent manner in MCF-7 cells through triggering ROS generation. Pretreatment of NAC prevented hesperetin-induced apoptosis, which is under control of ASK1/JNK pathway. In addition, hesperetin also induced apoptosis in triple-negative breast cancer MDA-MB-231 cells *via* intrinsic apoptotic pathway [53, 61–64]. In the light of previous findings, both naringenin and hesperetin are known as promising therapeutic candidates in breast cancer due to their sensitizing effect of HER2-positive breast cancer cells.

3.4. Flavan-3-ols

The most important member of flavan-3-ols (catechins) is abundantly present in green and black tea, red wine and chocolate. Catechins, which are generally found in green tea, comprise epigallocatechin gallate (EGCG), epicatechin (EC), gallocatechin (GC), epigallocatechin (EGC), catechin gallate (CG), epicatechin gallate (ECG), gallocatechin gallate (GCG), and catechin (C). Although green tea is a favorable catechin source, it is required to design more bioavailable structures to treat various cancer types, including breast cancer. The detailed investigation for EGCG was established in different studies. According to xenograft model studies, EGCG with tamoxifen has potential in ER-negative breast cancer models. The MDA-MB-231-mediated tumor volume was decreased following 25 mg/kg treatment of EGCG and/or EGCG + tamoxifen in athymic nude female mice model [65–68]. The potentiation of green tea catechins is generally acted on mTOR and EGFR pathways. Similar to these findings, studies indicated that EGCG produces anticancer effect by modulating the activity of MAPKs, IGF/IGF-1 receptor, Akt, NF-κB, and HIF-1α [69–73]. Although catechins have multiple molecular targets in the cells, it is required to improve their structural properties to achieve powerful treatment results.

3.5. Anthocyanins

Anthocyanins confer the bright red, blue, and purple colors to plants such as berries, grapes, and apples. Anthocyanidins lack the sugar component of the anthocyanin [74]. Six anthocyanidins occurred most commonly in nature are pelargonidin, cyanidin, peonidin, delphinidin, petunidin, and malvidin. It has been suggested that the consumption of cyanidin lowers the risk of cardiovascular disease, diabetes, and cancer due to the antioxidant and anti-inflammatory activities [75]. The phenolic structure is responsible for the antioxidant activity such as the ability to scavenge superoxide ($O_2 \cdot^-$), singlet oxygen ($^1O_2$), peroxide (ROO^-), hydrogen peroxide (H_2O_2), and hydroxyl radical (OH·), members of ROS [76], in in vitro cell lines including colon, liver, and breast cancer cells [77].

3.5.1. *Cyanidin*

The anticancer effect of cyanidin-rich extracts of different plant has been shown in MCF-7 ERα (+), MDA-MB-231 ER α (−), and MDA-MB-453 ER α (−) breast cancer cell lines. Moreover, apoptotic induction in MDA-MB-453 cells through the intrinsic pathway of apoptosis by activating caspase cascade, cleaving poly (ADP-ribose) polymerase (PARP), depolarizing mitochondrial membrane potential, and releasing cytochrome C has been shown [78]. In addition, in the same study, 100 mg/kg/day oral administration of cyanidin has been shown to reduce tumor growth and angiogenesis by affecting the expression of angiogenic factors MMP-9, MMP-2, and cell/extracellular matrix (ECM) interaction in nude mice bearing MDA-MB-453 cell xenografts [78]. Furthermore, inhibition of proliferation and cell cycle arrest were induced in MCF-7 human breast cancer cells after the treatment of bilberry extract, which contains high amount of cyanidin [79]. The same study also compared the effect of cyanidin with a well-known antioxidant Trolox, a vitamin E analog, and showed that cyaniding induced apoptosis and cell cycle arrest as much as Trolox [80]. In another study, pycnogenol, derived from pine bark, which contains high amounts of procyanidins, has been shown to induce cell death in breast cancer cells (derived from human fibrocystic mammary tissue) but not in normal human mammary MCF-10A cells [81].

Human epidermal growth factor receptor 2 (HER2) is overexpressed in 20% cases of breast cancer. Therefore, HER2-targeted therapies have been evaluated in recent years. In Liu et al.'s [82] study, cyanidin-3-glucoside, extracted from black rice, inhibited phospho-HER2 and phospho-AKT and induced apoptosis both in vitro and in vivo HER2-positive breast cancer cells and tissues. Another study also revealed that anthocyanidin-rich extracts from berries and grapes have been shown to exhibit proapoptotic effects in multiple cell types in vitro [83]. They induce apoptosis through both intrinsic (mitochondrial) and extrinsic (FAS) pathways.

3.5.2. Delphinidin

Delphinidin is a member of anthocyanins mainly found in pomegranate extract and found in many dietary supplements as complementary cancer medicine. A recent study showed that delphinidin treatment inhibited cell proliferation and induced apoptosis in ER-positive, triple-negative, and HER2-overexpressing breast cancer cell lines without any toxic effect in normal breast epithelial cells [84]. In addition, the same study also indicated that MAPK signaling was inhibited in both triple-negative and ER-negative breast cancer cells but not in MCF-10A normal epithelial cells.

Breast cancer cells overexpressing p65, the unit of NF-κB responsible from cell survival and proliferation, underwent apoptosis following delphinidin treatment. The possible explanation to this process was shown as the inhibition of phosphatidylinositol 3,4,5-trisphosphate (PI3K)-dependent phosphorylation of AKT in vitro and inhibition of the activation of NF-κB in vivo [85]. The same study also pointed out that miR-27a and miR-155 were able to inhibit PI3K and NF-κB and responsible from the anti-inflammatory and cytotoxic activity of delphinidin in MDA-MB-231 breast cancer cell line [86]. Delphinidin has been also shown to inhibit hepatocyte growth factor (HGF)-mediated tyrosyl phosphorylation of focal adhesion kinase (FAK), Src, paxillin, Gab-1, and GRB-2, which are inducers of cell proliferation upon phosphorylation by growth factor signaling. Delphinidin, in the same study, was found to repress Ras-ERK MAPKs and PI3K/AKT/mTOR/p70S6K pathways [16]. The compound also has anti-angiogenic and anti-invasive properties by decreasing MMP-9 activity in ER+ MCF-7 cells. Im et al. showed that delphinidin inhibited MMP-9 transcription by blocking NF-κB through MAPK signaling pathways [87].

3.5.3. *Pelargonidin*

Pelargonidin, a subclass of anthocyanin with estrogenic activity, was tested in MCF-7 breast cancer cells. The cytotoxic dose (5 μg/ml) of strawberry extract containing pelargonidin-3-O-glucoside caused 50% decrease in cell proliferation [88]. A study performed in breast cancer tissue of rats showed that pelargonidin could inhibit the synthesis of cytochrome c p450 family 1 subfamily A member 1 (CYP1A1) enzyme which converts estradiol into 2-hydroxy-estradiol that can cause DNA damage [89]. The inhibition of the estrogenic activity by 55% was also indicated following pelargonidin containing pomegranate seed oil in ER+ MCF-7 cells. On the other hand, pelargonidin treatment induced apoptosis in both MCF-7 and MDA-MB-231 (ER-). Seventy-five percent inhibition of invasion across a Matrigel was also observed in MCF-7 cells at 10 μg/ml pomegranate seed oil concentration. Studies suggest that further investigations on chemopreventive and therapeutic applications of pelargonidin should be performed against human breast cancer [90].

3.6. Isoflavonoids

3.6.1. *Daidzein*

Daidzein, is one of the isoflavonoid present in various plants and herbs such as soybeans, tofu, kwao krua (*Pueraria mirifica*), kudzu (*Pueraria lobata*), and also isolated from *Maackia amurensis* cultures [91]. Breast tumor growth inhibition by lower concentration of daidzein (10 μM) treatment in *in vitro* and *in vivo* has been reported. Daidzein prevented T47D breast cancer cell proliferation and acted as antiestrogenic agent [92]. Fifty micrometer daidzein concentration decreased the cell viability in MDA-MB-231 and MCF-7 breast cancer cells by 50 and 42%, respectively, for 48 h. Moreover, daidzein inhibited cell migration and invasion in breast cancer cells by using MicroRaman techniques [93]. As a soybean extract, daidzein stabilized proto-oncogene BRF2 mRNA and decreases BRF2 promoter methylation in ERα and ERβ breast cancer cells and female breast cancer mice models [94]. Antiproliferative effect of daidzein on breast cancer cells was reported by acting on TNF-α expression, down-regulating MMP-9 mRNA expression, and suppressing hedgehog signaling through preventing the Gli1 nuclear translocation. In in vivo MCF-7 athymic nude mice breast cancer models, fed daidzein prevented tumor growth through suppressing ATP2A3 and BLNK expression and decreased MYC oncogene expression [95]. However, no significant association between breast cancer risk and plasma equol and/or equol: daidzein concentrations have been reported in the Chinese population [96].

3.6.2. *Genistein*

Soybean is one of the dietary components, which contains phytoestrogens and genistein acting as a chemopreventive agent against various cancer cells such as prostate and breast cancer. As a predominant isoflavone, genistein inhibits growth and proliferation of ER-positive and ER-negative breast cancer cells by inhibiting receptor-associated tyrosine kinase (RTK) signaling [97]. Genistein inhibited cell proliferation, growth, invasion, and metastasis and acted as anticarcinogenic and anti-angiogenic compound on breast cancer in vitro and in vivo models

[98]. The molecular mechanism of anticarcinogenic effect of genistein on breast cancer cells is due to DNA topoisomerase, 5-reductase enzyme inhibition, suppressing the NF-κB, Akt and MAPK signaling pathways [99]. Genistein is one of the flavonoids that has been shown to effect on chronic diseases such as atherosclerosis and hereditary hemorrhagic telangiectasia. The molecular target of genistein was reported to enhance the action of transforming growth factor-β (TGF-β) [77]. Like other plant secondary metabolites (tocopherols, curcumin), flavonoids reported to regulate VEGF in breast tumors in vivo and in vitro studies. The anti-angiogenic, anticarcinogenic effect of genistein target VEGF receptor-2 (VEGFR-2) mediated PI3K/Akt/mTOR signaling pathway [100]. Angiogenesis is the formation of new blood vessels and sprouting of circulation by activation of VEGF family member, VEGF-A, leading to endothelial cell proliferation, migration, and destruction of matrix metalloproteins. Although the anti-angiogenic effect of isoflavonoids has been reported in various studies, the exact molecular inhibition mechanism has not been clarified yet. One of the anti-angiogenic effects of genistein is the inhibition of VEGF and its receptor secretion. Ten to fifty micrometer genistein prevented basal VEFG expression both in breast cancer and human umbilical vein endothelial cells (HUVECs) [101]. Moreover, under hypoxia conditions genistein has been shown to induce both VEGF downregulation and inhibition of hypoxia-inducible factor 1 (HIF-1) activation. The anti-angiogenic effect of genistein has been accelerated with curcumin-combined treatment in HUVEC cells by VEGFR-1 and VEGFR-2 downregulation [102]. According to in vivo experiments such as xenografts, chick chorioallantoic membrane or zebra fish experimental models showed the reduction of microvessel density due to genistein treatment mediated by plasminogen activator inhibitor-1, endostatin, angiostatin, and thrombospondin-1 activation. Pretreatment with genistein leads to the reduction of MMP-2, MMP-3, MMP-13, and MMP-15 mRNA expression and VEGF-mediated plasminogen activator (PA) and PAI1 expression blockage. However, no significant effect has been determined on MMP-2 and MMP-9 activity. Antiproliferative and anti-angiogenic effect of genistein is also shown by inhibition of cadherin, integrin V, connexin 43 mRNA expression, and genistein (40 mmol/L), or daidzein (110 μm/L) treatment suppresses epidermal growth factor (EGF) and insulin-like growth factor (IGF-I) [103]. NF-κB signaling pathway plays an important role in not only angiogenesis but also cell growth apoptosis, inflammation, and invasion. Thus, genistein treatment inhibited MMP-9 by NF-κB nuclear translocation-induced NF-κB signaling inactivation [104]. In addition, genistein induced cell proliferation suppression by acting on MAPKs such as ERK-1/2, c-Jun N-terminal kinases (JNK), and p38 dephosphorylation. In order to clarify the anti-angiogenic effect of flavonoids, genistein, one of the major catalytic enzymes of prostaglandin production [cyclooxygenase-2 COX-2], associated VEGF production was investigated [105]. COX isoenzyme catalyzes the production of prostaglandins, VEGF production, and angiogenesis induction. In MCF-7 breast cancer cells, genistein alone or combined treatment with capsaicin leads anti-angiogenic and anticarcinogenic effect *via* acting on reduced COX-2 expression. According to in vivo studies, in TPA-treated animals, genistein or daidzein suppresses NF-κB and COX-2 activity [77]. During cancer progression, various molecules have been involved in various steps such as cell proliferation, differentiation, migration, and extracellular matrix formation. Moreover, some tumor microenvironment modulators such as immunosuppressive and/or angiogenic-inducing factors play essential roles. One of the key targets during these hypoxic breast tumors is galectin-3 that

is involved by overexpression in cancer niche. Soy compound isoflavonoid genistein chemopreventive effect has been reported due to potential action on galectin-3 expression inhibition in breast cancer. The phytoestrogen genistein, which induced G2/M arrest due to galentin-3 downregulation, has been determined in human breast carcinoma cell lines [106]. As shown in **Figure 3**, analysis of transcriptomic profile of mammary epithelial cells of rat females fed a diet containing the soy isoflavone genistein or soy protein isolate showed that soy consumption is associated with reduced breast cancer risk in women. Results provide insight into the molecular basis of the beneficial effect of soy-rich diets.

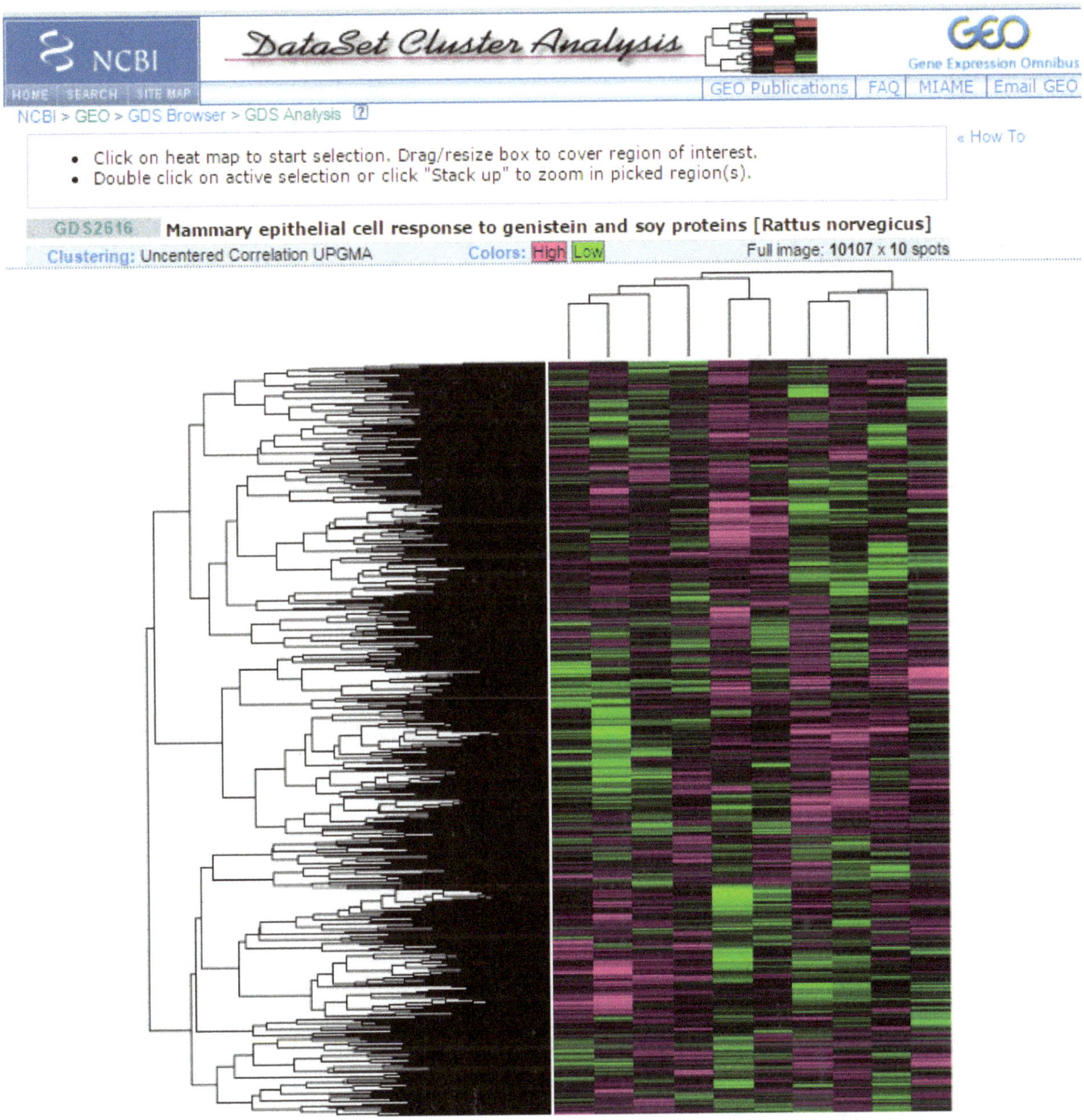

Figure 3. GEO Dataset (GDS2616) demonstration for soy protein genistein protective effect against mammary epithelial cells in *Rattus norvegicus*.

4. Conclusion

In summary, flavonoids can potentially contribute to breast cancer prevention and treatment either by antioxidant or apoptotic activity (**Table 1**). Previous studies highlighted that plant-derived flavonoids are promising when their bioavailability is increased to provide better therapeutic approach in the treatment of disease. However, elucidation of their molecular targets in cell type-specific manner may increase their potential therapeutic effects. Noteworthy that consumption of dietary flavonoids in diet types might be advised to control disease and poor prognosis.

		The effect caused by flavonoid treatment in breast cancer models		
Group of flavonoid	**Subgroup**	**Apoptotic**	**Anti-angiogenic**	**Antioxidant**
Flavanols	Quercetin	+		+
	Kaempferol	+	+	+
	Myricetin			+
	Isorhamnetin	+	+	
	Silymarin	+	+	
Flavanes	Luteolin		+	+
	Apigenin	+	+	
Flavanones	Naringenin	+		
	Eriodictyol			+
	Hesperetin	+		
Flavan-3-ols	Cyanidin	+	+	+
	Delphinidin	+		
	Pelargonidin	+		
Isoflavonoids	Daidzein	+		
	Genistein	+	+	

Table 1. The summary of the effects of flavonoids in breast cancer.

Author details

Pinar Obakan-Yerlikaya*, Elif Damla Arisan, Ajda Coker-Gurkan and Narcin Palavan-Unsal

*Address all correspondence to: p.obakan@iku.edu.tr

Department of Molecular Biology and Genetics, Istanbul Kultur University, Bakirkoy-Istanbul, Turkey

References

[1] Zhang, C.X., et al., Greater vegetable and fruit intake is associated with a lower risk of breast cancer among Chinese women. Int J Cancer, 2009. 125(1): pp. 181-8.

[2] Hui, C., et al., MicroRNA-34a and microRNA-21 play roles in the chemopreventive effects of 3,6-dihydroxyflavone on 1-methyl-1-nitrosourea-induced breast carcinogenesis. Breast Cancer Res, 2012. 14(3): p. R80.

[3] Ni, F., et al., Flavonoid ampelopsin inhibits the growth and metastasis of prostate cancer in vitro and in mice. PLoS One, 2012. 7(6): p. e38802.

[4] Ramos, S., Effects of dietary flavonoids on apoptotic pathways related to cancer chemoprevention. J Nutr Biochem, 2007. 18(7): pp. 427-42.

[5] Aune, D., et al., Fruits, vegetables and breast cancer risk: a systematic review and meta-analysis of prospective studies. Breast Cancer Res Treat, 2012. 134(2): pp. 479-93.

[6] Sak, K., Cytotoxicity of dietary flavonoids on different human cancer types. Pharmacogn Rev, 2014. 8(16): pp. 122-46.

[7] Aune, D., et al., Fruits, vegetables and breast cancer risk: a systematic review and meta-analysis of prospective studies. Breast Cancer Res Treat, 2012. 134(2): pp. 479-93.

[8] Martinez-Perez, C., et al., Novel flavonoids as anti-cancer agents: mechanisms of action and promise for their potential application in breast cancer. Biochem Soc Trans, 2014. 42(4): pp. 1017-23.

[9] Das, D.K., Naturally occurring flavonoids: Structure, chemistry, and high-performance liquid chromatography methods for separation and characterization. Methods Enzymol, 1994. 234: pp. 410-20.

[10] Harborne, J.B., The flavonoids: advances in research since 1980, 2013: Springer, London, UK.

[11] Wagner, H. and L. Farkas, Synthesis of flavonoids, in The Flavonoids, 1975. pp. 127-213: Springer, Dordrecht, Netherlands.

[12] Cermak, R., S. Landgraf, and S. Wolffram, Quercetin glucosides inhibit glucose uptake into brush-border-membrane vesicles of porcine jejunum. Br J Nutr, 2004. 91(6): pp. 849-55.

[13] Gonzales, G.B., et al., Flavonoid interactions during digestion, absorption, distribution and metabolism: a sequential structure-activity/property relationship-based approach in the study of bioavailability and bioactivity. Drug Metab Rev, 2015. 47(2): pp. 175-90.

[14] Passamonti, S., et al., Bioavailability of flavonoids: a review of their membrane transport and the function of bilitranslocase in animal and plant organisms. Curr Drug Metab, 2009. 10(4): pp. 369-94.

[15] Kroon, P.A., et al., How should we assess the effects of exposure to dietary polyphenols in vitro? Am J Clin Nutr, 2004. 80(1): pp. 15-21.

[16] Hertog, M.G., et al., Intake of potentially anticarcinogenic flavonoids and their determinants in adults in The Netherlands. Nutr Cancer, 1993. 20(1): pp. 21-9.

[17] Scalbert, A. and G. Williamson, Dietary intake and bioavailability of polyphenols. J Nutr, 2000. 130(8): pp. 2073S-85S.

[18] Seelinger, G., et al., Anti-carcinogenic effects of the flavonoid luteolin. Molecules, 2008. 13(10): pp. 2628-51.

[19] Okushio, K., et al., Absorption of tea catechins into rat portal vein. Biol Pharm Bull, 1996. 19(2): pp. 326-9.

[20] Stoclet, J.C. and V. Schini-Kerth, Dietary flavonoids and human health. Ann Pharm Fr, 2011. 69(2): pp. 78-90.

[21] Ranganathan, S., D. Halagowder, and N.D. Sivasithambaram, Quercetin suppresses twist to induce apoptosis in MCF-7 breast cancer cells. PLoS One, 2015. 10(10): p. e0141370.

[22] Deng, X.H., et al., Effects of quercetin on the proliferation of breast cancer cells and expression of survivin in vitro. Exp Ther Med, 2013. 6(5): pp. 1155-58.

[23] Dechsupa, S., et al., Quercetin, Siamois 1 and Siamois 2 induce apoptosis in human breast cancer MDA-mB-435 cells xenograft in vivo. Cancer Biol Ther, 2007. 6(1): pp. 56-61.

[24] Duo, J., et al., Quercetin inhibits human breast cancer cell proliferation and induces apoptosis via Bcl-2 and Bax regulation. Mol Med Rep, 2012. 5(6): pp. 1453-6.

[25] Kim, S.H. and K.C. Choi, Anti-cancer effect and underlying mechanism(s) of kaempferol, a phytoestrogen, on the regulation of apoptosis in diverse cancer cell models. Toxicol Res, 2013. 29(4): pp. 229-34.

[26] Luo, H., et al., Kaempferol inhibits VEGF expression and in vitro angiogenesis through a novel ERK-NFkappaB-cMyc-p21 pathway. Food Chem, 2012. 130(2): pp. 321-328.

[27] Choi, E.J. and W.S. Ahn, Kaempferol induced the apoptosis via cell cycle arrest in human breast cancer MDA-MB-453 cells. Nutr Res Pract, 2008. 2(4): pp. 322-5.

[28] Kim, B.W., et al., Sustained ERK activation is involved in the kaempferol-induced apoptosis of breast cancer cells and is more evident under 3-D culture condition. Cancer Biol Ther, 2008. 7(7): pp. 1080-9.

[29] Noolu, B., et al., In Vivo Inhibition of Proteasome Activity and Tumour Growth by Murraya koenigii Leaf Extract in Breast Cancer Xenografts and by its active flavonoids in breast cancer cells. Anticancer Agents Med Chem, 2016. 16:12 (1605-1614).

[30] Kim, S.H., K.A. Hwang, and K.C. Choi, Treatment with kaempferol suppresses breast cancer cell growth caused by estrogen and triclosan in cellular and xenograft breast cancer models. J Nutr Biochem, 2016. 28: pp. 70-82.

[31] Astin, J.W., et al., An in vivo antilymphatic screen in zebrafish identifies novel inhibitors of mammalian lymphangiogenesis and lymphatic-mediated metastasis. Mol Cancer Ther, 2014. 13(10): pp. 2450-62.

[32] Rodgers, E.H. and M.H. Grant, The effect of the flavonoids, quercetin, myricetin and epicatechin on the growth and enzyme activities of MCF7 human breast cancer cells. Chem Biol Interact, 1998. 116(3): pp. 213-28.

[33] Jayakumar, J.K., et al., Evaluation of protective effect of myricetin, a bioflavonoid in dimethyl benzanthracene-induced breast cancer in female Wistar rats. South Asian J Cancer, 2014. 3(2): pp. 107-11.

[34] Maggiolini, M., et al., The red wine phenolics piceatannol and myricetin act as agonists for estrogen receptor alpha in human breast cancer cells. J Mol Endocrinol, 2005. 35(2): pp. 269-81.

[35] Kim, B., Y.E. Choi, and H.S. Kim, Eruca sativa and its flavonoid components, quercetin and isorhamnetin, improve skin barrier function by activation of peroxisome proliferator-activated receptor (PPAR)-alpha and suppression of inflammatory cytokines. Phytother Res, 2014. 28(9): pp. 1359-66.

[36] Li, C., et al., Inhibitory effects of isorhamnetin on the invasion of human breast carcinoma cells by downregulating the expression and activity of matrix metalloproteinase-2/9. Nutr Cancer, 2015. 67(7): pp. 1191-200.

[37] Bruning, A., Inhibition of mTOR signaling by quercetin in cancer treatment and prevention. Anticancer Agents Med Chem, 2013. 13(7): pp. 1025-31.

[38] Zhu, X.X., et al., Silibinin: a potential old drug for cancer therapy. Expert Rev Clin Pharmacol, 2016: 18: 1-8.

[39] Singh, R.P., et al., Silibinin strongly inhibits growth and survival of human endothelial cells via cell cycle arrest and downregulation of survivin, Akt and NF-kappaB: implications for angioprevention and antiangiogenic therapy. Oncogene, 2005. 24(7): pp. 1188-202.

[40] Manna, S.K., et al., Silymarin suppresses TNF-induced activation of NF-kappa B, c-Jun N-terminal kinase, and apoptosis. J Immunol, 1999. 163(12): pp. 6800-9.

[41] Deep, G., et al., Angiopreventive efficacy of pure flavonolignans from milk thistle extract against prostate cancer: targeting VEGF-VEGFR signaling. PLoS One, 2012. 7(4): p. e34630.

[42] Zheng, N., et al., ER beta up-regulation was involved in silibinin-induced growth inhibition of human breast cancer MCF-7 cells. Arch Biochem Biophys, 2016. 591: pp. 141-9.

[43] Birt, D.F., S. Hendrich, and W. Wang, Dietary agents in cancer prevention: flavonoids and isoflavonoids. Pharmacol Ther, 2001. 90(2-3): pp. 157-77.

[44] Lien, E.J., et al., Quantitative structure-activity relationship analysis of phenolic antioxidants. Free Radic Biol Med, 1999. 26(3-4): pp. 285-94.

[45] Markaverich, B.M., K. Shoulars, and M.A. Rodriguez, Luteolin regulation of estrogen signaling and cell cycle pathway genes in MCF-7 human breast cancer cells. Int J Biomed Sci, 2011. 7(2): pp. 101-11.

[46] Chen, P.Y., et al., Up-Regulation of miR-34a Expression in Response to the Luteolin-Induced Neurite Outgrowth of PC12 Cells. J Agric Food Chem, 2015. 63(16): pp. 4148-59.

[47] Harrison, M.E., et al., Exposure of breast cancer cells to a subcytotoxic dose of apigenin causes growth inhibition, oxidative stress, and hypophosphorylation of Akt. Exp Mol Pathol, 2014. 97(2): pp. 211-7.

[48] Scherbakov, A.M. and O.E. Andreeva, Apigenin inhibits growth of breast cancer cells: the role of ERalpha and HER2/neu. Acta Naturae, 2015. 7(3): pp. 133-9.

[49] Choi, E.J. and G.H. Kim, Apigenin induces apoptosis through a mitochondria/caspase-pathway in human breast cancer MDA-MB-453 cells. J Clin Biochem Nutr, 2009. 44(3): pp. 260-5.

[50] Seo, H.S., et al., Apigenin induces apoptosis via extrinsic pathway, inducing p53 and inhibiting STAT3 and NFkappaB signaling in HER2-overexpressing breast cancer cells. Mol Cell Biochem, 2012. 366(1-2): pp. 319-34.

[51] Lee, W.J., et al., Apigenin inhibits HGF-promoted invasive growth and metastasis involving blocking PI3K/Akt pathway and beta 4 integrin function in MDA-MB-231 breast cancer cells. Toxicol Appl Pharmacol, 2008. 226(2): pp. 178-91.

[52] Abaza, M.S., et al., Growth inhibitory and chemo-sensitization effects of naringenin, a natural flavanone purified from Thymus vulgaris, on human breast and colorectal cancer. Cancer Cell Int, 2015. 15: p. 46.

[53] Chandrika, B.B., et al., Hesperetin and naringenin sensitize HER2 positive cancer cells to death by serving as HER2 tyrosine kinase inhibitors. Life Sci, 2016.

[54] Zhang, F., et al., Naringenin prevents TGF-beta1 secretion from breast cancer and suppresses pulmonary metastasis by inhibiting PKC activation. Breast Cancer Res, 2016. 18(1): p. 38.

[55] Zierau, O., et al., Naringenin-type flavonoids show different estrogenic effects in mammalian and teleost test systems. Biochem Biophys Res Commun, 2005. 326(4): pp. 909-16.

[56] Chung, S.Y., et al., Inhibition of P-glycoprotein by natural products in human breast cancer cells. Arch Pharm Res, 2005. 28(7): pp. 823-8.

[57] Hatkevich, T., et al., A naringenin-tamoxifen combination impairs cell proliferation and survival of MCF-7 breast cancer cells. Exp Cell Res, 2014. 327(2): pp. 331-9.

[58] Meiyanto, E., A. Hermawan, and Anindyajati, Natural products for cancer-targeted therapy: citrus flavonoids as potent chemopreventive agents. Asian Pac J Cancer Prev, 2012. 13(2): pp. 427-36.

[59] Jing, X., et al., Eriodictyol-7-O- glucoside activates Nrf2 and protects against cerebral ischemic injury. Toxicol Appl Pharmacol, 2013.

[60] Lou, H., et al., Eriodictyol protects against H(2)O(2)-induced neuron-like PC12 cell death through activation of Nrf2/ARE signaling pathway. Neurochem Int, 2012. 61(2): pp. 251-7.

[61] Guthrie, N. and K.K. Carroll, Inhibition of mammary cancer by citrus flavonoids. Adv Exp Med Biol, 1998. 439: pp. 227-36.

[62] Palit, S., et al., Hesperetin induces apoptosis in breast carcinoma by triggering accumulation of ROS and activation of ASK1/JNK pathway. J Cell Physiol, 2015. 230(8): pp. 1729-39.

[63] So, F.V., et al., Inhibition of proliferation of estrogen receptor-positive MCF-7 human breast cancer cells by flavonoids in the presence and absence of excess estrogen. Cancer Lett, 1997. 112(2): pp. 127-33.

[64] So, F.V., et al., Inhibition of human breast cancer cell proliferation and delay of mammary tumorigenesis by flavonoids and citrus juices. Nutr Cancer, 1996. 26(2): pp. 167-81.

[65] Farabegoli, F., A. Papi, and M. Orlandi, (−)-Epigallocatechin-3-gallate down-regulates EGFR, MMP-2, MMP-9 and EMMPRIN and inhibits the invasion of MCF-7 tamoxifen-resistant cells. Biosci Rep, 2011. 31(2): pp. 99-108.

[66] Parvez, S., et al., Catechin prevents tamoxifen-induced oxidative stress and biochemical perturbations in mice. Toxicology, 2006. 225(2-3): pp. 109-18.

[67] Scandlyn, M.J., et al., A new role for tamoxifen in oestrogen receptor-negative breast cancer when it is combined with epigallocatechin gallate. Br J Cancer, 2008. 99(7): pp. 1056-63.

[68] Stuart, E.C., R.M. Jarvis, and R.J. Rosengren, In vitro mechanism of action for the cytotoxicity elicited by the combination of epigallocatechin gallate and raloxifene in MDA-MB-231 cells. Oncol Rep, 2010. 24(3): pp. 779-85.

[69] Butt, M.S., et al., Green tea and anticancer perspectives: updates from last decade. Crit Rev Food Sci Nutr, 2015. 55(6): pp. 792-805.

[70] Delgado, L., et al., Anti-proliferative effects of quercetin and catechin metabolites. Food Funct, 2014. 5(4): pp. 797-803.

[71] Rathore, K., et al., Green tea catechin intervention of reactive oxygen species-mediated ERK pathway activation and chronically induced breast cell carcinogenesis. Carcinogenesis, 2012. 33(1): pp. 174-83.

[72] Rathore, K. and H.C. Wang, Green tea catechin extract in intervention of chronic breast cell carcinogenesis induced by environmental carcinogens. Mol Carcinog, 2012. 51(3): pp. 280-9.

[73] Sen, T. and A. Chatterjee, Epigallocatechin-3-gallate (EGCG) downregulates EGF-induced MMP-9 in breast cancer cells: involvement of integrin receptor alpha5beta1 in the process. Eur J Nutr, 2011. 50(6): pp. 465-78.

[74] Singletary, K.W., K.J. Jung, and M. Giusti, Anthocyanin-rich grape extract blocks breast cell DNA damage. J Med Food, 2007. 10(2): pp. 244-51.

[75] Prior, R.L. and X. Wu, Anthocyanins: structural characteristics that result in unique metabolic patterns and biological activities. Free Radic Res, 2006. 40(10): pp. 1014-28.

[76] Wang, S.Y. and H. Jiao, Scavenging capacity of berry crops on superoxide radicals, hydrogen peroxide, hydroxyl radicals, and singlet oxygen. J Agric Food Chem, 2000. 48(11): pp. 5677-84.

[77] Kim, H., T.G. Peterson, and S. Barnes, Mechanisms of action of the soy isoflavone genistein: emerging role for its effects via transforming growth factor beta signaling pathways. Am J Clin Nutr, 1998. 68(6 Suppl): pp. 1418S-1425S.

[78] Hui, C., et al., Anticancer activities of an anthocyanin-rich extract from black rice against breast cancer cells in vitro and in vivo. Nutr Cancer, 2010. 62(8): pp. 1128-36.

[79] Tang, J., et al., Delphinidin and cyanidin exhibit antiproliferative and apoptotic effects in MCF7 human breast cancer cells. Integr Cancer Sci Ther, 2015. 2: pp. 82-86.

[80] Rimm, E.B., et al., Relation between intake of flavonoids and risk for coronary heart disease in male health professionals. Ann Intern Med, 1996. 125(5): pp. 384-9.

[81] Yao, L.H., et al., Flavonoids in food and their health benefits. Plant foods for human nutrition, 2004. 59(3): pp. 113-122.

[82] Liu, W., et al., Selective anti-proliferation of HER2-positive breast cancer cells by anthocyanins identified by high-throughput screening. PLoS One, 2013. 8(12): p. e81586.

[83] Bunea, A., et al., Anthocyanin determination in blueberry extracts from various cultivars and their antiproliferative and apoptotic properties in B16-F10 metastatic murine melanoma cells. Phytochemistry, 2013. 95: pp. 436-44.

[84] Ozbay, T. and R. Nahta, Delphinidin inhibits HER2 and Erk1/2 signaling and suppresses growth of HER2-overexpressing and triple negative breast cancer cell lines. Breast Cancer (Auckl), 2011. 5: pp. 143-54.

[85] Martin, S., et al., Delphinidin inhibits endothelial cell proliferation and cell cycle progression through a transient activation of ERK-1/-2. Biochem Pharmacol, 2003. 65(4): pp. 669-75.

[86] Syed, D.N., et al., Delphinidin inhibits cell proliferation and invasion via modulation of Met receptor phosphorylation. Toxicol Appl Pharmacol, 2008. 231(1): pp. 52-60.

[87] Im, N.K., et al., Delphinidin suppresses PMA-induced MMP-9 expression by blocking the NF-kappaB activation through MAPK signaling pathways in MCF-7 human breast carcinoma cells. J Med Food, 2014. 17(8): pp. 855-61.

[88] Weaver, J., et al., Strawberry polyphenols are equally cytotoxic to tumourigenic and normal human breast and prostate cell lines. Int J Oncol, 2009. 34(3): pp. 777-86.

[89] Jeyabalan, J., et al., Chemopreventive and therapeutic activity of dietary blueberry against estrogen-mediated breast cancer. J Agric Food Chem, 2014. 62(18): pp. 3963-71.

[90] Kim, N.D., et al., Chemopreventive and adjuvant therapeutic potential of pomegranate (*Punica granatum*) for human breast cancer. Breast Cancer Res Treat, 2002. 71(3): pp. 203-17.

[91] Fedoreyev, S.A., et al., Isoflavonoid production by callus cultures of *Maackia amurensis*. Fitoterapia, 2000. 71(4): pp. 365-72.

[92] de Lemos, M.L., Effects of soy phytoestrogens genistein and daidzein on breast cancer growth. Ann Pharmacother, 2001. 35(9): pp. 1118-21.

[93] Medeiros, P.S., et al., Raman microspectroscopy for probing the impact of a dietary antioxidant on human breast cancer cells. Food Funct, 2016. 7(6): pp. 2800-10.

[94] Koo, J., et al., Induction of proto-oncogene BRF2 in breast cancer cells by the dietary soybean isoflavone daidzein. BMC Cancer, 2015. 15: pp. 905.

[95] Bao, C., et al., Daidzein suppresses tumor necrosis factor-alpha induced migration and invasion by inhibiting hedgehog/Gli1 signaling in human breast cancer cells. J Agric Food Chem, 2014. 62(17): pp. 3759-67.

[96] Atkinson, C., et al., Plasma equol concentration is not associated with breast cancer and fibrocystic breast conditions among women in Shanghai, China. Nutr Res, 2016. 36(8): pp. 863-71.

[97] Akiyama, T., et al., Genistein, a specific inhibitor of tyrosine-specific protein kinases. J Biol Chem, 1987. 262(12): pp. 5592-5.

[98] Hsieh, C.Y., et al., Estrogenic effects of genistein on the growth of estrogen receptor-positive human breast cancer (MCF-7) cells in vitro and in vivo. Cancer Res, 1998. 58(17): pp. 3833-8.

[99] Li, Z., et al., Genistein induces cell apoptosis in MDA-MB-231 breast cancer cells via the mitogen-activated protein kinase pathway. Toxicol In Vitro, 2008. 22(7): pp. 1749-53.

[100] Morgan, T.M., T.D. Koreckij, and E. Corey, Targeted therapy for advanced prostate cancer: inhibition of the PI3K/Akt/mTOR pathway. Curr Cancer Drug Targets, 2009. 9(2): pp. 237-49.

[101] Yu, X., et al., Anti-angiogenic genistein inhibits VEGF-induced endothelial cell activation by decreasing PTK activity and MAPK activation. Med Oncol, 2012. 29(1): pp. 349-57.

[102] Buchler, P., et al., Antiangiogenic activity of genistein in pancreatic carcinoma cells is mediated by the inhibition of hypoxia-inducible factor-1 and the down-regulation of VEGF gene expression. Cancer, 2004. 100(1): pp. 201-10.

[103] Sounni, N.E., et al., Up-regulation of vascular endothelial growth factor-A by active membrane-type 1 matrix metalloproteinase through activation of Src-tyrosine kinases. J Biol Chem, 2004. 279(14): pp. 13564-74.

[104] Gupta, S.C., et al., Regulation of survival, proliferation, invasion, angiogenesis, and metastasis of tumor cells through modulation of inflammatory pathways by nutraceuticals. Cancer Metastasis Rev, 2010. 29(3): pp. 405-34.

[105] Chung, M.H., et al., Genistein inhibits phorbol ester-induced NF-kappaB transcriptional activity and COX-2 expression by blocking the phosphorylation of p65/RelA in human mammary epithelial cells. Mutat Res, 2014. 768: pp. 74-83.

[106] Lin, H.M., et al., Galectin-3 mediates genistein-induced G(2)/M arrest and inhibits apoptosis. Carcinogenesis, 2000. 21(11): pp. 1941-5.

12

Management of Hormone Receptor-Positive Metastatic Breast Cancer

Joanne W. Chiu

Abstract

Hormone-receptor positive HER2-negative breast cancer constitutes about 2/3 of breast cancer. Hormonal therapy such as tamoxifen and aromatase inhibitors has been the main stay of treatment which gives favorable quality of life compared with traditional chemotherapy. However, the efficacy of subsequent hormonal therapy declines rapidly after the patients develops resistance to first line hormonal therapy. In recent years, there have been many breakthrough in the treatment of this cancer. A number of targeted agents including CDK4/6 inhibitor and mTOR inhibitor are now part of standard treatment paradigm to help prolong the use of hormonal therapy. New understanding in potential biomarker of resistance such as *ESR1* mutation or *PIK3CA* mutation has also empowered us to develops personalized approach in treatment. This article will explain the treatment logistic for this cancer, current knowledge in hormonal resistance, findings of key clinical trials that define the current treatment paradigm, efficacy and major side effect precaution of the targeted agents, and the unmet needs.

Keywords: metastatic breast cancer, hormone-receptor positive, CDK4/6 inhibitor, SERD, mTOR inhibitor

1. Introduction

Breast cancer is a common cancer in female with a high chance of recurrence even after curative treatment. The goal for treatment in metastatic disease is life prolongation and preservation of quality of life. Breast cancer is defined by the overexpression of hormone receptor (HR), either estrogen and/or progesterone receptors, and human epidermal growth factor receptor 2 (HER2) receptor. HR-positive HER2-negative ($HR^{+ve}/HER2^{-ve}$) breast cancer accounts for 70% of breast cancer [1]. For patients with $HR^{+ve}/HER2^{-ve}$ metastatic breast cancer (MBC), the choice between chemotherapy versus endocrine therapy depends on the disease load especially the presence of visceral crisis – patients with impending visceral crisis should be treated with systemic chemotherapy, whereas patients with stable condition should be given endocrine therapy. As hormonal stimulation is known to be the underlying driving force and these tumors tend to be slow growing, endocrine therapy is considered the mainstay of treatment for most patients.

The first endocrine therapy described for treatment of MBC was tamoxifen which dated back in year 1971 [2]. It is a selective estrogen receptor modulator (SERMs) that binds competitively to estrogen receptors, and can have both antagonistic and agonistic effect depending on the tissue of action. Nowadays tamoxifen and raloxifen are the most commonly used SERMs clinically. SERMs can be used in both pre- and post-menopausal women. These drugs are well tolerated and have favorable toxicity profile. The use of aromatase inhibitor (AI) was started in early 2000s for post-menopausal women. AI blocks the action of peripheral aromatase, preventing conversion of androgens to estrogen. Letrozole and anastrozole are non-steroidal reversible AIs, whereas exemestane is a steroidal irreversible AI. The initial evidence to support the use of AI was by the TARGET trial, which showed equivalent efficacy of anastrozole and tamoxifen in the first line treatment of HR-positive MBC but with lower incidence of side effects such as thromboembolic events and vaginal bleeding [3]. Subsequently letrozole was demonstrated to have superior time to progression (9.4 versus 6.0 months, $p < 0.0001$), improved objective response rate (ORR) (32 versus 21%, p −0.0002) and a trend toward longer overall survival (OS) (34 versus 30 months) compared with tamoxifen [4]. The third class of endocrine therapy is selective estrogen-receptor degrader (SERD), and fulvestrant is the only SERD approved by the U.S. Food and Drug Administration (FDA) so far. In the CONFIRM trial, it has been defined that fulvestrant should be given at a higher dose of 500 mg instead of 250 mg for its better benefit in overall survival [5]. In the recently published phase 3 FALCON trial in which endocrine therapy-naïve patients were randomized to receive fulvestrant 500 mg monthly or anastrozole 1 mg daily [6]. The progression-free survival (PFS) in the fulvestrant group was 16.6 months compared with that of 13.8 months in the anastrozole group. The p-value was at a borderline of 0.0486 and the overall survival data is not available yet. As such, both AI and fulvestrant are acceptable option for initial treatment of $HR^{+ve}/HER2^{-ve}$ MBC, yet the use of fulvestrant is often limited by the need for monthly intramuscular injection and its high cost.

Traditional endocrine therapy at the frontline setting achieves an overall response rate in the range of 25–45% and median PFS around 8–10 months [3, 4, 7]. Second line endocrine therapy often yields unfavorable response. With improving understanding in this disease, more and more evidence suggests that combining endocrine therapy with targeted therapy could overcome endocrine resistance and significantly prolong the time on endocrine therapy, delaying the needs for chemotherapy. This chapter will discuss the latest development in the targeted therapy for $HR^{+ve}/HER2^{-ve}$ MBC and the future direction.

2. Endocrine resistance

Endocrine resistance is a major obstacle for treatment of $HR^{+ve}/HER2^{-ve}$ MBC. Multiple mechanisms have been implicated. Based on these knowledge we now have a number of targeted therapy that can help overcome this problem. The more clinically relevant mechanisms are discussed as below.

2.1. Dysregulation of cell cycle checkpoints

In mammalian cells, cell cycle progression is determined by the checkpoint regular retinoblastoma protein (Rb), which itself is controlled by a number of cyclin-dependent kinases (CDK) [8]. In quiescent state, Rb in its hypo-phosphorylated state suppresses the cell cycle progression from G1 phase into S (synthesis) phase. In proliferative state, CDK subtypes 4 and 6 complexes with cyclin D1, D2, or D3, triggering Rb phosphorylation [9]. Hyperphosphorylation of Rb leads to increased activity of the E2F family of transcription factors and promotes cell cycle progression. Cyclin D1 amplification is common in HR-positive breast cancer. Cyclin D1 is encoded by *CCDN1*. *CCND1* and cyclin D1 have been found to be amplified in 15–20 and 28–58% of luminal breast cancer respectively [10, 11]. Preclinical research suggested dysregulated cell cycle checkpoint regulation could lead to abnormal cell cycle progression and loss of endocrine responsiveness. Treatment of antiestrogen in breast cancer cells was associated with suppressed cyclin D1 expression, and emergence of endocrine resistance was accompanied by persistent cyclin D1 expression and Rb phosphorylation [12, 13]. Subsequent *in vitro* study further demonstrated that in breast cancer cell lines, CDK4/6 inhibitor palbociclib had preferential activity in reversing treatment resistance in luminal cells [14]. A number of CDK4/6 inhibitors have been tested clinically, and have become standard treatment of HR^{+ve}/$HER2^{-ve}$ MBC.

2.2. Crosstalk growth factor receptor and PI3K/AKT/mTOR pathway

Phosphatidylinositol-3-kinasd (PI3K)-Akt-mammalian target of rapamycin (mTOR) pathway is an important signal transduction system on which many growth factor receptors pathways converge. Crosstalk between the PI3K/Akt/mTOR pathway and growth factor receptors such as EGFR, HER2, HER2, FGFR1, and IGF1R have been described in endocrine resistance [15–18].

Abnormal activation of the PI3K pathway could result in factitious cell proliferation. The PI3K complex is composed of a regulatory subunit and a catalytic subunit p110. P110 has four isoforms – α, β, γ, and δ. *PIK3CA* mutation is found in up to 40% of breast cancer and is likely to be present in early cancer development [19, 20]. Abnormal PK3K signaling was found in up to 70% of breast cancers [21]. Besides *PIK3CA* mutation, hyperactivation of this pathway can result from aberration other PI3K subunits, mutation or phosphorylation of effectors Akt, loss of inhibitory signal from PTEN or INPPR4B, leading to activation of downstream effector mTOR protein. As hyperactivation of PI3K pathway could promote estrogen-independent ER transcriptional activation, inhibition of PI3K or its downstream effectors is an attractive target to overcome endocrine resistance [21, 22].

2.3. Changes in the estrogen receptor (ER) and HER2 status

Loss of HR expression, although uncommon, has been reported in hormone-resistant breast cancer. Study of paired primary and metastatic HR-positive breast cancer found a positive-to-negative change in HR status in 10% of metastatic breast tumor [23]. In the P024 neoadjuvant endocrine therapy trial that recruited 228 post-menopausal women with HR-positive stage 2 or 3 breast cancer, those who lost ER status after AI treatment had worse recurrence-free survival compared with those who had no change in ER status (HR of relapse = 2.4, $p = 0.03$) [24]. Another study of paired sample analysis of primary cancer and liver metastases post-treatment showed ER status and HER2 status change in 30% and 10% of patients [25]. How these changes in receptor status affect management and outcome is not well understood.

2.4. Molecular changes secondary to the use of aromatase inhibitor

Molecular changes in the target receptors after treatment causing treatment failure is a well-known phenomenon in many malignancies. For HR-positive breast cancer, the target of interest is *ESR1*, which encodes for ERα. *ESR1* mutation has not been detected in sequencing analysis of 390 treatment-naïve primary breast cancer tissues in the Cancer Genome Atlas project [11]. In another study, tissue of patients with hormone-resistance breast cancer were sequenced, and showed 14 or 80 these cases showed *ESR1* mutations affecting the ligand-binding domain [26]. The mutations were the highly recurrent mutations encoding p.Tyr537Ser, p.Tyr537Asn and p.Asp538Gly alterations. p.Tyr537Ser and p.Asp538Gly play a role in hydrogen bonding of the mutant amino acid with Asp351 and favors the agonist conformation of the ER receptor. As a result the mutant ER becomes active in the absence of hormonal stimulation, and renders ER antagonists ineffective. The clinical significance of *ESR1* mutation will be further discussed in Section 3.4.

3. New clinical therapy and emerging treatment

3.1. CDK4/6 inhibitor is now a new standard treatment

3.1.1. Palbociclib

Palbociclib is a first-in-class CDK4/6 inhibitor [27]. Based on the impressive PFS found in the phase 2 study PALOMA-1 [28], palbociclib was granted accelerated approval in 2015 by the Food and Drug Administration (FDA) for treatment of $HR^{+ve}/HER2^{-ve}$ MBC in the first line setting.

3.1.1.1. Key results of phase 3 PALOMA studies

PALOMA-2, is a double-blind, placebo-controlled, randomized phase 3 study of palbociclib plus letrozole in women with $HR^{+ve}/HER2^{-ve}$ MBC patients who had no prior treatment for advanced disease [29]. Patients were randomized to receive palbociclib plus letrozole or placebo plus letrozole. The primary end point was PFS. Secondary end points included OS, objective response rate (ORR), clinical benefit response (CBR) and safety. The study recruited 666 women within 17 months. The primary endpoint was met – the addition of palbociclib to letrozole, as compared with placebo-letrozole, increased the median PFS from 14.5 months (95% confidence interval [CI], 12.9–17.1) to 24.8 months (95% CI, 22.1 to not estimable) (hazard ratio [HR] 0.58, 95% CI, 0.46–0.72; $p < 0.001$). Subgroup analyses of PFS confirmed a consistent benefit across all subgroups evaluated including different race, prior disease-free survival, visceral involvement, prior hormonal therapy, the type of recent hormonal therapy, or prior chemotherapy (HR ranges, 0.35–0.67). The ORR for all randomly assigned patients in palbociclib-letrozole group versus placebo-letrozole group was 42.1% (95% CI, 37.5–46.9) and 34.7% (95% CI, 28.4–41.3) (odds ratio 1.4, 95% CI, 0.98–2.01; $p = 0.06$). CBR among all patients randomized was 84.9% (95% CI, 81.2–88.1) for palbociclib-letrozole group and 70.3% (95% CI, 63.8–76.2) for placebo-letrozole group (odds ratio 2.39 (95% CI, 1.58–3.59; $p < 0.0010$). The most frequent grade 3 and 4 adverse event (AE) in the palbociclib-letrozole group was neutropenia (66%), but febrile neutropenia occurred in 1.8% of patients only. Other common AE included fatigue (37%), nausea (35%), arthralgia (33%), alopecia (33%) and diarrhea (26%) and all these were mild.

PALAMO-3 is another indication-defining phase 3 study of palbociclib [30]. Patients with $HR^{+ve}/HER2^{-ve}$ HER2-negative MBC who had relapsed or progressed during prior endocrine therapy were randomized to receive fulvestrant with placebo or fulvestrant with palbociclib. A total of 521 patients were randomized. The median PFS was 9.2 and 3.8 months in the fulvestrant-palbociclib and fulvestrant-placebo groups respectively (95% CI, 2.5–5.5) (HR 0.42, 95% CI, 0.32–0.56; $p < 0.001$). ORR was 10.4% with fulvestrant-palbociclib and 6.3% with fulvestrant-placebo, and the CBR was 34% with fulvestrant-palbociclib and 19% with fulvestrant-placebo. In the fulvestrant-palbociclib group, grade 3 or 4 neutropenia was found in 62%. Other common AEs were fatigue (38%), nausea (29%), anemia (26%), and headache (21%).

The results of PALOMA-2 echo those of PALOMA-1 that led to FDA approval. PALOMA-1 differs from PALOMA-2, besides being a phase 2 trial, in that it adopted a 1:1 randomization. There were also small differences in the subgroup analysis, such as inclusion of the newly diagnosed metastatic disease subgroup. Nevertheless, both studies showed significant survival benefit of palbociclib and similar toxicity profiles.

3.1.2. *Ribociclib*

Ribociclib is the second CDK 4/6 inhibitor received the U.S. FDA approval in March 2017. The first approval study was MONOLEESA-2 for first line setting. MONOLEESA-7, which is also a first line trial, had special interest in pre- and peri-menopausal women. The data also became available recently.

3.1.2.1. *Key results of phase 3 MONOLEESA studies*

MONOLEESA-2 is a double-blind, placebo-controlled, phase 3 study of ribociclib plus letrozole [31]. It mirrors PALOMA-2 for the target patient population. Patients were randomized 1:1 to ribociclib-letrozole or placebo-letrozole. The study demonstrated that the addition of ribociclib to letrozole significantly improved PFS from 14.5 months to over 25 months giving a HR of 0.56 for disease progression or death (95% CI, 0.43–0.72; $p < 0.001$). The ORR was 40.7% in the ribociclib group and 27.5% in the placebo group in the intention-to-treat population. The CBR was 79.6% in the ribociclib group and 72.8% in the placebo group ($p = 0.02$) respectively in the intention-to-treat population. The most common grade 3 and 4 AEs were neutropenia (60%), elevated alanine aminotransferase (9%), elevated aspartate aminotransferase (6%), infection (4%) and vomiting (4%). Other common AEs were minor and mild.

The results of MONOLEESA-7 was first released in the San Antonio Breast Cancer Symposium (SABCS) 2017 [32]. Unlike other studies of CDK4/6 inhibitors, this study recruited pre- or perimenopausal $HR^{+ve}/HER2^{-ve}$ MBC patients who had received no prior endocrine therapy for advanced disease, but allowed up to 1 line of chemotherapy. Patients were randomized to receive standard treatment of goserelin, plus either tamoxifen or AI, together with ribociclib or placebo. The median age of recruited patients were 44 years old, and 40% had *de novo* metastatic disease. For those who developed metastasis after primary resection, more than 50% had disease-free interval for more than 12 months. Median PFS turned out to be 13.0 months for the placebo group and 23.8 months for the ribociclib group (HR 0.553; 95% CI, 0.441–0.694; $p < 0.001$). About ¼ of the patients received tamoxifen, and there was no difference from those who received AI in term of PFS benefit gained with addition of ribociclib. Goserelin was an effective method for ovarian suppression for treatment of pre/peri-menopausal $HR^{+ve}/HER2^{-ve}$ MBC, and tamoxifen was as good as AI partnering with ribociclib.

3.1.3. *Abemaciclib*

In September 2017, abemaciclib was approved by the U.S. FDA to be used in combination with fulvestrant for HR-positive MBC progressed following endocrine therapy. It was also approved as monotherapy for HR-positive MBC with disease progression following endocrine therapy and chemotherapy in the metastatic setting.

3.1.3.1. *Important clinical trials of abemaciclib*

MONARCH-2 is a randomized placebo-controlled trial to study the combination of abemaciclib with fulvestrant in patients with $HR^{+ve}/HER2^{-ve}$ MBC who have progressed on or had less than 12 months from end of adjuvant endocrine therapy [33]. Patient received abemaciclib daily without resting period. The original study dose was 200 mg BD, but the protocol amended to reduce the dose to 150 mg BD as there were many clinically significant diarrheas. Abemaciclib plus fulvestrant significantly prolonged median PFS versus fulvestrant alone (16.4 versus 9.3 months; HR 0.553; 95% CI, 0.449–0.681; $p < 0.001$). In the intention-to-treat population, abemaciclib plus fulvestrant achieved an ORR of 35.2% compared with 16.1% in the control arm ($p < 0.001$), and it included 14 patients with complete response (3.1%). The treatment gave durable response with 12-month duration of response rate of 67.8 and 66.9% in the abemaciclib and the placebo arm respectively. After 12 cycles of treatment, the mean change in tumor size for the abemaciclib arm and placebo arm were − 62.5% and − 32.8% respectively. The most common adverse events in the abemaciclib arm were diarrhea (all grade 86.4%, grade 3 & 4 13.4%), neutropenia (all grade 46.0%, grade 3 & 4 26.5%), nausea (all grade 45.1%, grade 3 2.7%), and fatigue (all grade 39.9%, grade 3 2.7%).

The results of MONARCH-3 came after MONARCH-2. MONARCH-3 is a double-blind randomized phase 3 study of abemaciclib or placebo plus a non-steroid AI in $HR^{+ve}/HER2^{-ve}$ MBC patients who had no prior systemic therapy in the advanced setting [34]. Patients were randomized to receive either abemaciclib 150 mg BD continuously or placebo with anastrozole 1 mg or letrozole 2.5 mg daily. Median PFS was significantly longer in the abemaciclib arm compared with placebo arm (HR 0.54; 95% CI, 0.41–0.72; $p < 0.001$). The ORR in the intention-to-treat population was 48.2% and 34.5% for abemaciclib and placebo arms respectively ($p = 0.002$). Diarrhea was reported in 81.3% but most was grade 1. The most common grade 3 or 4 toxicity was neutropenia (21.1%) and diarrhea (9.5%).

While most clinical trials of palbociclib and ribociclib focused on first or early line treatment for metastatic disease, abemaciclib is the only CDK4/6 inhibitor that has proven to have meaningful activity in refractory disease. MONARCH-1 is a phase II single-arm open-label study for $HR^{+ve}/HER2^{-ve}$ MBC patients who had progressed on or after endocrine therapy, and had 1 or 2 chemotherapy regimens [35]. Abemaciclib was given at 200 mg BD continuously as monotherapy. The primary objective was ORR. Other endpoints included CBR, PFS, and OS. This study recruited 132 patients. Median line of treatment was 3. ORR was 19.7%, CBR was 42.4%, median PFS was 6.0 months, and median OS was 17.7 months. Major treatment-related AEs were diarrhea (all grade 90.2%, grade 3 & 4 19.7%), fatigue (all grade 65.2%, grade 3 12.9%), and nausea (all grade 64.4%, grade 3 4.5%). Neutropenia was reported in 87.5% of patients of which 26.9% were grade 3 or 4.

3.1.4. Biomarker of response

At the age of precision medicine, we aim to understand the potential biomarker of response that can guide us on treatment. For palbociclib, investigated biomarkers include cyclin D1 amplification and p16 loss, ER expression, Rb level, and Ki67 index [28, 36], as well as hormone-receptor expression level, *PIK3CA* mutation status, and plasma circulating tumor DNA *ESR1* mutation status [37, 38]. No biomarker of response has been identified for palbociclib.

As to ribociclib, ctDNA was collected for MONALEESA-2 study at baseline. Although patient with *PIK3CA* variants had shorted PFS compared with those with wild-type *PIK3CA*, they derived similar PFS benefit to the addition of ribociclib (Altered *PIK3CA* HR 0.53, wild-type *PIK3CA* HR 0.44) [31]. Similarly, altered *TP53* was a poor prognostic factor, yet both wild-type *TP53* and altered *TP53* had similar response to added benefit of ribociclib. There was a week trend toward limited PFS benefit with ribociclib was observed in patients with alteration in CDH1 and FGFR1/ZNF7–3. The incidence of these genetic events was found in only 5–11% of patients, thus the results still inconclusive. A better understanding in biology of endocrine resistance and obtaining study biopsy at the time of starting treatment or upon disease recurrence or progression might provide valuable insight in this field.

3.1.5. Discussion for CDK4/6 inhibitor

PALOMA-2 showed superior efficacy of adding palbociclib to letrozole in first line treatment of $HR^{+ve}/HER2^{-ve}$ MBC with an unprecedented PFS of over 2 years. This benefit extended to all subgroups, including those with prior exposure to hormonal therapy or chemotherapy. This study confirms the new standard of adding CDK4/6 inhibitor in this disease.

The most concerning toxicity of palbociclib and ribociclib was neutropenia. It happened in 80–90% of patients of which grade 3 or 4 neutropenia was reported in 60%. Patients who developed neutropenic fever, grade 4 neutropenia, or prolonged neutropenia would require dose reduction. The significance of dose reduction is not clear. PALOMA-3 is a study of palbociclib in combination with fulvestrant in patients who progressed on first line hormonal therapy [30]. Detailed analysis showed that dose modification of palbociclib for grade 3 and 4 neutropenia had no adverse effect on PFS [39]. Together with improved quality of life (QoL), and low incidence of neutropenic fever of less than 2%, palbociclib and ribociclib are drugs very well tolerated.

While PALOMA-1, PALOMA-2, and MONALEESA-2 provided the evidence to the use of CDK4/6 inhibitor in the first line setting, all these trials were done in post-menopausal women. In fact the last randomized trial dedicated to premenopausal women with MBS was published almost 2 decades ago. It is estimated that around 1/5 of newly diagnosed breast cancer in the U.S. was found in women younger than 50 years old [40]. In Asia-Pacific region, 40% of breast cancer patients were of age less than 50 years [41]. Breast cancer in young patients is believe to be more aggressive and has distinct tumor biology. MONALEESA-7 is the first of the series to explore the activity of CDK 4/6 inhibitor in these patients. It extended the use of CDK4/6 inhibitor in pre/peri-menopausal women in combination with GHRH agonist as the mean of ovarian suppression. It also proved that tamoxifen was an as effective hormonal partner as AI with CDK4/6 inhibitor.

The hazard ratios for all first line trials of CDK4/6 inhibitor were similar, ranging between 0.49 and 0.58. It appeared that these drugs had comparable efficacy. The choice of drug would probably depend on their toxicity profile, dosing regimen, or dosage form. The 3 CDK4/6 inhibitors were not made equal. Palbociclib and ribociclib are structurally similar, basing off a pyrido [2,3-d]pyrimidin-7-one scaffold that was optimized for selectivity toward CDK4/6 [42, 43]. Abemaciclib, on the other hand, derived from a 2-anilino-2,4-pyrimidine-[5-benzimidazole] scaffold. This compound not only has potent activity against CDK4 and 6, it also inhibits multiple kinases *in vitro* a concentration less than 100 nM [44]. Neutropenia is the most common side effect of palbociclib and ribociclib. It appeared that anemia, thrombocytopenia and possibly stomatitis were more common in patients given palbociclib. For ribociclib, results from MONOSEESA-2 showed grade 3 or 4 elevated alanine aminotransferase (ALT) and aspartate aminotransferase (AST) in up to 9% of the patients. Prolonged QTcF was also a concern for a small proportion of patients in the study. Although palbociclib and ribociclib have comparable spectrum of CDK activity [45], the small disparities in their chemical structure might explain the differences in their toxicities. Abemaciclib, being structurally distinct from the other 2 CDK4/6 inhibitors, has diarrhea being the most reported adverse event. Grade 3 and 4 neutropenia was at around 21–25%, half of that reported in the PALOMA or MONALEESA trials. Due to the lower incidence of bone marrow toxicity, this drug is taken twice per day continuously without the need for a resting week. It is also the only CDK4/6 inhibitor with an indication in heavily pretreated patients as a monotherapy.

Although $HR^{+ve}/HER2^{-ve}$ breast cancer is regarded as a less aggressive form of breast cancer, a significant proportion of patients after curative resection ultimately relapse. The impressive response in metastatic setting and decent QoL data of palbociclib suggest that this drug might have a role as adjuvant therapy and help prevent recurrence. A number of adjuvant trials are ongoing. For instance, PALLAS evaluates the outcome of adding 2 years of palbociclib to standard endocrine therapy [NCT02513394]. PENELOPE-B studies the role of adding palbociclib to standard endocrine therapy in patients with high risk of relapse after neoadjuvant chemotherapy [NCT01864746]. MonarchE [NCT03155997] is also recruiting. It studied the effect of adding 2 years of abemaciclib to standard adjuvant endocrine therapy in high-risk node-positive early stage patients post-resection.

CDK4/6 inhibitors revolutionized how $HR^{+ve}/HER2^{-ve}$ MBC should be treated. There is an unmet need for biomarker of response to guide management decision. Further studies on the benefit of continuing CDK 4/6 inhibitors beyond progression or the optimal time to add these targeted agents would also be needed.

3.2. Traditional mTOR inhibitor remains a standard treatment

mTOR is a downstream effector of the PI3K/AKT pathway. Targeting mTOR is a rational strategy to reverse endocrine resistance. TAMRAD is a phase 2 study that explored the combination of oral mTOR inhibitor everolimus with tamoxifen versus tamoxifen in patients with $HR^{+ve}/HER2^{-ve}$ MBC who have progressed on AI [46]. The dosage of everolimus was 10 mg daily. This primary end point was CBR. Everolimus significantly improved the CBR from 42–61%. Time to progression increased from 4.5 months with tamoxifen alone to 8.6 months with addition of everolimus (HR 0.54; 95% CI, 0.36–0.81). Significant adverse reaction included fatigue (72%), stomatitis (56%), rash (44%), anorexia (43%), and diarrhea (39%). Second line AI is a common strategy upon progression on first line AI. BOLERO-2 is a phase 3 trial which randomized patients who have receive exemestane plus everolimus or everolimus alone [47]. Patients had recurrence or progression while on previous endocrine therapy with a nonsteroidal AI in the adjuvant setting or to treat advance disease. The primary end point was PFS. The study stopped early after the interim analysis, as median PFS was 6.9 months with everolimus plus exemestane, versus 2.8 months with exemestane alone (HR 0.43; 95% CI, 0.35–0.54; $p < 0.001$) based on assessments by local investigators. These patients were heavily pretreated – besides nonsteroidal AI, 57% had received an antiestrogen, 26% had chemotherapy in the advance setting, and 54% had 3 or more lines of therapies. Stomatitis was the most frequent and debilitating adverse events (all grades 56%, grade 3 8%), followed by rash (add grades 36%, grade 3 1%), fatigue (all grades 33%, grade 3 3%), and diarrhea (all grades 30%, grade 3 2%). As everolimus is an immunosuppressant, the incidence of infection cannot be under-estimated and there were 2 cases of deaths from sepsis. Other class-specific severe toxicities included anemia (grade 3 5%), hyperglycemia (grade 3 4%), pneumonitis (grade 3 3%), and elevated AST (grade 3 3%) and elevated ALT (grade 3 3%). The study was not powered to detect a difference in OS, and the analysis of OS was negative [48]. Subsequent molecular analysis of archival tissue showed that the mutational status of *PIK3A*, amplification of *FGFR1*, or P3K/AKT/mTOR pathway alteration did not affect treatment response to everolimus [49]. This analysis reviewed some potential quantitative differences in the efficacy of everolimus among tumors of specific *PIK3CA* exons, *FGFR2*, *mTOR*, and chromosomal instabilities. These remains to be further investigated. BOLERO-2 also included analysis of plasma cell-free DNA (cfDNA) for 2 *ESR1* mutations [50]. *ESR1* D538G mutation was detected in 21% and *ESR1* Y537S mutation was found in 13%. Interestingly, patients with D538G mutation had PFS benefit with addition of everolimus (HR 0.34; 95 CI, 0.02–0.57), while those carrying Y537S mutation did not.

Everolimus is an inhibitor of mTORC1. It is postulated that mTORC1 inhibition by everolimus set off negative feedback mechanism via AKT signaling, and leads to treatment resistance. Vistusertib is a small molecule ATP competitive dual inhibitor of mTORC1 and mTORC2. Preclinical model demonstrated that vistusertib had superior activity to everolimus in suppressing tumor growth [51]. MANTA is a randomized phase 2 study of fulvestrant in combination with vistusertib or everolimus or fulvestrant alone in HR-positive HER2-negative MBC patients who have disease resistance to AI [52]. No more than 1 line prior chemotherapy was allowed in advanced setting. Primary end point was PFS. At median follow up of 17 months, it showed that addition of vistusertib did not add PFS benefit compared with fulvestrant alone (7.6 versus 5.4 months; HR 0.88; 95% CI, 0.63–1.24, $p = 0.46$). In fact, the fulvestrant-everolimus arm had superior PFS compared with the fulvestrant-vistusertib arm (12.3 versus 7.6 months; HR 0.63; 95% CI, 0.45–0.9, $p = 0.01$). Stomatitis and rash were the most common adverse effects of this dual mTOR inhibitor, and the frequency was comparable to that of everolimus. In summary, dual inhibition of mTOR did not derive superior effect. Everolimus remains the only mTOR inhibitor approved by the U.S. FDA for $HR^{+ve}/HER2^{-ve}$ MBC.

3.3. PI3K inhibitors as an emerging treatment

Intracellular signaling pathways have complex interaction. Targeted inhibition of a particular component in the pathway might cause relief of upstream feedback inhibition. Inhibition of the effector mTOR in the PI3K/AKT/mTOR pathway, could result in adaptive hyperactivation of the upstream AKT activity and leads to treatment failure [53]. As *PIK3CA* mutation is the most common genetic changes in breast cancer and represents a more proximal target, targeting *PIK3CA* might exert upstream halt of growth signaling. A number of PI3K inhibitors have been developed. Pictilisib is an orally active pan-inhibitor of class 1 PIK3K. FERGI is a randomized phase 2 study which recruited $HR^{+ve}/HER2^{-ve}$ MBC patients who have progressed on or after AI [54]. Patients were given either fulvestrant or fulvestrant with pictilisib. The primary end point was PFS. There was no difference between 2 groups, both in the intention-to-treat population or patients with *PIK3CA* mutation. Pictilisib-associated serious adverse events in the original study dose of 340 mg per day were reported in 16%, whereas those leading to discontinuation were rash, pneumonitis, diarrhea, abdominal pain, stomatitis or elevated AST or ALT. Close to half the patients required dose modification. Toxicities greatly limited drug exposure of the patients. Although in the second part of the study dosage has been reduced and toxicity profile improved, the drug was not further developed due to its lack of PFS benefit.

Another extensively studied PI3K inhibitor is buparlisib. It is also a pan-class I PI3K inhibitor. It showed encouraging results in early clinical studies and it was ultimately brought to a number of phase 3 trials. BELLL-2 combined fulvestrant with buparlisib or placebo in $HR^{+ve}/HER2^{-ve}$ MBC patients who have progressed on or after AI, and had received up to 1 line of chemotherapy in the advanced setting [55]. The median PFS was 6.9 months in the buparlisib group versus 5.0 months in the placebo group (HR 0.78; 95% CI, 0.67–0.189; one sided $p < 0.001$). In patients with PI3K pathway-activation, median PFS was 6.8 months in the buparlisib group versus 4.0 months in the placebo group (HR 0.76; one sided PFS p –0.014). The most common grade 3 or 4 toxicities in the buparlisib group was increased ALT (25%), increased AST (18%), hyperglycemia (15%), and rash (8%). As preclinical data showed that buparlisib in combination with fulvestrant can reverse resistance mTOR inhibitor (Novartis data), BELLE-3 studied the combination of fulvestrant with or without buparlisib in HR^{+ve}/$HER2^{-ve}$ MBC patients who have progressed on or after mTOR inhibition [56]. It demonstrated that addition of buparlisib to fulvestrant prolonged the median PFS 1.8 months to 3.9 months (HR 0.67; 95% CI, 0.53–0.84, one-sided p < 0001). Circulating tumor DNA (ctDNA) analysis of *PIK3CA* status was available. Of the 432 subjects, 34% carried PIK3CA mutation. Among these patients, the median PFS was 4.7 months for those in the buparlisib arm versus 1.6 months for those in the placebo arm, thus those who received the PI3K inhibitor were 50% less likely to have disease progression. Despite these encouraging findings, grade 3 or 4 adverse events related to buparlisib were alarming – they included elevated ALT (22%), elevated AST (18%), and hyperglycemia (12%). Other toxicities potentially related to the drug such as depression, anxiety, and rash were also concerning. The company decided not to pursue further development of the drug due to its safety profile.

On the other hand, the company has turned its focus to a α-specific PI3K inhibitor alpelisib. Early phase study showed preliminary preferential antitumor activity in *PIK3CA*-altered tumor treated with alpelisib [57]. A presentation of the preliminary results for the combination of alpelisib and fulvestrant demonstrated encouraging early efficacy [58]. The study recruited 87 patients with HR^{+ve}/$HER2^{-ve}$ MBC. Alpelisib was given at 300 mg on a continuous daily schedule. In the PIK3A-altered population, the CBR was 45%. Median PFS was 9 and 5 months in the *PIK3CA*-altered groups and *PIK3CA* wild-type group respectively. This drug appeared to be better tolerated than pan-PI3K inhibitors. At the moment, the phase III SOLAR-1 trial [NCT02437318] studying the same combination in patients who have progressed on or have failed AI is ongoing. First PFS analysis is expected to be available later the year.

3.4. SERDS and its new role

Fulvestrant is the only clinically available SERD. It targets the ER for proteasomal degradation and halts the action of estrogen. It is capable of binding to the ligand-binding domain of ERα, converting it to a form incapable with transcriptional activity [59, 60]. Fulvestrant is given by intramuscular injection on day 1, 15, 29, then every 28 days. The initial studied and market dose was 250 mg. At first line setting, as in the FACT study (SWOG S0226 trial), fulvestrant at 250 mg did not demonstrate survival advantage over AI [61]. As second line treatment, fulvestrant at 250 mg showed similar time to progression (TTP) to anastrozole. Yet the later CONFIRM study demonstrated that doubling the dose to 500 mg gave a superior PFS and OS compared with 250 mg [5, 62]. FALCON is a phase 3 study which further brings fulvestrant at 500 mg to first line setting in comparison with anastrozole. The PFS was 16.6 and 13.8 months for the fulvestrant and anastrozole groups respectively with a p value of 0.0486 [6].

Given the special property of SERD on receptor degradation and conformation, it would be interesting to explore if patients with *ESR1* mutation respond differently from those with *ESR1* wild type. SoFEA is a study comparing exemestane with fulvestrant-containing regimens in patients with prior sensitivity to nonsteroidal AI. Prospective-retrospective analysis of plasma ctDNA from SoFEA found *ESR1* mutation in 39% of patients, of which half were polyclonal [63]. Those with *ESR1* mutation had better PFS after giving fulvestrant compared with exemestane (HR 0.52, p = 0.02). Patients with *ESR1* wild type had similar benefit given either drug. PALOMA3 is a study that compared fulvestrant plus placebo with fulvestrant plus palbociclib in patients with progression after prior endocrine therapy. Plasma ctDNA analysis showed *ESR1* mutation rate of 25%, of which 28% where polyclonal. Fulvestrant plus palbociclib gave rise to better PFS compared with fulvestrant alone in both *ESR1* mutant (HR 0.43, p = 0.002) and *ESR1* wild type patients (0.49, p < 0.001) [63]. Analysis of ctDNA from the BOLERO2 study also supported that *ESR1* mutation can be found in around 30% of patients who have failed prior endocrine therapy [50]. Patients with *ESR1* mutation had shorted OS compared with wild type. This study did not involve the use of fulvestrant.

While fulvestrant is non-inferior to AI in the first line setting, more data on OS is awaited. Yet emerging evidence suggest that testing of *ESR1* mutation could probably guide us in the choice of hormonal therapy in patients who have failed prior endocrine therapy. The approach is limited by the availability of ctDNA analysis, sensitivity of different ctDNA methodology, often difficult-to-obtain tissue biopsy upon the time of progression, and accessibility to *ESR1* test in local laboratory as it is still not a standard practice.

4. The sequence of endocrine therapy and targeted drugs

AI has been the standard of care for first line treatment of patients with $HR^{+ve}/HER2^{-ve}$ MBC. The role of fulvestrant has been controversial. Due to the high cost, the need for monthly injection, and similar efficacy in the first line setting, fulvestrant is often an option rather than the preferred choice. Yet much remained to be learnt from this SERD. In the phase 3 FALCON trial, patients given monthly injection of fulvestrant at 500 mg had borderline statistically longer median PFS of 16.6 months (95% CI, 13.83–20.99) compared with those of 13.8 months (95% CI, 11.99–16.59) given oral anastrozole 1 mg daily (HR 0.797, 95% CI, 0.637–0.999; p = 0.0486) [6]. This approach showed that the ceiling PFS ceiling of hormonal therapy could be stretched to 20 months in some patients. More interestingly, subgroup analysis suggested that most of the survival benefit was derived from patients who had bone-only metastatic disease, with a median PFS of 22.3 month in the fulvestrant group versus 13.8 months in the anastrozole group (HR 0.59; 95 CI, 042–0.84). Reanalysis of SOG S0226 according to prior exposure to adjuvant adjuvant tamoxifen, showed that those without prior endocrine exposure had longer median PFS when given fulvestrant compared with anastrozole (16.7 versus 12.7 months; HR 0.73; 95% CI, 0.60–0.89, p = 0.002), which further translated into improved median OS by 1 year (40.3 versus 52.2 months, p = 0.0067) [64]. With the emergence of new treatment option of multiple CDK4/6 inhibitors, and the increasing financial burden associated with them, the practical questions would be how to choose the first line hormonal therapy. There have been international guidelines to lay the general clinical principle that treatment recommendation should be based on if the patient is naïve to endocrine therapy, the type of adjuvant therapy, length of disease free interval and if disease relapsing less than 12 months from the end of adjuvant AI [65, 66]. More updated and detailed guidelines are anticipated in light of new findings.

As to the choice of agent in the second line setting or beyond, the choice would largely depend on prior treatment. Some general principles are becoming apparent. First of all, there is enough data to suggest that CDK4/6 inhibitor should be part of standard treatment in patients with $HR^{+ve}/HER2^{-ve}$ MBC, be it first line (PALOMA-2, MONALEESA-2, MONARCH-3, MONALEESA-7), second line (PALOMA-3, MONARCH-2), or later line in refractory cases (MONARCH-1). Since PI3K/AKT/mTOR plays an important role in hormonal resistance, mTOR inhibitor should also be considered in all patients. The only approved choice currently is everolimus. For the choice of hormonal partner in patients who have progressed on or failed prior AI, testing of *ESR1* mutation status might provide some guidance as to if switching to SERD would be helpful. It is still not clear if patients who progress on first line CDK4/6 inhibitors should be continued this targeted agent with a switch of hormonal partner. Chemotherapy should be reserved for patients who have exhausted the options for hormonal therapy and these targeted therapies, or patients with impending visceral crisis.

5. Conclusion

Although we are becoming increasingly equipped to overcome resistance to hormonal therapy, these treatment would fail nevertheless. The preliminary OS data for the phase II PALOMA-1 trial was presented in June 2017. It showed that the median OS was 37.5 months in patients who received palbociclib and AI versus 34.5 months in those who received AI (HR 0.897) [67], suggesting the impressive gain in median PFS after adding palbociclib might not translate into long term survival. Interestingly, analysis of OS for BELL2 appears to be trending toward similar observation. The median OS for patients who received buparlisib and fulvestrant versus those who received placebo and fulvestrant was 33.2 and 30.4 months respectively (HR 0.87; 95% CI, 0.74 to 1.02; $p = 0.045$) [68]. Even in patients who had PI3K pathway activated or PIK3CA mutation, the improvement in median PFS with addition of buparlisib did not translate into better median OS (HR 0.81, $p > 0.05$). These might be explained by two reasons. Firstly, post-progression survival can be affected by availability and effectiveness of subsequent therapy. Second, progression on CDK4/6 inhibitor might have selected out patients who then became refractory to other treatment especially chemotherapy. More understanding in the mechanism of resistance to hormonal therapy and targeted therapy is needed to overcome these barriers.

$HR^{+ve}/HER2^{-ve}$ MBC is the most common type of breast cancer. The main stay of treatment is hormonal therapy, and the choice of hormonal therapy includes SERM, AI, and SERD. SERD might play a more important role in selected patients, as development of *ESR1* mutation could render patients resistant to AI. Addition of targeted therapy such as CDK4/6 inhibitor or mTOR inhibitor can help prolong the use of hormonal therapy, and should be part of standard treatment for all patients in their treatment journey. Future research would focus on strategies to overcome resistance to these therapies.

Conflict of interest

Dr. Chiu has no conflict of interest to declare.

Author details

Joanne W. Chiu

Address all correspondence to: jwychiu@hku.hk

Department of Medicine, Medical Oncology, Queen Mary Hospital, The University of Hong Kong, Hong Kong

References

[1] Anderson WF, Chatterjee N, Ershler WB, Brawley OW. Estrogen receptor breast cancer phenotypes in the surveillance, epidemiology, and end results database. Breast Cancer Research and Treatment. 2002;**76**(1):27-36

[2] Cole MP, Jones CT, Todd ID. A new anti-oestrogenic agent in late breast cancer. An early clinical appraisal of ICI46474. British Journal of Cancer. 1971;**25**(2):270-275

[3] Bonneterre J, Thurlimann B, Robertson JF, Krzakowski M, Mauriac L, Koralewski P, et al. Anastrozole versus tamoxifen as first-line therapy for advanced breast cancer in 668 postmenopausal women: Results of the tamoxifen or arimidex randomized group efficacy and tolerability study. Journal of Clinical Oncology. 2000;**18**(22):3748-3757

[4] Mouridsen H, Gershanovich M, Sun Y, Perez-Carrion R, Boni C, Monnier A, et al. Phase III study of letrozole versus tamoxifen as first-line therapy of advanced breast cancer in postmenopausal women: Analysis of survival and update of efficacy from the international Letrozole breast Cancer group. Journal of Clinical Oncology. 2003;**21**(11):2101-2109

[5] Di Leo A, Jerusalem G, Petruzelka L, Torres R, Bondarenko IN, Khasanov R, et al. Final overall survival: Fulvestrant 500 mg vs 250 mg in the randomized CONFIRM trial. Journal of the National Cancer Institute. 2014;**106**(1):djt337

[6] Robertson JFR, Bondarenko IM, Trishkina E, Dvorkin M, Panasci L, Manikhas A, et al. Fulvestrant 500 mg versus anastrozole 1 mg for hormone receptor-positive advanced breast cancer (FALCON): An international, randomised, double-blind, phase 3 trial. Lancet. 2016;**388**(10063):2997-3005

[7] Paridaens RJ, Dirix LY, Beex LV, Nooij M, Cameron DA, Cufer T, et al. Phase III study comparing exemestane with tamoxifen as first-line hormonal treatment of metastatic breast cancer in postmenopausal women: The European Organisation for research and treatment of cancer breast cancer cooperative group. Journal of Clinical Oncology. 2008;**26**(30):4883-4890

[8] Satyanarayana A, Kaldis P. Mammalian cell-cycle regulation: Several Cdks, numerous cyclins and diverse compensatory mechanisms. Oncogene. 2009;**28**(33):2925-2939

[9] Sherr CJ. D-type cyclins. Trends in Biochemical Sciences. 1995;**20**(5):187-190

[10] Barnes DM, Gillett CE. Cyclin D1 in breast cancer. Breast Cancer Research and Treatment. 1998;**52**(1-3):1-15

[11] Cancer Genome Atlas Network. Comprehensive molecular portraits of human breast tumours. Nature. 2012;**490**(7418):61-70

[12] Watts CK, Brady A, Sarcevic B, deFazio A, Musgrove EA, Sutherland RL. Antiestrogen inhibition of cell cycle progression in breast cancer cells in associated with inhibition of cyclin-dependent kinase activity and decreased retinoblastoma protein phosphorylation. Molecular Endocrinology. 1995;**9**(12):1804-1813

[13] Thangavel C, Dean JL, Ertel A, Knudsen KE, Aldaz CM, Witkiewicz AK, et al. Therapeutically activating RB: Reestablishing cell cycle control in endocrine therapy-resistant breast cancer. Endocrine-Related Cancer. 2011;**18**(3):333-345

[14] Finn RS, Dering J, Conklin D, Kalous O, Cohen DJ, Desai AJ, et al. PD 0332991, a selective cyclin D kinase 4/6 inhibitor, preferentially inhibits proliferation of luminal estrogen receptor-positive human breast cancer cell lines in vitro. Breast Cancer Research. 2009;**11**(5):R77

[15] Ellis MJ, Tao Y, Young O, White S, Proia AD, Murray J, et al. Estrogen-independent proliferation is present in estrogen-receptor HER2-positive primary breast cancer after neoadjuvant letrozole. Journal of Clinical Oncology. 2006;**24**(19):3019-3025

[16] Frogne T, Benjaminsen RV, Sonne-Hansen K, Sorensen BS, Nexo E, Laenkholm AV, et al. Activation of ErbB3, EGFR and Erk is essential for growth of human breast cancer cell lines with acquired resistance to fulvestrant. Breast Cancer Research and Treatment. 2009;**114**(2):263-275

[17] Turner N, Pearson A, Sharpe R, Lambros M, Geyer F, Lopez-Garcia MA, et al. FGFR1 amplification drives endocrine therapy resistance and is a therapeutic target in breast cancer. Cancer Research. 2010;**70**(5):2085-2094

[18] Fox EM, Miller TW, Balko JM, Kuba MG, Sanchez V, Smith RA, et al. A kinome-wide screen identifies the insulin/IGF-I receptor pathway as a mechanism of escape from hormone dependence in breast cancer. Cancer Research. 2011;**71**(21):6773-6784

[19] Campbell IG, Russell SE, Choong DY, Montgomery KG, Ciavarella ML, Hooi CS, et al. Mutation of the PIK3CA gene in ovarian and breast cancer. Cancer Research. 2004; **64**(21):7678-7681

[20] Saal LH, Holm K, Maurer M, Memeo L, Su T, Wang X, et al. PIK3CA mutations correlate with hormone receptors, node metastasis, and ERBB2, and are mutually exclusive with PTEN loss in human breast carcinoma. Cancer Research. 2005;**65**(7):2554-2559

[21] Fu X, Osborne CK, Schiff R. Biology and therapeutic potential of PI3K signaling in ER+/HER2-negative breast cancer. Breast. 2013;**22**(Suppl 2):S12-S18

[22] Miller TW, Hennessy BT, Gonzalez-Angulo AM, Fox EM, Mills GB, Chen H, et al. Hyperactivation of phosphatidylinositol-3 kinase promotes escape from hormone

dependence in estrogen receptor-positive human breast cancer. The Journal of Clinical Investigation. 2010;**120**(7):2406-2413

[23] Sighoko D, Liu J, Hou N, Gustafson P, Huo D. Discordance in hormone receptor status among primary, metastatic, and second primary breast cancers: Biological difference or misclassification? The Oncologist. 2014;**19**(6):592-601

[24] Ellis MJ, Tao Y, Luo J, A'Hern R, Evans DB, Bhatnagar AS, et al. Outcome prediction for estrogen receptor-positive breast cancer based on postneoadjuvant endocrine therapy tumor characteristics. Journal of the National Cancer Institute. 2008;**100**(19):1380-1388

[25] Liu J, Deng H, Jia W, Zeng Y, Rao N, Li S, et al. Comparison of ER/PR and HER2 statuses in primary and paired liver metastatic sites of breast carcinoma in patients with or without treatment. Journal of Cancer Research and Clinical Oncology. 2012;**138**(5):837-842

[26] Toy W, Shen Y, Won H, Green B, Sakr RA, Will M, et al. ESR1 ligand-binding domain mutations in hormone-resistant breast cancer. Nature Genetics. 2013;**45**(12):1439-1445

[27] Roberts PJ, Bisi JE, Strum JC, Combest AJ, Darr DB, Usary JE, et al. Multiple roles of cyclin-dependent kinase 4/6 inhibitors in cancer therapy. Journal of the National Cancer Institute. 2012;**104**(6):476-487

[28] Finn RS, Crown JP, Lang I, Boer K, Bondarenko IM, Kulyk SO, et al. The cyclin-dependent kinase 4/6 inhibitor palbociclib in combination with letrozole versus letrozole alone as first-line treatment of oestrogen receptor-positive, HER2-negative, advanced breast cancer (PALOMA-1/TRIO-18): A randomised phase 2 study. The Lancet Oncology. 2015; **16**(1):25-35

[29] Finn RS, Martin M, Rugo HS, Jones S, Im SA, Gelmon K, et al. Palbociclib and Letrozole in advanced breast cancer. The New England Journal of Medicine. 2016;**375**(20):1925-1936

[30] Turner NC, Ro J, Andre F, Loi S, Verma S, Iwata H, et al. Palbociclib in hormone-receptor-positive advanced breast cancer. The New England Journal of Medicine. 2015; **373**(3):209-219

[31] Hortobagyi GN, Stemmer SM, Burris HA, Yap YS, Sonke GS, Paluch-Shimon S, et al. Ribociclib as first-line therapy for HR-positive, advanced breast cancer. The New England Journal of Medicine. 2016;**375**(18):1738-1748

[32] Tripathy D, Sohn J, Im S-A, et al. First-line ribociclib or placebo combined with goserelin and tamoxifen or a non-steroidal aromatase inhibitor in premenopausal women with hormone receptor-positive, HER2 negative advanced breast cancer: Results from the randomized phase III MONALEESA-7 trial. In: Presented in San Antonio Breast Cancer Symposium (SABCS) 2017. 2017

[33] Sledge Jr GW, Toi M, Neven P, Sohn J, Inoue K, Pivot X, et al. MONARCH 2: Abemaciclib in combination with fulvestrant in women with HR+/HER2-advanced breast cancer who had progressed while receiving endocrine therapy. Journal of Clinical Oncology. 2017;**35**(25):2875-2884

[34] Goetz MP, Toi M, Campone M, Sohn J, Paluch-Shimon S, Huober J, et al. MONARCH 3: Abemaciclib as initial therapy for advanced breast cancer. Journal of Clinical Oncology. 2017;**35**(32):3638-3646

[35] Dickler MN, Tolaney SM, Rugo HS, Cortes J, Dieras V, Patt D, et al. MONARCH 1, a phase II study of abemaciclib, a CDK4 and CDK6 inhibitor, as a single agent, in patients with refractory HR(+)/HER2(−) metastatic breast cancer. Clinical Cancer Research. 2017;**23**(17):5218-5224

[36] Finn R, Jiang Y, Rugo H, et al. Biomarker analyses from the phase 3 PALOMA-2 trial of palbociclib (P) with letrozole (L) compared with placebo (PLB) plus L in postmenopausal women with ER+/HER2-advanced breast cancer (ABC). Annals of Oncology. 2016;**27**(suppl_6):LBA15

[37] Cristofanilli M, Turner NC, Bondarenko I, Ro J, Im SA, Masuda N, et al. Fulvestrant plus palbociclib versus fulvestrant plus placebo for treatment of hormone-receptor-positive, HER2-negative metastatic breast cancer that progressed on previous endocrine therapy (PALOMA-3): Final analysis of the multicentre, double-blind, phase 3 randomised controlled trial. The Lancet Oncology. 2016;**17**(4):425-439

[38] Turner N, Jiang Y, O'Leary B, et al. Efficacy of palbociclib plus fulvestrant (P+F) in patients (pts) with metastatic breast cancer (MBC) and ESR1 mutations (mus) in circulating tumor DNA (ctDNA). Journal of Clinical Oncology. 2016;**34**(supp; abstr 512)

[39] Verma S, Bartlett CH, Schnell P, DeMichele AM, Loi S, Ro J, et al. Palbociclib in combination with fulvestrant in women with hormone receptor-positive/HER2-negative advanced metastatic breast cancer: Detailed safety analysis from a multicenter, randomized, placebo-controlled, phase III study (PALOMA-3). The Oncologist. 2016;**21**(10):1165-1175

[40] DeSantis CE, Ma J, Goding Sauer A, Newman LA, Jemal A. Breast cancer statistics, 2017, racial disparity in mortality by state. CA: A Cancer Journal for Clinicians. 2017; **67**(6):439-448

[41] Youlden DR, Cramb SM, Yip CH, Baade PD. Incidence and mortality of female breast cancer in the Asia-Pacific region. Cancer Biology & Medicine. 2014;**11**(2):101-115

[42] VanderWel SN, Harvey PJ, McNamara DJ, Repine JT, Keller PR, Quin 3rd J, et al. Pyrido [2,3-d]pyrimidin-7-ones as specific inhibitors of cyclin-dependent kinase 4. Journal of Medicinal Chemistry. 2005;**48**(7):2371-2387

[43] Asghar U, Witkiewicz AK, Turner NC, Knudsen ES. The history and future of targeting cyclin-dependent kinases in cancer therapy. Nature Reviews. Drug Discovery. 2015; **14**(2):130-146

[44] Gelbert LM, Cai S, Lin X, Sanchez-Martinez C, Del Prado M, Lallena MJ, et al. Preclinical characterization of the CDK4/6 inhibitor LY2835219: In-vivo cell cycle-dependent/independent anti-tumor activities alone/in combination with gemcitabine. Investigational New Drugs. 2014;**32**(5):825-837

[45] Chen P, Lee NV, Hu W, Xu M, Ferre RA, Lam H, et al. Spectrum and degree of CDK drug interactions predicts clinical performance. Molecular Cancer Therapeutics. 2016; **15**(10):2273-2281

[46] Bachelot T, Bourgier C, Cropet C, Ray-Coquard I, Ferrero JM, Freyer G, et al. Randomized phase II trial of everolimus in combination with tamoxifen in patients with hormone receptor-positive, human epidermal growth factor receptor 2-negative metastatic breast cancer with prior exposure to aromatase inhibitors: A GINECO study. Journal of Clinical Oncology. 2012;**30**(22):2718-2724

[47] Baselga J, Campone M, Piccart M, Burris 3rd HA, Rugo HS, Sahmoud T, et al. Everolimus in postmenopausal hormone-receptor-positive advanced breast cancer. The New England Journal of Medicine. 2012;**366**(6):520-529

[48] Piccart M, Hortobagyi GN, Campone M, Pritchard KI, Lebrun F, Ito Y, et al. Everolimus plus exemestane for hormone-receptor-positive, human epidermal growth factor receptor-2-negative advanced breast cancer: Overall survival results from BOLERO-2dagger. Annals of Oncology. 2014;**25**(12):2357-2362

[49] Hortobagyi GN, Chen D, Piccart M, Rugo HS, Burris 3rd HA, Pritchard KI, et al. Correlative analysis of genetic alterations and everolimus benefit in hormone receptor-positive, human epidermal growth factor receptor 2-negative advanced breast cancer: Results from BOLERO-2. Journal of Clinical Oncology. 2016;**34**(5):419-426

[50] Chandarlapaty S, Chen D, He W, Sung P, Samoila A, You D, et al. Prevalence of ESR1 mutations in cell-free DNA and outcomes in metastatic breast cancer: A secondary analysis of the BOLERO-2 clinical trial. JAMA Oncology. 2016;**2**(10):1310-1315

[51] Guichard SM, Curwen J, Bihani T, D'Cruz CM, Yates JW, Grondine M, et al. AZD2014, an inhibitor of mTORC1 and mTORC2, is highly effective in ER+ breast Cancer when administered using intermittent or continuous schedules. Molecular Cancer Therapeutics. 2015; **14**(11):2508-2518

[52] Schmid P, Zaiss M, Harper-Wynne C, et al. MANTA – A randomized phase II study of fulvestrant in combination with the dual mTOR inhibitor AZD2014 or everolimus or fulvestrant alone in ER-positive advanced or metastatic breast cancer. In: Presented in San Antonio Breast Cancer Symposium 2017. 2017

[53] Chandarlapaty S. Negative feedback and adaptive resistance to the targeted therapy of cancer. Cancer Discovery. 2012;**2**(4):311-319

[54] Krop IE, Mayer IA, Ganju V, Dickler M, Johnston S, Morales S, et al. Pictilisib for oestrogen receptor-positive, aromatase inhibitor-resistant, advanced or metastatic breast cancer (FERGI): A randomised, double-blind, placebo-controlled, phase 2 trial. The Lancet Oncology. 2016;**17**(6):811-821

[55] Baselga J, Im SA, Iwata H, Cortes J, De Laurentiis M, Jiang Z, et al. Buparlisib plus fulvestrant versus placebo plus fulvestrant in postmenopausal, hormone receptor-positive,

HER2-negative, advanced breast cancer (BELLE-2): A randomised, double-blind, placebo-controlled, phase 3 trial. The Lancet Oncology. 2017;**18**(7):904-916

[56] Di Leo A, Johnston S, Lee KS, Ciruelos E, Lonning PE, Janni W, et al. Buparlisib plus fulvestrant in postmenopausal women with hormone-receptor-positive, HER2-negative, advanced breast cancer progressing on or after mTOR inhibition (BELLE-3): A randomised, double-blind, placebo-controlled, phase 3 trial. The Lancet Oncology. 2018; **19**(1):87-100

[57] Mayer IA, Abramson VG, Formisano L, Balko JM, Estrada MV, Sanders ME, et al. A phase Ib study of alpelisib (BYL719), a PI3Kalpha-specific inhibitor, with letrozole in ER+/HER2-metastatic breast cancer. Clinical Cancer Research. 2017;**23**(1):26-34

[58] Juric D, Andre F, Rugo H, et al. Combined alpelisib (BYL719) and fulvestrant in PIK3CA-altered or wild-type estrogen receptor-positive/human epidermal growth factor receptor 2-negative advanced breast cancer. In: Presented in Miami Breast Cancer Conference. 2016

[59] Pike AC, Brzozowski AM, Walton J, Hubbard RE, Thorsell AG, Li YL, et al. Structural insights into the mode of action of a pure antiestrogen. Structure. 2001;**9**(2):145-153

[60] Fawell SE, White R, Hoare S, Sydenham M, Page M, Parker MG. Inhibition of estrogen receptor-DNA binding by the "pure" antiestrogen ICI 164,384 appears to be mediated by impaired receptor dimerization. Proceedings of the National Academy of Sciences of the United States of America. 1990;**87**(17):6883-6887

[61] Bergh J, Jonsson PE, Lidbrink EK, Trudeau M, Eiermann W, Brattstrom D, et al. FACT: An open-label randomized phase III study of fulvestrant and anastrozole in combination compared with anastrozole alone as first-line therapy for patients with receptor-positive postmenopausal breast cancer. Journal of Clinical Oncology. 2012;**30**(16):1919-1925

[62] Di Leo A, Jerusalem G, Petruzelka L, Torres R, Bondarenko IN, Khasanov R, et al. Results of the CONFIRM phase III trial comparing fulvestrant 250 mg with fulvestrant 500 mg in postmenopausal women with estrogen receptor-positive advanced breast cancer. Journal of Clinical Oncology. 2010;**28**(30):4594-4600

[63] Fribbens C, O'Leary B, Kilburn L, Hrebien S, Garcia-Murillas I, Beaney M, et al. Plasma ESR1 mutations and the treatment of estrogen receptor-positive advanced breast cancer. Journal of Clinical Oncology. 2016;**34**(25):2961-2968

[64] Mehta RS, Barlow WE, Albain KS, et al. A phase III randomized trial of anastrozole and fulvestrant versus anastrozole or sequential anastrozole and fulvestrant as first-line therapy for postmenopausal women with metastatic breast cancer: Final survival outcome of SWOG S0226. In: Presented in San Antonio Breast Cancer Symposium. 2017

[65] Rugo HS, Rumble RB, Macrae E, Barton DL, Connolly HK, Dickler MN, et al. Endocrine therapy for hormone receptor-positive metastatic breast Cancer: American Society of Clinical Oncology guideline. Journal of Clinical Oncology. 2016;**34**(25):3069-3103

[66] Cardoso F, Costa A, Senkus E, Aapro M, Andre F, Barrios CH, et al. 3rd ESO-ESMO international consensus guidelines for advanced breast cancer (ABC 3). Breast. 2017; **31**:244-259

[67] Finn RS, Crown JP, Lang I, et al. Overall survival resutls from the randomized phase II study of palbociclib in combination with letrozole versus letrozole alone for frontline treatment of ER+/HER2 advanced breast cancer (PALOMA-1; TRIO-18). In: Presented in American Society of Clinical Oncology Annual Meeting. 2017

[68] Campone M, Im SA, Iwata H, et al. Buparlisib or placebo plus fulvestrant in postmenopausal patients with hormone receptor-positive, human epidermal growth factor receptor 2-negative advanced breast cancer: Overal survival results from BELL2, a randomized phase III study. In: Presented in San Antonio Breast Cancer Symposium. 2017

Permissions

All chapters in this book were first published in BCS, by InTech Open; hereby published with permission under the Creative Commons Attribution License or equivalent. Every chapter published in this book has been scrutinized by our experts. Their significance has been extensively debated. The topics covered herein carry significant findings which will fuel the growth of the discipline. They may even be implemented as practical applications or may be referred to as a beginning point for another development.

The contributors of this book come from diverse backgrounds, making this book a truly international effort. This book will bring forth new frontiers with its revolutionizing research information and detailed analysis of the nascent developments around the world.

We would like to thank all the contributing authors for lending their expertise to make the book truly unique. They have played a crucial role in the development of this book. Without their invaluable contributions this book wouldn't have been possible. They have made vital efforts to compile up to date information on the varied aspects of this subject to make this book a valuable addition to the collection of many professionals and students.

This book was conceptualized with the vision of imparting up-to-date information and advanced data in this field. To ensure the same, a matchless editorial board was set up. Every individual on the board went through rigorous rounds of assessment to prove their worth. After which they invested a large part of their time researching and compiling the most relevant data for our readers.

The editorial board has been involved in producing this book since its inception. They have spent rigorous hours researching and exploring the diverse topics which have resulted in the successful publishing of this book. They have passed on their knowledge of decades through this book. To expedite this challenging task, the publisher supported the team at every step. A small team of assistant editors was also appointed to further simplify the editing procedure and attain best results for the readers.

Apart from the editorial board, the designing team has also invested a significant amount of their time in understanding the subject and creating the most relevant covers. They scrutinized every image to scout for the most suitable representation of the subject and create an appropriate cover for the book.

The publishing team has been an ardent support to the editorial, designing and production team. Their endless efforts to recruit the best for this project, has resulted in the accomplishment of this book. They are a veteran in the field of academics and their pool of knowledge is as vast as their experience in printing. Their expertise and guidance has proved useful at every step. Their uncompromising quality standards have made this book an exceptional effort. Their encouragement from time to time has been an inspiration for everyone.

The publisher and the editorial board hope that this book will prove to be a valuable piece of knowledge for researchers, students, practitioners and scholars across the globe.

List of Contributors

Viveka Hammelin, Luz María Tejada-Tayabas, Dulce María Galarza-Tejada and Joel Monárrez-Espino
Department of Public Health Sciences, Karolinska Institutet, Stockholm, Sweden

Shahnorbanun Sahran, Ashwaq Qasem, Khairuddin Omar, Afzan Adam, Siti Norul Huda Sheikh Abdullah and Azizi Abdullah
Center for Artificial Intelligence Technology, Faculty of Information Science and Technology, Universiti Kebangsaan Malaysia, Bangi, Malaysia

Dheeb Albashih
Computer Science Department, Prince Abdullah Bin Ghazi Faculty of Information Technology, Al-Balqa Applied University, Jordan

Rizuana Iqbal Hussain
Department of Radiology, Universiti Kebangsaan Malaysia Medical Center, Malaysia

Fuad Ismail
Department of Oncology, Universiti Kebangsaan Malaysia Medical Center, Malaysia

Norlia Abdullah
Department of Surgeon, Universiti Kebangsaan Malaysia Medical center, Malaysia

Suria Hayati Md Pauzi and Nurdashima Abd Shukor
Department of Pathology, Universiti Kebangsaan Malaysia Medical Center, Malaysia

Anna Maria Badowska-Kozakiewicz and Michał Piotr Budzik
Department of Biophysics and Human Physiology, Medical University of Warsaw, Warsaw, Poland

Nilufer Bulut
Department of Medical Oncology, Kanuni Sultan Suleyman Education and Research Hospital, Kucukcekmece, Istanbul, Turkey

Shadia Al-Bahlani
Department of Allied Health Sciences, College of Medicine and Health Sciences, Sultan
Qaboos University, Muscat, Oman

Samiya Al-Jaaidi
Department of Applied Sciences, Higher College of Technology, Muscat, Oman

Josie Todd
Department of Surgery, CDHB, Christchurch, New Zealand
Royal College of Surgeons of Edinburgh, UK
University of Otago, New Zealand
Health Disability and Ethics Commission (HDEC), New Zealand
Accident Compensation Corporation (ACC), New Zealand

Heidi Abrahamse and Ivan Sosthene Mfouo Tynga
Laser Research Centre, Faculty of Health Sciences, University of Johannesburg, Doornfontein, South Africa

Malgorzata Banys-Paluchowski
Department of Gynecology and Obstetrics, Marienkrankenhaus Hamburg, Hamburg, Germany

Florian Reinhardt and Tanja Fehm
Department of Gynecology and Obstetrics, University Hospital Duesseldorf, University of Duesseldorf, Duesseldorf, Germany

Fatma Sen
Avrasya Hospital, Medical Oncology Unit, Zeytinburnu, Istanbul, Turkey

Anggorowati Anggorowati
Nursing Department, Medical Faculty, Diponegoro University, Semarang, Indonesia

Ibrahim O. Alanazi
National Center for Biotechnology, King Abdulaziz City for Science and Technology (KACST), Saudi Arabia

Zahid Khan
Genome Research Chair, Department of Biochemistry, College of Science, King Saud University, Riyadh, Kingdom of Saudi Arabia

Pinar Obakan-Yerlikaya, Elif Damla Arisan, Ajda Coker-Gurkan and Narcin Palavan-Unsal
Department of Molecular Biology and Genetics, Istanbul Kultur University, Bakirkoy- Istanbul, Turkey

Joanne W. Chiu
Department of Medicine, Medical Oncology, Queen Mary Hospital, The University of Hong Kong, Hong Kong

Index

www.ingramcontent.com/pod-product-compliance
Lightning Source LLC
LaVergne TN
LVHW081024210926
848485LV00004B/944